SMART
Obstetrics and Gynecology Handbook

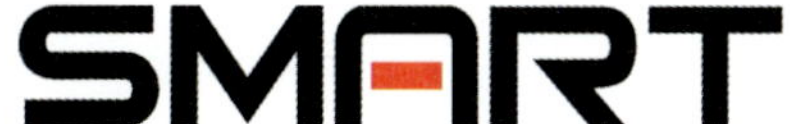

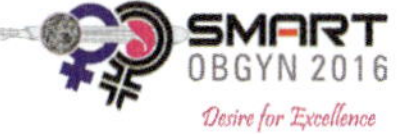

SMART Obstetrics and Gynecology Handbook

Editors

Nandita Palshetkar MD FCPS FICOG
Professor of Gynecology
Dr DY Patil Medical College
Navi Mumbai, Maharashtra, India
Organizing Chairperson
President MOGS (2016)

Rishma Dhillon Pai MD DNB FCPS DGO FICOG
Consultant Gynecologist
Jaslok and Lilavati Hospitals
Mumbai, Maharashtra, India
Organizing Secretary
All India Congress of Obstetrics and Gynaecology (AICOG) 2013, Mumbai
President Elect FOGSI
Secretary
Indian Society for Assisted Reproduction
Joint Clinical Secretary
Mumbai Obstetric and Gynecological Society

Pratik Tambe MD FICOG
ART Consultant and Gynec-Endoscopic Surgeon
Executive Council Member, MOGS, IAGE and AMC
Mentor, MOGS Youth Council
National Coordinator, FOGSI Endocrinology Committee

Deepali Kale MBBS DGO FCPS DNB FMAS
Assistant Professor of Obstetrics and Gynecology
Nowrosjee Wadia Maternity Hospital
Seth GS Medical College
Mumbai, Maharashtra, India

Rohan Palshetkar MBBS MS (OBGY)
Lecturer
Dr DY Patil Hospital and Research Center
Nerul, Navi Mumbai, Maharashtra, India

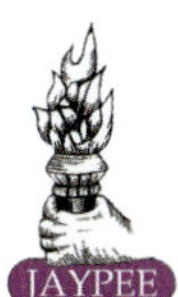

The Health Sciences Publisher

New Delhi | London | Philadelphia | Panama

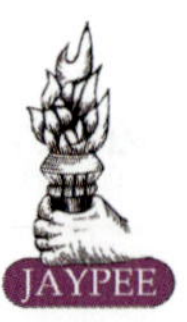

Jaypee Brothers Medical Publishers (P) Ltd.

Headquarters
Jaypee Brothers Medical Publishers (P) Ltd
4838/24, Ansari Road, Daryaganj
New Delhi 110 002, India
Phone: +91-11-43574357
Fax: +91-11-43574314
E-mail: jaypee@jaypeebrothers.com

Overseas Offices

J.P. Medical Ltd
83, Victoria Street, London
SW1H 0HW (UK)
Phone: +44 20 3170 8910
Fax: +44 (0)20 3008 6180
E-mail: info@jpmedpub.com

Jaypee Medical Inc.
325, Chestnut Street
Suite 412, Philadelphia,
PA 19106, USA
Phone: +1 267-519-9789
E-mail: support@jpmedus.com

Jaypee Brothers Medical Publishers (P) Ltd
Bhotahity, Kathmandu, Nepal
Phone: +977-9741283608
E-mail: kathmandu@jaypeebrothers.com

Jaypee-Highlights Medical Publishers Inc.
City of Knowledge, Building 235, 2nd Floor Clayton
Panama City, Panama
Phone: +1 507-301-0496
Fax: +1 507-301-0499
E-mail: cservice@jphmedical.com

Jaypee Brothers Medical Publishers (P) Ltd
17/1-B, Babar Road, Block-B, Shaymali
Mohammadpur, Dhaka-1207
Bangladesh
Mobile: +08801912003485
E-mail: jaypeedhaka@gmail.com

Website: www.jaypeebrothers.com
Website: www.jaypeedigital.com

Inquiries for bulk sales may be solicited at: jaypee@jaypeebrothers.com

SMART ***Obstetrics and Gynecology Handbook***

First Edition: 2016
ISBN: 978-93-85999-72-7
Printed at: Samrat Offset Pvt. Ltd.

Dedicated to

Our elders and teachers,
a continual source of inspiration ...

Dedicated to

Chairpersons' Message

Dear friends,

Clinical practice in the past was based on the clinical experience of our peers and teachers. Today, it is based on the evidence accumulated from very diligent and precise research. Our morality and our principles dictate how ethically we practice. Keeping the best interest of our patients in mind and following the ethical principles of "do not harm" are uppermost in our minds.

As science rapidly progresses, so does excellence in the art of this science. Hence, to bring together these various aspects of our subject together, we have organized this meeting in collaboration with the SAFOG. During this meeting, we proposed to review the evidence which will lead to the best practices, debate the ethics of various problems, and learn from the excellence of our colleagues, thus "clarifying the gray zone in obstetrics and gynecology".

We sincerely hope that the scientific program of this conference will evoke a great interest in the field of Obstetrics and Gynecology and will enrich all of us with the newer thoughts, ideas and technology that will be beneficial in our clinical practice.

This manual has been put together to give you a comprehensive insight into the important topics from high-risk Obstetrics, Infertility, Endoscopic Surgery and Urogynecology, which would be of interest to the delegates and faculty attending from the SAARC countries and which may be of relevance to their day-to-day practice. This has made it necessary for all of us to keep abreast with these changes to give the best to our patients.

We look forward to seeing you at "SMART OBGYN 2016" organized by MOGS (Mumbai Obstetric and Gynaecological Society) in association with SAFOG (South Asia Federation of Obstetrics and Gynaecology). Imbibe the evidence, ethics, the excellence of the scientific program and enjoy our hospitality. We know that you will enjoy being part of this brilliant meeting, just as we have enjoyed putting it together.

"Learning is a treasure that will follow its owner everywhere".

Nandita Palshetkar
Organizing Chairperson
President, MOGS (2016)
Mumbai Obstetric and
Gynecological Society

Shyam Desai
Organizing Chairperson
Trustee, MOGS
Chairperson, International
Affairs, SAFOG

Alka Kriplani
President, FOGSI

Ashma Rana
President, SAFOG

Scientific Committee

Organizing Secretaries		
Rishma Dhillon Pai President Elect, FOGSI Second Vice President, ISAR	**Jaydeep Tank** Dy Secretary General, FOGSI Secretary, MOGS 2016	**Narendra Malhotra** President, ISAR Past President, FOGSI
Scientific Chairpersons		
Hrishikesh Pai Secretary General, FOGSI	**Nozer Sheriar** Past Secretary General, FOGSI Past President, MOGS	**Rubina Sohail** President Elect, SAFOG
Jaideep Malhotra Vice Chairman, ICOG Past Vice President, FOGSI		
Joint Organization Secretaries		
Ameet Patki Past President, MOGS	**Arun Nayak** President, MOGS 2015	**Bipin Pandit** Secretary, MOGS 2015
Madhuri Patel Treasurer, FOGSI	**Yousuf Latif** Joint Secretary, SAFOG	
Treasurers		
Sarita Bhalerao Treasurer, MOGS	**Marlene Abeyawardene** Treasurer, SAFOG	**Suvarna Khadilkar** Joint Treasurer, MOGS
Advisors		
Suchitra Pandit	**Ameet Patki**	
Editors		
Nandita Palshetkar	**Rishma Dhillon Pai**	**Pratik Tambe**
Deepali Kale	**Rohan Palshetkar**	

South Asia Federation of Obstetrics and Gynaecology

List of Contributors

Aaradhana Wagh
Adi E Dastur
Ameet Patki
Ameya Purandare
Animesh Gandhi
Anupama Rao
Bipin Pandit
CV Hegde
Deepali Kale
Ganpat Sawant
Gayatri Rao
Hrishikesh Pai
Jaideep Malhotra
Nagendra Sardeshpande
Nandita Palshetkar
Narendra Malhotra
Neerja Bhatla
Neeta Warty
Neharika Malhotra Bora
Neha Saxena
Nikhil Purandare
Nozer K Sheriar
Pooja Bandekar
Prakash Trivedi
Pratik Tambe
Rajendra Sankpal
Rajkishor Sawant
Rakesh Sinha
Rishma Dhillon Pai
Rohan Palshetkar
Sandeep Patil
Shailesh Kore
Shirish S Sheth
Shweta Raje
S Krishnakumar
Soumil Trivedi
Vandana Bansal
Vinita Salvi
Zenab Tambawala

Preface

It gives me a great pleasure to write the Preface for the *SMART Obstetrics and Gynecology Handbook* on behalf of my co-editors. This book is meant as an accompaniment to the SMART Obstetrics and Gynecology SAFOG Conference to be held at the Grand Hyatt, Mumbai from 15th–17th April, 2016. We would like to thank Dr Hrishikesh Pai, Dr Rishma Dhillon Pai and Dr Nandita Palshetkar for entrusting us with such a monumental task.

The delegates who attend this event hail from the SAARC countries and are likely from a diverse range of geographical and socioeconomic backgrounds, including general gynecologists, high-risk obstetrics practitioners, endoscopic surgeons and ART consultants. Considering the target audience, we have included a broad range of topics from the subspecialties of gynecologic surgery, infertility, high-risk obstetrics and endoscopic surgery.

This book is meant to supplement the proceedings of the conference by offering, at a glance, the current state of evidence and practice guidelines for the busy practitioners. You may use it as a ready-reckoner or a reference text to look up, when confronted with the issues we have attempted to address.

Many of the authors are renowned stalwarts; whom we, in our formative years, have been fortunate enough to be guided by and we have been directly under their tutelage or have been the silent witnesses to their surgical mastery.

We hope it gives you as much pleasure to read and refer to as it gave us to compile, edit and put together.

Pratik Tambe
(On behalf of the Editors)

Acknowledgments

We would like to acknowledge the efforts of all the authors in preparation of the manuscript, especially Dr Deepali Kale and Dr Rohan Palshetkar for the painstaking proofreading, the editorial team at M/s Jaypee Brothers Medical Publishers (P) Ltd., New Delhi, India, for their kind cooperation and Mr Sabarish Menon (Commissioning Editor), Mumbai Branch, Jaypee Brothers, for his pivotal role in the smooth coordination towards the release of this book in time.

Contents

Intrauterine Insemination: Patient Selection and Workup

1

Rishma Dhillon Pai

DEFINITION

The deposition of spermatozoa in the uterus at any point above the internal os is considered as intrauterine insemination (IUI).

RATIONALE

The rationale of IUI performed using either husband's or donor spermatozoa is to overcome the problems of (i) Vaginal acidity; (ii) Cervical mucus hostility and (iii) Deposition of a good number of highly motile and morphologically normal sperms in the uterus near the fundus at the anticipated time of ovulation.

INDICATIONS OF INTRAUTERINE INSEMINATION

Unexplained Infertility

In this condition, there is no definite cause for infertility, even after subjecting the patient to complete workup. The complete workup includes routine lab investigations, hormonal investigations (T3, T4, TSH, prolactin, T, DHEAS, day 2 LH, FSH and E2 and day 21 progesterone) semen analysis, assessment of tubal status (HSG or laparoscopy-hysteroscopy) and assessment of ovulation (serial vaginal USG, daily urinary LH or day 21 progesterone). The average incidence of unexplained infertility is around 10–15%.

The pregnancy rates in these patients are as follows:

- Natural cycle + IUI: 6%
- Clomiphene (CC) and/or gonadotropins + IUI: 18–19% Zeyneloglu et al. demonstrated that superovulation with IUI gave the best chance of pregnancy.

A Cochrane systematic review in 2016 did not find conclusive evidence of a difference in live birth or multiple pregnancy in most of the comparisons for couples with unexplained subfertility treated with intrauterine insemination (IUI) when compared with timed intercourse (TI), both with and without ovarian hyperstimulation (OH). There were insufficient studies to allow for pooling of data on the important outcome measures for each of the comparisons.[1]

Cervical Factor

The following are some common causes of cervical factor:
- Insufficient mucus production
- Altered quality of mucus
- *Abnormal cervix*: Stenosis, injury, malformation, infection, erosion
- Abnormal postcoital test (the general consensus is that PCT has nonpredictive value in terms of pregnancy).

The pregnancy rate is as follows:
- Natural cycle + IUI: 14%
- CC and/or HMG/FSH: 17%.

Male Factor

Zayed et al[2] reported a PR of 19% per cycle in patients with mild male factor. *Mild male factor was defined as follows:*
- Patient with only one abnormal male parameter
- Total motile sperm concentration of more than 5 million and morphology greater than 5%.

Sperm quality has to be one of the main determinants to predict IUI success. Clinical practice would benefit from the establishment of threshold levels for sperm parameters above which IUI pregnancy outcome is significantly improved and below which a successful outcome is unlikely. There is a lack of standardization in semen-testing methodology and the huge heterogeneity of patient groups and IUI treatment strategies. The four sperm parameters most frequently examined were: (i) inseminating motile count after washing: cut-off value between 0.8 million and 5 million; (ii) sperm morphology using strict criteria: cut-off value >4% normal morphology; (iii) total motile sperm count in native sperm sample: cut-off value of 5–10 million; and (iv) total motility in native sperm sample: threshold value of 30%.[3] Patients with severe male factor infertility should go directly for IVF/ICSI.

Ejaculatory Failure

Causes

Anatomical: Severe hypospadias: In this the semen is collected by masturbation and IUI is performed.

Neurological: Retrograde ejaculation and paraplegics: In retrograde ejaculation, urine is centrifuged and then washed to isolate sperms and IUI performed. In paraplegics, the semen is collected by electroejaculation. In electroejaculation, a probe is inserted into the rectum and a stimulus is given to the seminal vesicles to bring about ejaculation. The semen is collected and IUI performed. In both these conditions, the sperm quality especially its motility is hampered. Good results are obtained in whom the progressive motility is more than 20–30%.

Psychological conditions: Impotence and erectile dyfunction: In this, the patient is given sex-psychotherapy. Drugs such as viagra, muse, or papaverine may be given to bring about a good erection. Some patients benefit with the use of mechanical vibrators. Very occasionally the patients may have be subjected to general anesthesia and electroejaculation. Following this IUI may be performed.

Immunological

Infertile couples suffer infertility by immunological mechanisms mainly by the presence of antisperm antibodies (ASA) in blood, semen or cervicovaginal secretions; the formation of ASA in men and women may be associated with disturbance in immunomodulatory mechanisms that result in functional impairment of sperm and thus its inability to fertilize the oocyte. Immunological infertility caused by ASA is the result of interference of these antibodies in various stages of fertilization process, inhibiting the ability of interaction between sperm and oocyte.[4]

Endometriosis

Patients with mild to moderate endometriosis have good pregnancy rates of between 7% and 18% with IUI. However, as the pregnancy rates (3–5%) are very low with severe endometriosis, it is best to opt for IVF/ICSI.

Donor Semen IUI

When there is azoospermia due to testicular failure and high FSH.

When there is obstructive azoospermia but the couple does not want to undergo ICSI with sperm extraction.

Severe Oligoasthenospermia

Single woman or those are in a homosexual relationship. The following etiological factors of intrauterine insemination are elaborated in Figure 1.1.

PREREQUISITES FOR INTRAUTERINE INSEMINATION

- Age less than 40 years.
- Patient capable of spontaneous or induced ovulation.
- At least one patent fallopian tube with good tubo-ovarian relationship which would not hamper the egg collection by the tubal fimbria from Pouch of Douglas.

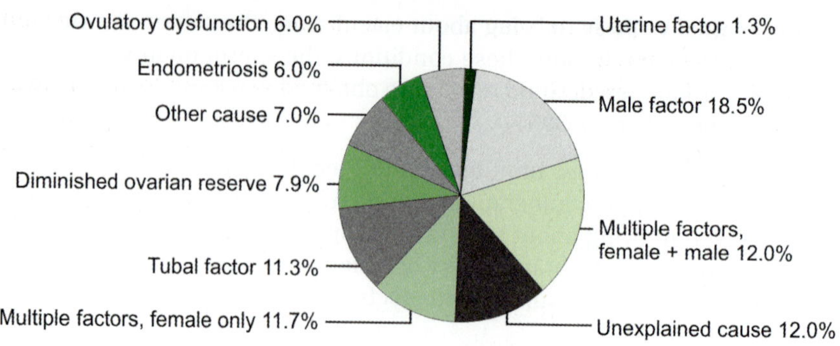

Note: Total does not equal 100% due to rounding.

Fig. 1.1: Etiological factors of intrauterine insemination

- Sperm count of more than 10 million/mL prewash or a postwash count of >5 million motile sperms.
- Easy access to the uterine cavity via a negotiable cervical canal.

Intrauterine Insemination: Steps

- Patient selection and workup
- Ovarian stimulation
- Semen wash
- Insemination
- Luteal support.

Patient Selection and Workup

The patients are selected based on their tubal, hormonal and seminal status. For further details one can look up the section on indications.

Patient Workup

- **Routine investigations of both husband and wife**
  - Hb, CBC, ESR, VDRL, HBSAG, HIV, HCV, blood sugars
- **Investigations of the husband**
  - Semen analysis after 3–4 days of abstinence
  - *Optional tests:* Semen culture
  - Kruger sperm morphology
  - *Sperm antibodies:* Immunobead and MAR test
  - Scrotal Doppler to rule out varicocele, FSH, testosterone, prolactin
- **Hormonal investigations of the wife**
  - Serum FSH, LH, estradiol on day 3 of cycle (FSH >10 mIU/mL and E2 >60 pg/mL indicates poor ovarian reserve LH/FSH >2/1 indicates PCOS. Low LH, FSH, E2 indicates hypogonadotrophic hypogonadism. FSH more than 17 mIU/mL on day 10 after CC indicates poor prognosis).

- In case of patients suspected to be poor responders, one can do additional tests:
  - *Anti-müllerian hormone (AMH):* AMH levels seem to have a positive correlation and patient's age and LH levels had a negative correlation with the outcome of IUI and controlled ovarian stimulation with gonadotropins. AMH concentration was significantly higher and LH was significantly lower in patients with a clinical pregnancy after three cycles of IUI treatment compared with those who did not achieve pregnancy.[5]
  - Serum inhibin-B test which is >45 pg/mL in poor responders
  - *Clomiphene challenge test:* CC 100 mg/day from day 5 to day 9 and FSH on day 10. A high FSH indicates poor response and poor prognosis.

Nowadays, inhibin and CC challenge test are rarely done.

- Serum prolactin and T3, T4, TSH
- In case of patients with PCOS diagnosed by USG, or symptomatology or having features of androgen excess one can do the following tests:
  - Fasting serum insulin level (>10 mIU/mL is significant)
  - Fasting and postprandial blood sugar
  - DHEAS, androstenedione and testosterone.
  - In obese patients a follicle phase 17-OHP level (to rule out congenital adrenal hyperplasia) and dexamethasone suppression test (to rule out Cushing's syndrome) should be carried out.
  - Rarely, serum alanine transaminase level is done in patients who are intolerant to metformin treatment and who need to be placed on Rosiglitazone
  - In women with past history of renal disease on metformin treatment, serum creatinine and/or 24 hour creatinine clearance may have to be done.
  - For screening and academic purposes a C peptide assay may be performed to pick up latent diabetes.

- **Tests to rule out tuberculosis:** These are especially important in developing countries.
  - CBC
  - ESR
  - Mantoux test
  - Serum IgG and IgM for tuberculosis
  - Plain X-ray of chest
  - Sputum acid fast bacilli on three consecutive days.
  - TMA or PCR on any tissue suspected of having tuberculosis
  - Guinea pig inoculation and culture
- **An USG of the abdomen and pelvis should be done.** It is preferable to perform a transvaginal USG.
- **Hysterosalpingography (Immediately after the menstrual period)**
  - It is normally indicated in the early phase of treatment when the couple has just started trying for a pregnancy. It is a relatively simple,

minimally invasive test which can give us a lot of information, however, it is painful. If HSG is normal, one can offer the couple few cycles of CC with planned relations. If that fails to achieve pregnancy, one can try few cycle of CC plus IUI before going for a thorough investigation by performing a laparoscopy, hysteroscopy and endometrial biopsy. It is prudent not to subject the patient to too many CC cycles before doing laparoscopy, as too many stimulation cycles may predispose to long term effects of increased incidence of ovarian cancer in the sixth and seventh decade of the patients life.
  - It can also be performed in patients who have already undergone laparoscopy in the past. It can be done to rule out any gross abnormalities in the uterus prior to starting IUI treatment.
  - It can also be done as a therapeutic procedure of fallopian tube recanalization (FTR) where the tubal blocks could be opened by guide wire under image intensifier HSG control. One of the prerequisites of this procedure is blocked tubes without having any major pathology seen on Laparoscopy.
- **Diagnostic cum operative laparoscopy—hysteroscopy—endometrial biopsy—histopathalogy**
- **Tests for classifying patients ovulatory status (ovulatory or anovulatory)**
  - Basal body temperature (Rarely done nowadays)
  - Serial vaginal ultrasound follicular scan in spontaneous cycle
  - Serum progesterone on Day 21 of cycle >4 ng/mL indicates ovulation and >10 ng/mL indicates adequate luteal phase
  - Endometrial biopsy—secretory premenstrual biopsy indicates ovulation.

REFERENCES

1. Veltman-Verhulst SM1, Hughes E, Ayeleke RO, Cohlen BJ. Intrauterine insemination for unexplained subfertility. Cochrane Database Syst Rev. 2016;2:CD001838.
2. Zayed F, Lenton EA, Cooke I. Comparison between stimulated in vitro fertilization and stimulated intrauterine insemination for the treatment of unexplained and mild male factor infertility. Hum Reprod. 1997;12(11):2408-13.
3. Ombelet W1, Dhont N2, Thijssen A3, Bosmans E2, Kruger T4. Semen quality and prediction of IUI success in male subfertility: a systematic review. Reprod Biomed Online. 2014;28(3):300-9.
4. Restrepo B1, Cardona-Maya W. Antisperm antibodies and fertility association. Actas Urol Esp. 2013;37(9):571-8.
5. Bakas P1, Boutas I1, Creatsa M1, Vlahos N1, Gregoriou O1, Creatsas G1, Hassiakos D1. Can anti-müllerian hormone (AMH) predict the outcome of intrauterine insemination with controlled ovarian stimulation? Gynecol Endocrinol. 2015;31(10):765-8. doi: 10.3109/09513590.2015.1025381. Epub 2015 Aug 18.

2

Ovulation Induction

Nandita Palshetkar

INTRODUCTION

Many patients who are unable to conceive after one year of unprotected intercourse are offered the option of intrauterine insemination (IUI). Ovulation induction is an important step in this process, as it aims at stimulating maturation of more than one oocyte at a time, which improves the chances of fertilization and pregnancy.

RATIONALE FOR INDUCING OVULATION WHILE CARRYING OUT INTRAUTERINE INSEMINATION

Ovarian stimulation has been shown to significantly improve the outcome in IUI cycles. Ovarian stimulation may improve the results of IUI by following two mechanisms:

1. By increasing the number of eggs available for fertilization
2. By overcoming a subtle defect in ovulatory function and luteal phase.

Numerous studies have highlighted the benefits of ovarian stimulation with IUI. From a retrospective analysis of 45 studies, Guzick et al. concluded that the combined pregnancy rates of ovulation induction with IUI were better than isolated ovulation induction without IUI or COH. The results of their study are summarized in Table 2.1.

Nulsen et al. compared the fertility rates among group of patients undergoing IUI alone with those undergoing IUI along with superovulation. They found that the cycle fecundity rate in the IUI with superovulation group was 12.2% as compared to 2.3% in the IUI only group.[3]

PROCEDURE OF OVARIAN STIMULATION AND INDUCTION

The key to success in ovulation stimulation is proper patient selection. The female partner of an infertile couple may either be ovulatory or anovulatory. When anovulation is the cause of infertility, ovarian stimulation is aimed at

TABLE 2.1: Results of a meta-analysis studying utility of ovulation induction in IUI[2]

Treatment group	*Observed pregnancy rates (%)*
No treatment	1.3–1.4
IUI	3.8
CC+IUI	8.3
HMG	7.7
HMG+IUI	17.1

TABLE 2.2: Various drugs used for ovulation induction

- Clomiphene citrate (CC)
  - Letrozole
- Gonadotrophins
- Clomiphene with gonadotrophins
  - Letrozole with gonadotrophins
- Gonadotrophins with GnRH analogues
- Gonadotrophins with GnRH antagonists
- CC/Letrozol with FSH with GnRH antagonist (the soft protocol)

achieving monofollicular response. On the other hand, in ovulating patients, the goal of therapy is mild stimulation of ovaries so as to induce development of 2–3 follicles. Various drugs and protocols are used for ovulation induction. They are enlisted below in Table 2.2.

Clomiphene Citrate

Clomiphene citrate is a selective estrogen receptor modulator with a structure that allows it to bind to hypothalamic estrogen receptors which interferes with estrogen receptor replenishment in the hypothalamus, resulting in increased pituitary release of FSH.[4] Increased FSH release drives folliculogenesis at the level of pituitary.[5] It is simple to use, cost effective and associated with fewer complications. It is the drug of choice for inducing ovulation in women with oligo-ovulatory and anovulatory cycles. In such patients, it has been reported to induce ovulation in 70–80% women with pregnancy rates varying from 30–50%.[6,7] In combination with IUI, it has been successfully used in ovulating patients also. The reported pregnancy rates in such patients varies from 12% to 35%.[2, 8] In a recent analysis of infertility treatment with a combination of clomiphene citrate and IUI, a total of 4100 cycles were studied. The results of this analysis in terms of the pregnancy rates achieved are summarized in Table 2.3.[9]

An analysis of these results also showed that younger patients have a higher pregnancy rates per cycle than older patients. The PR per cycle for

TABLE 2.3: Results of treatment of infertility with clomiphene citrate and IUI[9]

Age	*% of all pregnancies achieved within 3 cycles*	*% of all pregnancies achieved within 4 cycles*
<35	89.5	94.5
35–37	91.	92.3
38–40	95	97.5
41–42	66.7	83.3
>42	100	0

patients who initiate only one or only two treatment cycles is notably higher than the corresponding per cycle rates for cycles 3 through 9. The success rate is dismally low among patients in forth decade of their life. Such a low success rate above 40 years suggests that CC with IUI has virtually no role in treatment.

Dosage

Clomiphene citrate is administered in dosage varying from 50 to 250 mg per day for 5 days starting from the early follicular phase that is second to fifth day of cycle. The dose of CC is increased by 50 mg per cycle till ovulation is achieved. However it is seen that cumulative conception rate does not increase beyond 150 mg dosage, as the antiestrogenic properties of CC manifest more with greater dosage and in high doses CC interferes with implantation and pregnancy.[1,6] The antiestrogenic effects of CC may be in the form of:

- Poor cervical mucous
- Poor endometrial development seen as a thin hypoechoic lining on USG. The endometrial thickness is said to positively correlate with pregnancy rates and in one study it was found to be significantly lower in clomiphene cycles as compared with HMG cycles.[11]

So it is better to administer gonadotrophins along with low dose clomiphene, rather than increasing the dose of clomiphene beyond 150 mg per day.[10] Clomiphene should be used for a maximum of 6 consecutive months or 12 months in a patient's lifetime, as 75% patients respond favorably during the first 3 months of therapy and continuing the treatment beyond the above mentioned period does not yield any additional advantage.[10]

Protocol

- Baseline ultrasonography (USG) is performed on day 2 of cycle to rule out ovarian cyst
- Clomiphene citrate is administered from day 2 to day 6 in a dosage of 100 mg per day
- Serial USG monitoring is started from day 8 onwards, or urinary LH assay is performed from day 9 onwards

- Inj hCG 5000/10000 IU IM is administered when the leading follicle reaches a size of 18–20 mm and endometrial thickness is more than 8–9 mm
- IUI is performed after 36–40 hours of hCG administration
- Luteal support is given with oral or micronized progesterone.

Side Effects

- Hot flushes occur in upto 10% of patients
- Nausea and vomiting
- Breast discomfort and bloating
- Hair loss and dryness
- *Visual disturbances (1.6%):* Blurred vision, diplopia, scotoma, light sensitivity may occur and need cessation of drug and change of therapy
- Ovarian hyperstimulation
- *Ovarian cyst (6.4%):* These resolve without treatment in a few weeks
- *Multiple pregnancy (5–8%):* Most multiple pregnancies are twins. Triple pregnancies account for only 0.5% and quadruplets account for about 0.3%.
- *Ovarian cancer:* Though early studies had raised a concern for ovarian cancer, recent studies have found only a small increase in borderline serous tumors and no increase in invasive cancers. Additional studies have not even found increased risk of borderline tumors.[12]
- *Antiestrogenic effects:* These are more common with higher dosage of the drug and may need the following measures:
  - Oral supplementary estrogen can be started in late follicular phase.
  - CC to start on cycle day one (this can cause better rapid follicular growth and can give a longer CC free period before IUI, with better PR)
  - Introduce CC plus gonadotrophin sequence
  - Start pure gonadotrophin therapy

Outcomes

There are three outcomes of CC therapy

1. *Pregnancy:* The desired outcome.
2. *CC resistance:* No response to 150 mg of CC for 3 consecutive cycles.
3. *CC failures:* No response despite ovulation with CC for 6 months.

Treatment

Treatment of CC failure/resistance

- *Extended course of CC treatment:* It has been seen that up to 50% of clomiphene resistant patients may ovulate after longer duration of treatment (7 days).
- *Adjunctive treatment of clomiphene citrate with glucocorticoids:* Combining glucocorticoids with clomiphene citrate can successfully induce ovulation in many patients who fail to respond to CC alone.

Either prednisone (5 mg/d) or dexamethasone (0.5–2 mg/d) can be used in continuous or follicular phase treatment regimes (days 5–14). The exact mechanism of action of glucocorticoids is unclear. The effects can be due to androgen suppression, direct effect on developing oocyte and indirect effects on intrafollicular growth factors and cytokines that act synergistically with FSH.

- *Preliminary suppressive therapy with either OCP or a long acting GnRH agonist:* Their use helps to bring down the elevated LH levels and thus restore the disturbed harmony of the hypothalamo pituitary axis in patients with anovulation.
- *Surgical treatment:* In women with PCOS, surgical alternatives can be tried. Laparoscopic electrocauterization of ovarian surface (LEOS) has been shown to produce high rates of ovulation and pregnancy in women with PCOS who have failed with CC therapy. It is also said to correct the various endocrinological abnormalities associated with the disease. High ovulation (more than 13 80%) and pregnancy (60%) rates have been reported following LOS.

Gonadotrophins

Gonadotrophins have been the standard second line treatment for patients who failed to conceive with CC. Gonadotrophins are indicated for patients in whom both clomiphene citrate and letrozole have failed to induce ovulation. Gonadotrophins are the drugs of choice in WHO Group 1 patients (Hypogonadotrophic hypogonadism). They yield high pregnancy rate (17%) but their use is plagued by a high incidence of multiple gestation (30–40%).

A recent Cochrane review (2007) on the available results of gonadotrophins suggested that gonadotrophins might be the most effective drugs when IUI is combined with ovarian hyperstimulation. When gonadotrophins are used for ovarian stimulation low dose protocols are advised since pregnancy rates do not differ from pregnancy rates which result from high dose regimen, whereas the chances to encounter negative effects from ovarian stimulation such as multiples and OHSS are limited with low dose gonadotrophins.[13] Gonadotrophins may be applied on a daily basis.

Choice of Gonadotrophins

The choice of gonadotrophin to be used depends upon the day 2 plasma LH/FSH/E2 levels. If serum LH is elevated, FSH containing gonadotrophins are indicated, whereas if serum FSH is elevated (>10 mIU/mL), a combination of LH and FSH is used for ovarian stimulation. For ovarian stimulation in patients with hypogonadotropic hypogonadism, a combination of LH and FSH is used.

Various types of Gonadotrophin preparations available for clinical use are:

- Human menopausal gonadotrophins (Containing 75 IU FSH and 75 IU LH)
- Highly purified human menopausal gonadotrophins (Containing 75 IU FSH, 75 IU LH and less than 5% urinary proteins)

- Highly purified urinary FSH (Containing 75 IU FSH and less than 0.0017 IU LH)
- Recombinant FSH
- Recombinant LH

Factors influencing the dose of gonadotrophins:*
- *BMI:* Dosage is directly proportional to patient's BMI
- *Ovarian reserve:* FSH level above 10 IU/L indicates a need for higher dose
- *Age of the patient:* Patients above 35 years of age need higher dose
- *Cause of infertility:* Patients with PCOS need lower dosage whereas patients of unexplained infertility and hypogonadotrophic hypogonadism need higher doses
- Dose needed for stimulation in previous cycle

*Start with 150 IU in young women with no adverse factors. Poor responders may need 225 IU as starting dose.

Regimens

Three different regimes of gonadotrophins are used for ovulation induction. They include:

1. *Conventional regimen:* This regime has been used with success in clomiphene resistant and clomiphene failure cases. It has yielded acceptable pregnancy rates of up to 30%. The protocol is summarized as below:
   - Baseline USG on Day 1 or 2 of periods
   - Start with 75–150 IU/day on day 2–3 in the evening
   - Serial USG for follicular monitoring is performed from day 8 onwards
   - Serum estradiol (E2) is done on day 8
   - If serum E2 > 200 pg/mL and follicle >10 mm is seen, the daily dose of gonadotrophins is maintained
   - If serum E2 < 200 pg/mL and no follicle >10 mm, the daily dose is increased by 75 units per day till follicular growth is obtained
   - Inj hCG 5000/10000 units is given when leading follicle is >16–18 mm and endometrial thickness is > 7 mm.

   Supraphysiological doses of FSH lead to recruitment of excessive follicles, which increases the risk of OHSS and multiple pregnancies.

   Disadvantages of conventional regime include the following:
   - Although good pregnancy rates are achieved with this regime, it is associated with high rates of multiple gestations ranging from 35% to 15%. Multiple gestation is associated with high rates of abortion and maternal and neonatal morbidity. Age of the patient, number of days of gonadotropin treatment, total dose of gonadotropin, and number of follicles = 15 mm at the time of human chorionic gonadotropin administration have been found to be statistically significant predictors of multiple gestation in more than one studies.[14,15]

- OHSS conventional regime is associated with a potentially life threatening OHSS in 6–14% cases.[14, 22]
- Costly and requires strict monitoring.

2. *Low dose step-up regime:* This regimen has especially been useful in women with PCOS. The principle behind this regimen is to find the "threshold " level of FSH which will lead to the development of a single preovulatory follicle.[16, 17] The key feature of this regimen is the low starting dose of drug, persistence of treatment with the same dose for up to 14 days and a stepwise increase in subsequent doses, if necessary with an aim of achieving the development of a single dominant follicle rather than the development of many large follicles, so as to avoid the complications of OHSS and multiple pregnancy.[18]

   Protocol
   - Do a baseline USG on Day 2 rule out ovarian cyst
   - Start with a low dose (37.5–75 units/day) to be given for 7 days, starting from day 2 of the cycle
   - Measure serum E2 level and perform USG on day 7. If day 8 serum E2 is > 200 pg/mL or follicle size is above 10 mm, the same dose is continued. If, however, serum E2 level or the follicle size is inadequate, the dose is increased by 37.5 units/day every week till serum E2 level rises adequately
   - Continue follicular monitoring
   - Administer Inj hCG when leading follicle is more than 16–18 mm and endometrial thickness is 7 mm or above. The rest of the precautions are as per the conventional regime.

   Advantages
   - It is especially useful in patients with PCOS, who are at high risk for OHSS as it causes the recruitment of lesser number of follicles. In a number of studies, this regime has achieved a consistent uniovulatory development in up to 70% cycles and an acceptable cumulative pregnancy rate of 40% and 20% per cycle respectively.[18,19]
   - There is a decreased risk of multiple pregnancies. The multiple pregnancy rate are reported 5–6%.[19]

   Disadvantage
   - Extended duration of treatment is required.

3. *Step down regime:* Low dose step up regimen is a popular regimen for ovulation induction, as it is associated with acceptable success rate and decreased incidence of complications. However, this therapeutic approach is very unphysiological. Low dose regimen results in elevated levels of FSH during late follicular phase contrary to the natural cycles.

   In a natural cycle FSH promotes growth because of two events, the FSH threshold and FSH window.[21,22] FSH threshold is the level of FSH below which no follicular growth can be initiated. The FSH window is the number of days that FSH levels are above the threshold, which accounts for the total number of follicles that are activated. Since sensitivity of follicle increases with development, the required FSH for a follicle will decrease. Balance between the decreasing levels of FSH and increasing FSH sensitivity is responsible for the growth of the dominant follicle and atresia of remaining follicles. This is the principle behind step down regime, which mimics the hormonal pattern in normally ovulatory women and induces development of one follicle at a time in anovulatory women.[20]

Protocol: HMG/FSH therapy at a daily dose of 150 units is started on Day 2 and continued till a dominant follicle of > 10 mm is observed on TVS. After this, the dose is decreased to 112.5 units IM per day for 3 days, followed by 75 units IM per day for next 3 days. This dose is then continued till the day of hCG injection. Rest of the regimen is same as in the step up regime.

Advantages: The advantages of step down regime over step up regime have been confirmed in a number of studies.[23,24] In a randomized study, that compared low dose step up regime and step down regime in CC resistant women, monofollicular development was seen in 88% of the women treated with step down regimen, compared to 56% observed in women treated with step up regimen, thus reducing the risk of multiple pregnancy and hyperstimulation. The mean duration of treatment in patients treated with step down regimen was just 9 days, in comparison to 18 days for patients treated with step up regimen.[24]

Clomiphene Citrate with Gonadotrophins

Sequential use of CC and gonadotrophin (HMG or FSH) therapy has become an increasingly utilized method for COH for patients who fail CC therapy.[25,26]

Advantages

A combination of two has following advantages:
- Higher pregnancy rate than with CC alone[26,27]
- More cost effective, as the dosage of gonadotrophins is reduced[25-27]
- Lesser multiple pregnancy rate than with gonadotrophins alone[26, 28]
- Lower incidence of OHSS, as compared to the conventional regime.

Protocol

- Do a baseline scan on day 2 to rule out ovarian cyst
- Start CC 100 mg from day 2 to day 6
- Administer Inj FSH/HMG 150 units on day 6 and day 8
- Do serial transvaginal USG from day 8 onwards
- In case the follicle growth or number is inadequate, consider giving additional FSH/HMG injections from day 9 onwards
- Administer Inj hCG 5000/10000 units IM when leading follicle is 18–20 mm.

Disadvantage

The disadvantage of adding CC has been its antiestrogenic effect which has an adverse pregnancy outcome.[29,30]

GnRH Analog in Combination with Gonadotrophins

In almost 15–20% of cycles, which have been stimulated with gonadotrophins or CC, the exaggerated estradiol level due to the multifollicular development often provokes higher LH levels during the follicular phase or an untimely LH hormone surge, which leads to cycle cancellation.[31] Therefore, in order to avoid interference from endogenous gonadotrophin secretion, a combination of gonadotrophins and GnRH analogs has being used for ovulation induction. Although GnRH analogs are routinely used in IVF cycles, their routine use in IUI cycles is not recommended.[32] Cochrane review has concluded that GnRH analogs do not significantly improve pregnancy rates in IUI.

Indications

Some specific indications of its clinical use are:

- Patients undergoing IUI, wherein the standard stimulation with CC or gonadotrophins has failed to yield pregnancy after 2–4 attempts. Here, they may be tried as an alternative as they have been shown to improve the pregnancy rates.[33]
- In patients who have shown premature luteinization or premature LH surge while undergoing stimulation by gonadotrophin only. Normally 20–24% of these patients undergo premature LH surge, while being stimulated with gonadotrophins only.
- Patients with PCOS usually have highly elevated LH level, or a history of premature luteinization. Both these conditions are associated with an adverse effect on follicle and oocyte quality and also result in miscarriages.[34]
- In patients with endometriosis who require down-regulation. In these patients, depot preparations of GnRH are especially useful.

Mechanism of Action of GnRH Agonists

GnRH agonist administration leads to a prolonged agonistic action on the GnRH receptors due to their higher affinity to the receptors and their higher biological activity.[35] It leads to an initial agonistic action and increase in gonadotrophin secretion from the pituitary cells, a phenomenon called as "flare effect". However, prolonged administration of GnRH agonists leads to down-regulation of GnRH receptors and subsequently suppresses pituitary function and Gonadotrophin secretion.

Protocols

Depending on the duration of administration of GnRH agonist three protocols are described:

1. **Long protocol***:* This has two distinct phases. In the first phase, agonist is given for pituitary desensitization and 2nd phase is the stimulatory phase.

- Start GnRH agonist (e.g. Inj Lupride 20 IU, subcutaneously) from midluteal phase of previous cycle
- Continue the same dose till 1st day of menstruation
- Check for down-regulation (Serum E2 level below 50 pg/mL or endometrial thickness <5 mm)
- Dose of agonist is reduced to half and gonadotrophins are started on day 1or 2 of the period
- Continue follicular monitoring and adjust the dose of gonadotrophin according to the clinical response
- Administer Inj hCG 10,000 IU once the follicle is 18–20 mm in size

Disadvantages: Long protocol is an extremely useful protocol for patients with premature LH surge. However, it has the following disadvantages:

- Increased duration of therapy
- Higher cost of treatment
- Higher consumption of hormones with resultant higher risk of hyperstimulation syndrome (up to 0.6–14% per cycle) and higher multiple pregnancy rates
- High risk of cyst formation (6–25%)
- Pregnancy rates are not significantly better than with gonadotrophin only protocol.[32]
- Luteal support is necessary as it is associated with LPD and premature luteolysis

2. **Short protocol:** It utilizes both the initial flare response on adding agonist and the subsequent inhibitory effect of the agonist on pituitary gonadotrophes.
   - Start the GnRH agonist on day 1 of menstrual cycle
   - Start the gonadotrophin on day 3 of menstrual cycle
   - Start follicular monitoring from day 8 and adjust the dose of gonadotrophin according to the response
   - Administer Inj hCG when the follicle size is 18–20 mm
   - Perform IUI 36 hrs later

   Advantages
   - Shorter protocol
   - Less expensive
   - The flare effect increases the number of recruited follicles so is useful in poor responders and in patients of hypogonadotrophic hypogonadism

   Disadvantages: The suppression of LH levels is not complete and therefore, it is not useful in patients with PCOS, who have raised LH. Further, sometimes the LH surges cannot be avoided.[36]
3. **Ultra short protocol:** This was designed for poor responders but has not gained much popularity due to poor pregnancy rates. Here, the GnRH agonist is started on day 1 and given for only 3rd days, and gonadotrophin injection is started from 3rd day till the day of hCG inj.

GnRH Antagonists

Mechanism of Action

They act by competitive inhibition of GnRH receptors, which results in rapid decline in FSH/LH levels thus preventing premature LH surge. The drug can be given in a single dose or daily dose regimen.

Protocol

The two protocols for administering are:

1. *Lubeck protocol:* Gonadotrophins are started as usual and antagonist is started when the follicle reaches a size of 14 mm, or from 6th day of stimulation onwards in a dose of 0.25mg/day till the day of HCG injection.[37]
2. *French protocol:* Gonadotrophins are started as usual and a single dose (3 mg) of antagonist is given when serum E2 level is about 150–200 pg/mL and follicular size is around 14 mm.

Both these protocols are equally effective in preventing premature LH surge. Their efficacy in preventing LH surge and pregnancy outcome has been compared to GnRH agonist (Bryce Dietrich et al.). They studied the patients with unexplained infertility and mild male factor infertility and subjected them to COH/IUI with both the above mentioned regimens, and concluded that both regimens were equally effective. The ongoing pregnancy rates were 28.1% in agonist group and 30% in antagonist group.[38]

In another study by Sakhel et al. a similar comparison was done, and the authors reported clinical pregnancy rates of 48.1% vs 50% in the two groups.[39] No group had premature LH surge. It has also been shown that administration of antagonists to patients having COH cycles with multifollicular development, significantly improves the pregnancy rates.

Antagonist

A meta-analysis conducted in 2014 suggested that GnRH-ant can reduce the incidence of premature luteinization and increase the CPR when used in COS/IUI cycles, and it was especially useful for non-PCOS patients. However, evidence to support its use in PCOS patients is still insufficient.[41]

Another study states that the delayed administration of GnRH antagonists in MOH with IUI cycles when follicle size is ≥16 mm is beneficial in terms of preventing the occurrence of premature LH surge but with no improvement in pregnancy rates.[42]

Advantages

- Use of antagonist allows the manipulation of follicular development so that IUI can be avoided at weekends without any detrimental effect on PR.[40]

- When compared to agonist it is relatively simple and inexpensive. There is no suppression of oestrogen and the effects are easily reversible.
- Antagonists are associated with lower rates of OHSS. The preserved pituitary response with antagonist has opened new paths in the treatment of patients at high-risk of developing OHSS, as ovulation induction is possible by giving GnRH agonist and so the deleterious effects of hCG are avoided.[43]

Approach to Patients with Polycystic Ovary Syndrome and Metabolic Syndrome

In patients of polycystic ovary syndrome (PCOS), which is one of the most important causes of anovulation characterized by hyperandrogenism, insulin resistance and anovulation despite COH, certain other measures have been recommended which helps in ovulation induction and pregnancy.[44,45] These measures include:

- The first step in obese insulin resistant woman (BMI >30) is weight reduction. Obesity is associated with poor outcome in natural conception as well as assisted conception and also higher miscarriage rates. It also exaggerates the insulin resistance present in such females. Some recent studies have proved that even small weight loss of even 5–10% may lead to spontaneous ovulation and hence, increased spontaneous pregnancy rates. Weight loss can be achieved by exercise and a low caloric diet which has a low glycemic index.
- An endocrinological assessment to rule out other disorders of pancreas, thyroid, adrenal and pituitary is indicated. Appropriate treatment should be instituted.
- Patients with PCOS with signs and symptoms of insulin resistance are started on metformin.[46] It is a biguanide which is a class B drug in pregnancy. Metformin is known to decrease fasting insulin levels, blood pressure, low density lipoprotein levels and free testosterone. Spontaneous ovulation rates of 87% with pregnancy rates of 5-20% are achieved with metformin alone. A recent meta-analysis suggests that metformin increases the likelihood of ovulation and, in combination with clomiphene, increases the odds of both ovulation and pregnancy in women with polycystic ovarian syndrome.[6] However, the usefulness of metformin has been questioned by Bedaiwy et al. who found no improvement in pregnancy outcome in cotreatment with metformin.[47] We advocate metformin therapy for all patients of PCOS with or without associated metabolic disturbances. Oral metformin is given in a dose of 1500–2000 mg/day in two or three divided doses for 3-6 months.
- Laparoscopic ovarian drilling is now increasingly being used in these patients. It involves producing multiple holes on the ovarian surface using either electrocautery or laser. Electrosurgical reduction in the volume of ovarian stroma decreases ovarian androgen production and provides a better follicular environment. Reduction in androgen

production causes lesser peripheral aromatization and elevated FSH levels and re-establishment of HPO axis. Good ovulation (more than 80%) and pregnancy (60%) rates have been reported following LOS. It is also cheaper than Gonadotrophins and is not associated with risk of multiple pregnancy and hyperstimulation; however it carries with it the inherent risk of being a surgical procedure which might lead to adhesion formation and damage to the ovaries.

- Myoinositol is the another promising drug prescribed in PCOS cases. A study conducted recently in 2015 analyzed that myoinositol with DCI showed better results in terms of weight reduction, resumption of spontaneous ovulation and spontaneous pregnancy than metformin in PCOS patients. However, the effect of both modalities were comparable in decreasing either AMH or insulin resistance.

The study suggested that in future the studies should use different doses of MI + DCI and the use of a combination of both drugs in the same patients.[48]

SUMMARY

All the protocols have been used in COH with IUI with varying success rates. The drug most commonly used for ovulation induction is clomiphene citrate.[8] It alone successfully induces ovulation in upto 70% of patients. Gonadotrophins may be good alternative in women who fail to ovulate or get pregnant with clomiphene therapy.

REFERENCES

1. Fisch P, Casper, Brown SE, Wrixon W, Collins JA, Reid R L, Simpson C. Unexplained infertility: evaluation of treatment with clomiphene citrate human chorionic gonadotrophin or in vitro fertilization. Fertil Steril. 1989;51:828-33.
2. Guzick DS, Sullivan MW, Adamson GD, Cedars MI, Falk RJ, Peterson EP, Steinkampf MP. Efficacy of treatment for unexplained infertility. Fertil Steril. 1998;70(2):207.
3. Nulsen JC, Walsh S, DumezS, MetzgerAM. A randomized and longitudinal study of human menopausal gonadotrophin with intrauterine insemination in the treatment of infertility. Obstet Gynecol. 1993;82:780-6.
4. Practice committee of the American Society of Reproductive Medicine. Use of clomiphene citrate in women. Fertil Steril. 2004;82:S90-6.
5. Clark JH, Mardaverlch BM. The agonist antagonist properties of clomiphene citrate: A review. Pharmacol Ther. 1982;15:467-519.
6. Hammond MG, Halme JK, Talbert LM. Factors affecting the pregnancy rate in clomiphene citrate induction of ovulation. Obstet Gynecol. 1983;62:196-202.
7. Homburg R. Clomiphene citrate–the end of an era? A mini review. Human Reprod. 2005;20:2043-51.
8. Dickey RP, Taylor SN, Lu PY, Sartor BM, Rye PH, Pyrzak R. Effect of diagnosis, age, sperm quality and number of preovulatory follicles on the outcome of multiple cycles of clomiphene citrate-intrauterine insemination. Fertil Steril. 2002;78:1088-95.

9. Dovey S, Sneeringer RM, Penzias AS. Clomiphene citrate and intrauterine insemination: analysis of more than 4100 cycles. Fertil Steril; 2008.
10. Speroff L, Glass R, Kase N. In vitro fertilization in clinical gynaecological endocrinology and infertility (Eds). Speroff L, Glass R, Kase N, William and Wilkins Baltimore.
11. Adashi EY. Clomiphene citrate induced ovulation. Semin Reprod Endicrinol. 1986;4:255-76.
12. Sanner K, Conner P, Bergfeldt K, Dickman P, Sundfeldt K, Bergh T, Hagenfeldt K, Janson PO, Nilsson S, Persson I. Ovarian epithelial neoplasia after hormonal infertility treatment: long-term follow-up of a historical cohort in Sweden. Fertil Steril; 2008.
13. Cohlen BJ, Heineman MJ. Ovarian stimulation protocols (antiestrogens, gonadotrophins with and without GnRH agonist/antagonist) for intrauterine insemination in women with subfertility. Cochrane Database Systematic Review. 2007;(2):CD005356.
14. Hamilton-Fairley D, Franks S. Common problems in induction of ovulation. Ballie Áres Clin Obstet Gynaecol. 1996;4:609-25.
15. Paul F Kaplan, Misha Patel, Douglas J Austin, Richard Freund. Assessing the risk of multiple gestation in gonadotropin intrauterine insemination cycles. AJOG. 2002;186(6):1244-9.
16. Homburg R, Insler V. Ovulation induction in perspective. Human Reprod Update. 2002;8:449-62.
17. Homburg R, Howles CM. Low dose FSH therapy for anovulatory infertility associated with polycystic ovary syndrome: rationale. Human Reprod Update. 199;5:493-9.
18. Mathur R, Kailasam C, Jenkins J. Review of the evidence base of strategies to prevent ovarian hyperstimulation syndrome. Hum Fertil (Camb). 2007;10(2):75-85.
19. Homburg R, Howles CM. Low dose FSH therapy for anovulatory infertility associated with polycystic ovary syndrome: rationale, reflections and refinements. Human Reprod Update. 1999;5:493-9.
20. Schoot DC, Hop WC, De Jong FH, Van dessel HJ, Fauser BC. Growth of the ovarian follicle is similar to normal in gonadotrophin stimulated PCOS patients exhibiting monofollicular development. Acta Endicrinol. 1993;129:126-9.
21. Brown JB. Pituitary control of ovarian function—Concepts derived from gonadotrophin therapy. Aust NZ J Obstet Gynecol. 1978;52:553-9.
22. Fauser BC, Van Heusdan AM. Manipulation of human ovarian function: Physiologic concepts and clinical consequences. Endocr Rev. 1997;18:71-106.
23. Van Santbrink EJ, Donderwinkel PF, Van Diessel TJ, Fauser BC. Gonadotrophin induction of ovulation using step down regimen: Single centre clinical experience in 82 patients. Hum Reprod. 1995;10:1048-53.
24. Van Santbrink EJ, Fauser BC. Urinary follicle stimulating hormone for normogonadotrophic clomiphene resistant infertility: Prospective randomized comparison between low dose step up and step down dose regime. J Clin Endocrinol Metab. 1997;82:3597-602.
25. Lu PY, Chen AL, Atkinson EJ, Lee SH ,Erickson LD, Ory SJ. Minimal stimulation achieves pregnancy rates comparable to human menopausal gonadotropins in the treatment of infertility. Fertil Steril. 1996;65:583-7.

26. Kemmann E, Jones JR. Sequential clomiphene citrate menotrophin therapy for induction or enhancement of ovulation. Fertil Steril. 1983;39:772-9.
27. Dickey RP, Olar TT, Taylor SN, Curole DN, Rye PH. Sequential clomiphene citrate and human menopausal Gonadotrophin for ovulation induction: comparison to clomiphene citrate alone and human menopausal gonadotrophin alone. Human Reprod. 1993;8:56-9.
28. Ron-el R, Soffer Y, Langer R, Herman A, Weintraub Z, Caspi E. Low multiple pregnancy rate in combined clomiphene citrate—human menopausal gonadotrophin treatment for ovulation induction or enhancement. Human Reprod. 1989;4(5):495-50.
29. Mitwally MFM, Casper RF. Aromatase inhibition reduces gonadotrophin dose required for controlled ovarian stimulation in women with unexplained infertility. Hum Reprod. 2003;18:1588-97.
30. Gerardo B, Gerardo H, Hector F, Juan CRR, Murat A, Sergio O. Comparison of the efficacy of the aromatase inhibitor letrozole and clomiphene citrate as adjuvants to recombinant follicle-stimulating hormone in controlled ovarian hyperstimulation: a prospective, randomized, blinded clinical trial. Feril Steril. 2004;86(5):1428-31.
31. Cohlen BJ, Te Velde ER, Van Kooij RJ, Looman CWN, Habbema JDF. Controlled ovarian hyperstimulation and intrauterine insemination for treating male subfertility: a controlled study. Hum Reprod. 1998;13(6):1553-8.
32. Gagliardi CL. Utility of gonadotropin-releasing hormone agonists in programs of ovarian hyperstimulationv with intrauterine insemination. Clin Obstet Gynecol. 1993;36(3):711-8.
33. Nuojua-Huttunen S, Tuomivaara L, Juntunen K, Tomás C, Martikainen H. Long gonadotrophin releasing hormone agonist/human menopausal gonadotrophin protocol for ovarian stimulation in intrauterine insemination treatment. Eur J Obstet Gynecol Reprod Biol. 1997;74(1):83-7.
34. Balen A H, Tan SL, Jacobs HS. Hypersecretion of luteinising hormone: a significant cause of infertility and miscarriage. Br J Obstet Gynaecol. 1993;100:1082-9.
35. Henzl RM. Gonadotrophin releasing hormone and its analogues: from laboratory to bedside. Clin Obstet Gynecol. 1993;36:617-35.
36. Ho PC, Chan YF, So WK, Yering WS, Chan ST. Luteinising hormone surge in patients using Buserelin spray during ovarian stimulation for assisted reproduction. Gynecol Endocrinol. 1990;4(2):112-8.
37. Diedrich K, Diedrich C, Santos E, Zoll C, Al-Hasani S, Reissmann T, et al. Suppression of the endogenous luteinizing hormone surge by the gonadotrophin-releasing hormone antagonist Cetrorelix during ovarian stimulation. Hum Reprod. 1994;9:788-91.
38. Olivennes F, Fanchin R, Bouchard P, de Ziegler D, Taieb J, Selva J, et al. The single or dual administration of the gonadotropin-releasing hormone antagonist Cetrorelix in an in vitro fertilizationembryo transfer program. Fertil Steril. 1994;62:468.
39. Sakhel K, Abuzeid M. The effects of GnRH antagonist vs. GnRH agonist down regulation on the outcome of IUI cycles. 2007;88(1):286.
40. Miguel A Checa, María Prat, Ana Robles, Ramón Carreras. Use of gonadotropin-releasing hormone antagonists to overcome the drawbacks orf intrauterine insemination on weekends. Fertil Steril. 2006;85:573-7.

41. Shan Luo, Shangwei Li , Song Jin, Ya Li, Yaoyao Zhan. Effectiveness of GnRH antagonist in the management of subfertile couples undergoing controlled ovarian stimulation and intrauterine insemination: A meta-analysis; 2014. *http://dx.doi.org/10.1371/journal.pone.0109133.*
42. Wadehwa L, Khanna R, Gupta T, Gupta S, Arora S, Nandwani S. Evaluation of role of GnRH antagonist in intrauterine insemination (IUI) cycles with mild ovarian hyperstimulation (MOH): A prospective randomised study. J Obs Gyn. 2016. pp.1-7. *http://link.springer.com/journal/13224.*
43. Olivennes F, Fanchin R, Bouchard P, Taieb J, Frydman R. Triggering of ovulation by ae gonadotropin-releasing hormone (GnRH) agonist in patients pretreated with GnRH antagonist. Fertil Steril. 1996;66:151-3.
44. Kousta E, White DM, Cela E, McCarthy MI, Franks S. The prevalence of polycystic ovaries in women with infertility. Human Reproduction. 1999;14:2720-3.
45. Dunaifa. Hypergonadotrophic anovulation (PCOS): a unique disorder of insulin action associated with an increased risk of non insulin dependent diabetes mellitus. Am J Med. 1995;98:335-95.
46. Creanga AA, Bradley HM, McCormick C, Witkop CT. Use of metformin in polycystic ovary syndrome: a metaanalysis. Obstet Gynecol. 2008;111(4):959-68.
47. Bedaiwy MA, Shabaan OM, Ryan E, Casper RF. Pregnancy outcome after the use of metformin. Fertil Steril. 2007;88(1):185.
48. Amr Mohamed S, Abdel Hamid, Wael A, Ismail Madkour, Tamer F. Inositol versus metformin administration in polycystic ovary syndrome patients: a case control study. BORG. Evidence based Women's Health J. 2015,5:93-8.

BIBLIOGRAPHY

1. Begum MR, Quadir E, Begum A, Begum RA, Begum M. Role of aromatase inhibitor in ovulation induction in patients with poor response to clomiphene citrate. J Obstet Gynaecol Res. 2006;32(5):502-6.
2. Coelho C, Hannigan S, Growing DR. Effectiveness of letrozole for induction of ovulation in clomiphene citrate resistant polycystic ovarian syndrome (PCOS). Fertil Steril. 2005;8:163.
3. DeUgarte CM, Hayter K, Blacker CM, Wegienka G, Strickler RC. Clomiphene citrate vs. letrozole: comparison of cycle characteristics and pregnancy rates. Fertil Steril. 2007;88:292.
4. Gregoriou O, Vlahos NF, Konidaris S, Papadias K, Botsis D, Creatsas GK. Randomized controlled trial comparing superovulation with letrozole versus recombinant follicle-stimulating hormone combined to intrauterine insemination for couples with unexplained infertility who had failed clomiphene citrate stimulation and intrauterine insemination. Fertil Steril; 2007.
5. Kafy S, Tulandi T. New advances in ovulation induction. Curr Opin Obstet Gynecol. 2007;19(3):248.
6. Li TC, Saravelos H,Chow MS, Chisabingo R, Cookie ID. Factors affecting the outcome of laparoscopic ovarian drilling of polycystic ovarian syndrome in women with anovulatory infertility. Br J Obstet Gynaecol. 1998;105:338-44.

7. Mitwally MFM, Casper RF. Aromatase inhibition for ovarian stimulation: future avenues for infertility management. Curr Opin Obstet Gynecol. 2002;14:255-63.
8. Mitwally MFM, Casper RF. Aromatase inhibition improves ovarian response to follicle-stimulating hormone in poor responders. Fertil Steril. 2002;77:776-80.
9. Mitwally MF, Casper RF. Aromatase inhibitors in ovulation induction. Semin Reprod Med. 2004;22:61-78.
10. Mitwally MF, Casper RF. Single dose administration of aromatase inhibitors in ovulation stimulation. Fertil Steril. 2005;83:229-31.
11. Mitwally MFM, Casper RF. Use of an aromatase inhibitor for induction of ovulation in patients with an inadequate response to clomiphene citrate. Fertil Steril. 2001;75:305-9.
12. Quintero RB, Urban R, Lathi RB, Westphal LM, Dahan MH. A comparison of letrozole to gonadtropins for ovulation induction, in subjects who failed to conceive with clomiphene citrate. Fertil Steril. 2007;88(4):879-85.
13. Santen RJ. Inhibition of aromatase: insights from recent studies. Steroids. 2003;68:559-67.

The Luteal Phase

3

Hrishikesh Pai

LUTEAL PHASE SUPPORT

Following ovulation, the luteal phase of natural cycle is characterized by the formation of corpus luteum, which secretes steroid hormones including progesterone. Normal luteal function is essential for maintaining pregnancy.

Several studies have shown that removal of corpus luteum during early pregnancy results in complete abortion.[1,2]

A meta-analysis[3] of randomized trials indicated that luteal phase support led to significantly higher pregnancy rates than placebo in assisted reproduction techniques (ART) cycles. In another randomized study,[4] pregnancy rate after intrauterine insemination (IUI) was found to be significantly high in patients with luteal support. These data suggest that a good luteal phase support is necessary for the survival of the early pregnancy and it positively affects the success of controlled ovarian hyperstimulation (COH) and IUI cycles. After IUI, a good luteal phase must be ensured.

Why Luteal Support is Needed in Controlled Ovarian Stimulation with IUI?

Luteal support is needed after IUI because excessively high estrogen levels seen in controlled ovarian stimulation protocols may induce premature luteolysis. Some protocols may give only pure follicle-stimulation hormone (FSH), thus leading to relatively low luteinizing hormone (LH) values. Some protocols use gonadotropin-releasing hormone (GnRH) antagonist to prevent premature LH surge or to avoid IUI on weekends. Though they are administered for a short period and have a short duration of effect, their impact on corpus luteum is still not known. Luteal phase support is given to counter luteal insufficiency if any.

Initially, using human chorionic gonadotropin (hCG) or progesterone provided luteal phase support. Over the years, progesterone has become the agent of choice because hCG was found to be associated with a higher risk of ovarian hyperstimulation syndrome.[5-8]

Most treatment protocols advocate the use of progesterone throughout the first trimester of pregnancy, based on the findings of Shamma et al.[9] who used 17-hydroxy progesterone as a marker to demonstrate ongoing corpus luteum activity up to 10 weeks of pregnancy.

Types of Progesterone

Natural Progesterone-Micronized Progesterone

Various formulations of progesterone are now available, including oral, vaginal, intramuscular (IM) and rectal.

Progesterone administered orally is subjected to significant prehepatic and hepatic first pass metabolism resulting into its degradation to various metabolites and decreased bioavailability. In addition to erratic absorption, plasma levels also are poorly sustained and returns to baseline within six hours. Moreover, the metabolites formed act centrally and can cause sedation, headache and drowsiness. Patient may complain of urinary frequency and constipation also.

There is increased bioavailability and reduced variability when progesterone is administered vaginally. Plasma level remains elevated for up to 48 hours. This sustained level produces a more physiological endometrial response. It has a unique "uterine first pass" effect where the uterine tissue has a higher than expected progesterone level, despite a lower serum progesterone.[10] Furthermore, by bypassing the first hepatic pass, progesterone is not metabolized to by products that can cause dizziness and somnolence.

Several studies have compared oral versus vaginal progesterone. Levine and Watson[11] compared the pharmacokinetics of oral micronized progesterone (100 mg) with that of vaginal progesterone gel (crinone 8%, 90 mg). Results showed that vaginal gel was associated with a higher maximum concentration of progesterone. Furthermore, the 24 hours area under the curve for drug concentration versus time was higher in the group who had received vaginal progesterone. They concluded that the vaginal administration of progesterone results in a greater bioavailability with less relative variability than oral progesterone.

In another randomized study,[12] investigators compared vaginal progesterone gel (crinone 8%) 90 mg once daily with an oral progesterone preparation uterogestan 400 mg once daily, and IM progesterone in oil, 50 mg once daily.

The clinical and ongoing pregnancy rates were comparable between the vaginal gel and IM groups, but significantly lower with the oral formulation.

Intramuscular route is the most reliable route to achieve the desired concentration of progesterone. However, it has the disadvantage of inconvenience of daily injection and pain and abscess formation at injection site.

It has a rare risk of developing severe allergic reactions, acute respiratory distress syndrome (ARDS) and eosinophilic pneumonitis. Oil used in the preparation of IM progesterone is derived from sesame oil. In case of known allergies, it is recommended to switch over to peanut oil preparations. Cicinelli et al.[13] recently compared vaginal progesterone gel administration with IM injection. They found that the ratio of endometrial to serum progesterone concentrations was markedly higher in patients who had received vaginal progesterone gel. In another study,[14] histological changes on endometrium were same after vaginal and IM administration of progesterone.

This occurred despite the fact that serum levels were lower after vaginal gel administration than after IM administration.

All these studies strongly suggest that both vaginal and IM progesterone are effective, but vaginal administration is much easier and convenient for patients whereas orally administered progesterone appears to be inferior.

Vaginal route is the most preferred route of administration.

Other Progestogens

Dydrogesterone

Dydrogesterone has a dual advantage as it acts as immunomodulator also and thus, prevents rejection of paternal antigen by mother.

Doses of progesterone supplementation for early pregnancy support:

- Micronized progesterone 200–300 mg/day, orally or vaginally
  OR
- Injection progesterone 25–50 mg IM every day OR
- Oral dydrogesterone 20–30 mg/day.

Duration of Support

Support is started from the day of IUI. It is given initially for 14 days. At the end of 14 days, serum B hCG is done for detection of pregnancy. If patient is pregnant, luteal support is continued until 10–12 weeks when placenta takes over the role of progesterone production.

Luteal support should be continued for 10–12 weeks of pregnancy.

ROLE OF ANTIBIOTICS

The vagina is an area of the body that is abundant with normal bacterial flora.

Therefore, any procedure through the vagina may be considered to have added potential for resulting in postprocedure infection. Prophylactic antibiotics may play a role in the prevention of postprocedure transcervical intrauterine infections.

Many units like to give prophylactic antibiotic for 5–7 days after IUI. However, there have been no randomized controlled trials evaluating the usefulness of antibiotics for the prevention of infection after these procedures.[15]

Post IUI role of prophylactic antibiotics is still controversial.

REFERENCES

1. Gibson WE, Toner JP, et al. Experience with a novel progesterone preparation in a donor oocyte program. Fertil Steril. 1998;69:96-101.
2. Fatemi HM, Popovic-todorovic B, et al. An update of luteal phase support in stimulated IVF cycles. Hum Reprod Update. 2007;13(6):581-90.
3. Soliman S, Daya S, Collins J, Hughes EG. The role of luteal phase support in infertility treatment (a meta-analysis of randomized trials). Fertil Steril. 1994; 61:1068-76.
4. Atmaca S, Erdem M, et al. The impact of luteal phase support on pregnancy rates in intrauterine insemination cycles; a prospective randomized study. Fertil and steril. 2007(8);1:S-163.
5. Herman A, Ron-El R, Golan A, Raziel A, Soffer Y, Caspi E. Pregnancy rate and ovarian hyperstimulation after luteal human chorionic gonadotropin in in vitro fertilization stimulated with gonadotropin-releasing hormone analog and menotropins. Fertil Steril. 1990; 53:92-6.
6. Mochter MH, Hogerzeil HV, Mol BW. Progesterone alone versus progesterone combined with hCG as luteal support in GnRHa/HMG induced IVF cycles (a randomized trial). Hum Reprod. 1996;11:1602-5.
7. McClure N, Leya J, Radwanska E, Rawlins R, Haning RV. Luteal phase support and severe ovarian hyperstimulation syndrome. Hum Reprod. 1992; 7:758-64.
8. MacDougall MJ, Tan SL, Jacobs HS. In vitro fertilization and the ovarian hyperstimulation syndrome. Hum Reprod. 1992;7:597-600.
9. Shamma FN, Penzias AS, Thatcher S, DeCherney AH, Lavy G. Corpus luteum function in successful in vitro fertilization cycles. Fertil Steril. 1992;57:1107-9,10.
10. Bulletti C, de Ziegler D, et al. Targeted drug delivery in gynecology: the first uterine pass effect. Hum Reprod. 1997;12:1073-79.
11. Levine H, Watson N. Comparison of the pharmacokinetics of Crinone 8% administered vaginally versus Prometrium administered orally in postmenopausal women. Fertil Steril. 2000;73:516-21.
12. Saucedo LLE, Galache VP, Hernandez AS, Santos HR, Arenas ML, Patrizio P. Randomized trial of three different forms of progesterone supplementation. (abstract P-175) Fertil Steril. 2000;74(3S):S205.
13. Cicinelli E, DeZiegler D, Bulletti C, Matteo MG, Schonauer LM, Galantino P. Direct transport of progesterone from vagina to uterus. Obstet Gynecol. 2000;95: 403-6.
14. Tavaniotou A, Smitz J, Bourgain C, Devroey P. Comparison between different routes of progesterone administration as luteal phase support in infertility treatments. Hum Reprod Update. 2000;6:139-48.
15. Thinkhamrop J, Laopaiboon M, Lumbiganon P. Prophylactic antibiotics for transcervical intrauterine procedures. Cochrane Database of Systematic Reviews 2007, Issue 3. Art. No.: CD005637. DOI: 10.1002/14651858.CD005637.pub2.

4

Nuchal Translucency

Shailesh Kore, Neha Saxena

INTRODUCTION

Trisomy 21 is one of the most commonly observed chromosomal abnormalities. In 1866, Langdon Down described the phenotypic features of individuals with this syndrome, which was subsequently named after him.[1] He reported that the skin of an individual with trisomy 21 appears to be too large for their body.[1] More than a century later, Szabo and Gellen (1990) described the association between Down's syndrome and neck edema in the first trimester.[2] Nicolaides et al. (1992) referred to this as "Nuchal Translucency."

Nuchal translucency (NT) is the appearance of a collection of fluid under the skin behind the fetal neck in the first-trimester of pregnancy on ultrasound. The term translucency is used, irrespective of whether it is septated or not and whether it is confined to the neck or envelopes the whole fetus.

Many studies have shown established association between increased nuchal translucency measurement and fetal aneuploidies, fetal anomalies, rare genetic syndromes and spontaneous abortions.[3] In past, little was known of the overall long-term outcome of euploid children with increased NT.[4] However, according to the recent reports, it is shown that pregnancy outcomes are much more adverse with an NT that exceeds a set threshold of 3.5 mm, which represents 99th percentile or more for any gestational age window for first trimester screening.[5]

INCREASED NUCHAL TRANSLUCENCY— PATHOPHYSIOLOGY

Lymphatic system of fetus starts developing between 10–14 weeks of gestation. Thus, it was thought that, progressive increase in the width of the translucent area during this period may be indicative of congenital lymphedema.[6]

However, the heterogeneity of conditions associated with increased nuchal translucency indicates that there may more than one mechanism for abnormal collection of fluid below the skin of the fetus.[7]

The possible mechanisms are:
- Cardiac failure due to associated anomalies of the heart and great vessels.
- Altered composition of the extracellular matrix.
- Abnormal/delayed development of lymphatic system.
- Failure of lymphatic drainage due to impaired fetal movements associated with various neuromuscular disorders.
- Fetal anemia or hypoproteinemia.
- Congenital infections, acting through cardiac failure or anemia.
- Venous congestion in the heart or neck in conditions like diaphragmatic hernia or skeletal dysplasia.

MEASUREMENT OF NUCHAL TRANSLUCENCY

The 'Fetal Medicine Foundation' (London) has laid down following guidelines for correct measurement of 'Nuchal Translucency:[8]
- The gestational period must be 11–13 weeks and six days. At and after 14 weeks of gestation with fetus is often in a vertical position, which makes it difficult to obtain the appropriate image.
- The fetal crown-rump length should be between 45 and 84 mm.
- The magnification of the image should be such that the fetal head and thorax occupy the whole screen.
- A mid-sagittal view of the face should be obtained. This is defined by the presence of the echogenic tip of the nose and rectangular shape of the palate anteriorly, the translucent diencephalon in the center and the nuchal membrane posteriorly. Minor deviations from the exact midline plane would cause non-visualization of the tip of the nose and visibility of the zygomatic process of the maxilla (Fig. 4.1).
- The fetus should be in a neutral position, with the head in line with the spine. Failure to visualize sonolucent amniotic fluid between chin of the fetus and thorax indicates that fetus is in hyperflexed position. When the fetal neck is hyperextended the measurement can be falsely increased and when the neck is hyperflexed, the measurement can be falsely decreased.
- Care must be taken to distinguish between fetal skin and amnion. In case of doubt, sonographer should wait for fetal movement clearly away from the amnion.
- The widest part of translucency must always be measured.
- Measurements should be taken with the inner border of the horizontal line of the calipers placed on the line that defines the nuchal translucency thickness—the crossbar of the caliper should be such that it is hardly visible as it merges with the white line of the border, not in the nuchal fluid (Fig. 4.2).
- In magnifying the image (pre- or post-freeze zoom) it is important to turn the gain down. This avoids the mistake of placing the caliper on the fuzzy edge of the line which causes an underestimate of the nuchal measurement.

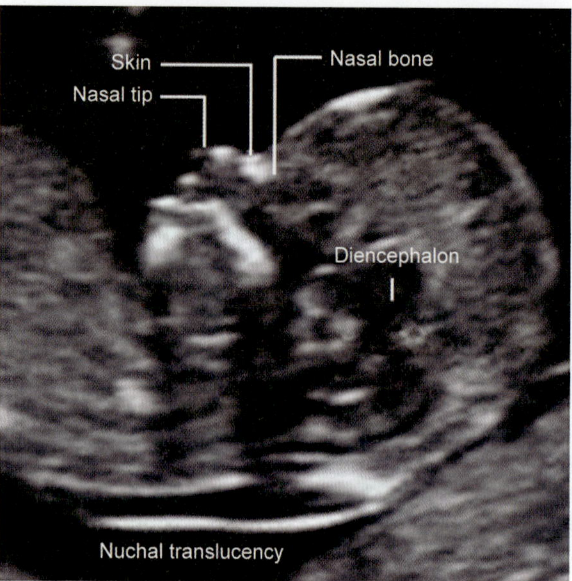

Fig. 4.1: Nuchal translucency measurement by ultrasound

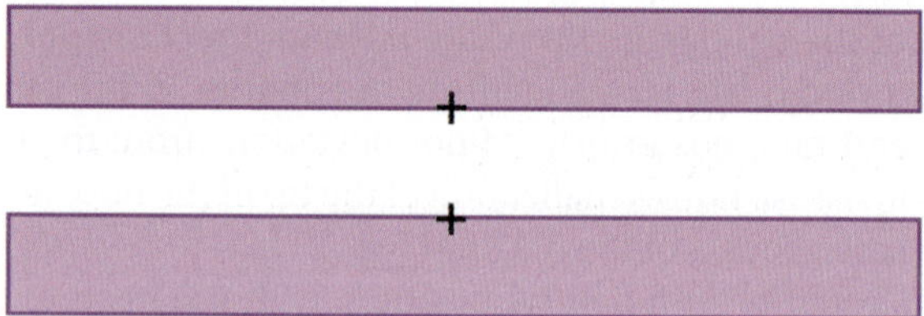

Fig. 4.2: Correct placement of calipers for measurement of nuchal translucency

- During the scan more than one measurement must be taken and the maximum one that meets all the above criteria should be recorded in the database.

The use of a semiautomated technique for the measurement of NT improves the accuracy of measurements. This measurement obtained is similar to that obtained manually and it is, therefore, applicable to the software of the Fetal Medicine Foundation.

Nuchal cord has clinical implications on the measurement of NT in the first trimesters of pregnancy.[9,10] In cases of loop of cord, the average of the two measurements of NT above and below the cord is taken to avoid a falsely increased NT.

According to the Fetal Medicine Foundation' (London) it was also found that:

- In 95% cases, NT can be measured successfully by transabdominal ultrasonography, while remaining 5% cases may require vaginal route.

The extremely obese women or patients with acutely retroverted uterus may require vaginal ultrasonography.

- To obtain optimum measurement, ultrasound machine should be of good quality, should have a video-loop function and the caliper should be able to provide measurements to one decimal point. The Doppler machine may be useful in certain cases.
- The sonographer performing scan should be capable of obtaining correct fetal sagittal view required for measurement of crown-rump length. After few hours of supervised training, such sonographer can acquire skill of measuring 'Nuchal Translucency'. The sonographer should take adequate time (approximately 10 minutes) to get proper image by adhering to standard guidelines.
- The ability to measure nuchal translucency and obtain reproducible results improves with training; good results are generally achieved after 80–100 supervised or audited scans.[11]
- The distribution of nuchal translucency measurements, quality of images in terms of adherence to standard guidelines like magnification, section, caliper placement, skin line and visualization of the amnion separate from the nuchal membrane are taken into account in the audit of the results.[12] (Herman A 1998)
- The ability to achieve reliable measurement of nuchal translucency is dependant on motivation of the sonographer. A study by Roberts LJ[13] (1995) comparing the results obtained from the hospitals where nuchal translucency was used in clinical practice for intervention to those from hospitals where they merely recorded the values but did not act on the results, reported that, in the interventional group, successful measurement of nuchal translucency was achieved in 100% of cases and measurement was more than 2.5 mm in only 2.3% of cases; while the respective percentages in the other group were 85% and 12%.
- It is necessary that all operators follow same standard criteria to achieve uniformity of results.
- The maximum thickness of subcutaneous translucency between the skin and the soft tissue overlying the cervical spine should be measured by placing the calipers on the lines as shown the Figure 4.1.

REPEATABILITY IN THE MEASUREMENT OF NUCHAL TRANSLUCENCY

A potential criticism of screening by ultrasound is that scanning not only requires highly skilled operators but it is also prone to operator variability. But various studies have confirmed the good repeatability in the NT measurement. The prospective study by Pandya et al.[14] has showed that the intraobserver variability was less than 0.54 mm and interobserver variability was less than 0.62 mm in 95% of the cases. The same study also demonstrated that the caliper placement repeatability was similar to the intraobserver and interobserver repeatability, suggesting that a large part of the variation in the measurement can be accounted for caliper placement rather than the generation of the image. Digital image processing and automation of caliper placement can reduce the variation of measurements.[15]

Ultrasound examination of the fetus is a subjective process that is highly dependent on operator skills and the quality of the ultrasonography equipment. These limitations militate against the deployment of ultrasound as a screening tool in the manner in which maternal serum biochemistry has been used.[16]

NUCHAL TRANSLUCENCY AND CHROMOSOMAL DEFECTS

Increased nuchal translucency (Fig. 4.3) can be associated with a number of anomalies, including:

- Aneuploidy—trisomies (including Down's syndrome) and Turner's syndrome
- Nonaneuploidy structural defects and syndromes—congenital diaphragmatic hernia, congenital heart disease, omphalocele, skeletal dysplasia, fetal infections, etc.[17-19]

There have been various researches to establish the association between increased NT and adverse pregnancy outcome in karyotypically normal fetuses.[20]

Sairam et al. reported the presence of an increased NT as an independent risk for fetal cardiac and extracardiac defects in patients with a normal karyotype.[21] Studies by Hyett et al. have also shown an increased prevalence of congenital heart diseases with raised NT thickness.[22]

In most of the women with increased NT, as gestation progresses, the region of nuchal translucency might either regress or evolve into nuchal edema or cystic hygroma.

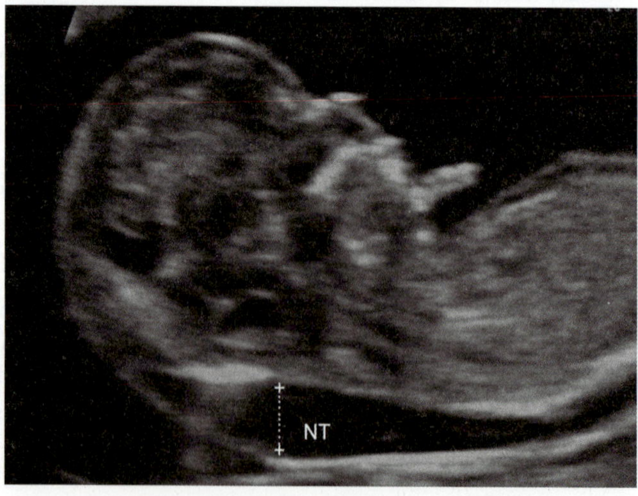

Fig. 4.3: Increased nuchal translucency (NT)

In chromosomally normal fetuses where NT regresses, a large proportion will have a normal outcome (but spontaneous regression does not however, mean a normal karyotype).

Other possibilities of erroneous reporting of increased NT can be incorrect measurement technique, chorioamniotic separation, fetal neck skin thickening due to first-trimester hydrops fetalis or presence of nuchal cord. These possibilities should be ruled out before deciding about further course of action. In few cases, repeat examination at higher center may be warranted.

ACCURACY OF NUCHAL TRANSLUCENCY AS A SCREENING MARKER

The detection rate of about 75–80% can be obtained by screening of fetuses by NT alone with maternal age for trisomy 21 and other major aneuploidies with a false positive rate of 5%. The detection rate can be improved to 90% by a combination of NT with maternal serum free β-hCG and pregnancy-associated plasma protein A (PAPP-A). However, the detection rate can further be increased up to 95% and the false positive rate can be reduced to 3% by taking into consideration the nasal bone, ductus venosus flow and tricuspid flow.

The measurement of nuchal transparency is a potentially useful 1st trimester screening tool, as 65–85% of trisomy fetuses and other, nontrisomy abnormal fetuses show increased NT. Abnormal findings warrant further evaluation on a targeted basis.

At 12 weeks of gestational age, an "average" nuchal thickness of 2.18 mm has been observed; however, up to 13% of chromosomally normal fetuses present with a nuchal translucency of greater than 2.5 mm. Thus, for even greater accuracy of predicting risks, the outcome of the nuchal scan may be combined with the results of simultaneous maternal blood tests. In pregnancies affected by Down's syndrome there is a tendency for the levels of hCG to be increased and PAPP-A to be decreased. There has been a reduction in false positive rates with the use of nuchal scanning over the previous use of just biochemical blood profiling alone.[23]

Since early 1990s, many studies demonstrated the association of increased nuchal translucency at 11–14 weeks and chromosomal defects, the sensitivities of various studies ranging from 20 to 80%. This variation in the results was probably because of difference in maternal age distribution of the population studied, 'cut off' value of abnormal translucency measurement, which ranged from 2 to 10 mm. Also difference in criteria or protocol in measurement of the nuchal translucency led to this variation. Subsequent larger study by Pandya PP[24] (1995) & Szabo & Gellen (1995) for screening of downs syndrome had sensitivities ranging from 75–80%, with acceptable false positive rate. Nicolaides et al.[25] in 1994 reported a series of 1273 pregnancies in which a nuchal translucency >= 2.5 mm was seen in 84% of fetuses with trisomy 21 and 4.5% of normal fetuses. Also, Comas C in their study reported the prenatal detection rates of trisomy 21 greater than 95% and a 5% false-positive rate with an early second trimester nuchal translucency measurement (Table 4.1).[26]

It must be remembered that mean measurement of nuchal translucency is around 1.5–2.0 mm. If 'cut off' value for screen positive is far above the mean, though the test will become more specific, but it will have very low sensitivity. Thus, it is essential to keep cut off value at level where test will give good sensitivity with acceptable (<5%) false positive rate. As NT increases with gestation, instead of using standard cut off, it is necessary to use gestation related multiple of the median (MoM) value/cut offs to decide whether patient is screen positive or not. Actual risk assessment by using software taking into consideration maternal age and other demographic/risk factors along with NT measurement with or without maternal serum dual markers values (MoM) is more appropriate method of screening and useful in counseling the couple.

Appropriate training, high motivation and adherence to a standard technique/criteria are required for successful screening program with good sensitivity with acceptable false positive rate. According to Monni et al.[27,28] detection rate of trisomy 21 in their study improved from 30 to 80% by following the standard guidelines. The accuracy and repeatability greatly depends on level of competence of the staff which can be achieved by proper and adequate training, certified by external agency. It should be subjected to quality control with high standard precision equipment and clinical protocol.[12]

One Stop Center for Assessment of Risk (OSCAR)

Fetal Medicine Foundation (FMF) recommends universal screening, that is, all women between 11 and 13^{+6} weeks should be offered combined first trimester screening (Age+ NT+ maternal serum PAPP-A and β-hCG). With technological advances, it is now possible to give report of screening and risk assessment in one visit. Actual risk assessment is done by using software using age, other risk factors along with NT and maternal serum markers (MoMs). Rather than saying patient as screen positive or negative, actual final risk is told to the patient/couple. The couple is then asked to take decision after nondirectional counseling about further testing. In many cases, women with increased risk are subjected to invasive testing with chorion villus sampling for definitive diagnosis. However, this procedure carries a small

TABLE 4.1: Results of studies of screening for trisomies using nuchal translucency measurement

Author	*Gestation (weeks)*	*N*	*Sensitivity*	*False-positive ratio*
Pandya et al[24]	10–14	1763	75%	3.6%
Nicolaides et al[25]	11–14	1273	84%	4.4%
Comas[26]	11–16	11, 281	95%	5%

risk of miscarriage. Thus, it is necessary to have screening done with good detection with low false positive rate. False positive rate can be reduced greatly by adding other markers like nasal bone, ductus venosus flow and tricuspid flow. Also non-invasive prenatal test (NIPT) which uses cell-free fetal DNA in maternal blood can be used in high risk/screen positive cases to select only those who will actually require invasive testing.

SUMMARY AND CONCLUSION

- Nuchal translucency is a promising first trimester screening tool for the detection of chromosomal anomalies and congenital malformations.
- Optimum time for successful measurement of nuchal translucency was 11 and 13^{+6} weeks.
- Prevalence of chromosomal defect is dependent on both nuchal translucency thickness and maternal age.
- All pregnant women between 11 and 13^{+6} weeks should be offered combined first trimester screening (Age+ NT+ Maternal serum PAPP-A and β-hCG).
- The risk of an adverse fetal outcome remains and increases with increasing NT even in a fetus with a normal karyotype.
- For reproducible and accurate measurements of NT, strict adherence to quality guidelines of the technique, training and supervision of the sonologist is of utmost importance.

REFERENCES

1. Langdon Down J. Observations on an ethnic classification of idiots. Clin Lectures and Reports, London Hospital. 1866;3:259-62.
2. Szabo J, Gellen J. Nuchal fluid accumulation in trisomy-21 detected by vaginal sonography in first trimester. Lancet. 1990;336:1133.
3. Pandya PP, Kondylios A, Hilbert L, Snijders RJM, Nicolaides KH. Chromosomal defects and outcome in1015 fetuses with increased nuchal translucency. Ultrasound Obstet Gynecol. 1995;5:15-9.
4. Pandya PP, Snijders RJM, Johnson SP, Brizot de Lourdes M, Nicolaides KH. Screening for fetal trisomies by maternal age and fetal nuchal translucency thickness at 10-14 weeks of gestation. Br J Obstet Gynaecol. 1995d;102:957-62.
5. Souka AP, von Kaisenberg CS, Hyett JA, Sonek JD, Nicolaides KH. Increased nuchal translucency with normal karyotype. American Journal of Obstetrics and Gynecology. 2005;192(4):1005-21.
6. Souka AP, Krampl E, Geerts L and Nicolaides KH. Congenital lymphedema presenting with increased nuchal translucency at 13 weeks of gestation. Prenat Diagn. 2002;22:91-2.
7. Nicolaides KH, Sebire NJ, Snijders RJM. Pathophysiology of increased nuchal translucency. In the 11-14 weeks scan: The diagnosis of fetal abnormalities. Carnforth, UK: Patherson publishing; 1999. pp. 95-113.

8. Nicolaides KH, Sebire NJ, Snijders RJM. Nuchal translucency and chromosomal defects. In the 11-14 weeks scan: The diagnosis of fetal abnormalities. Carnforth,UK: Patherson publishing. 1999; pp.1-63.
9. Lee P, Won H, Chung J, Shin H, Kim A. The variables affecting nuchal skin fold thickness in mid trimester. Prenatal diagnosis. 2003;23(1):60-4.
10. Scheier M, Egle D, Himmel I, Ramoni A, Viertl S, Huter O, et al. Impact of nuchal cord on measurement of fetal nuchal translucency thickness. Ultrasound in Obstetrics & Gynecology. 2007;30(2):197-200.
11. Braithwaite JM, Kadir RA, Pepera TA, Morris RW, Thomson PJ, Economides DL. Nuchal translucency measurement: training of potential examiners. Ultrsound Obstet Gynecol. 1996;8:192-5.
12. Herman A, Mayman R, Dreazen E, Caspi E, Bukovsky I, Weinraub Z. Nuchal translucency audit: a novel image-scoring method. Ultrsound Obstet Gynecol. 1998;12:398-403.
13. Roberts LJ, Bewley S, Mackinson AM, Rodeck Ch. First trimester fetal nuchal translucency: problem with screening the general population. Br J Obstet Gynecol. 1995;102:381-5.
14. Pandya PP, Altman D, Brizot ML, Pettersen H, Nicolaides KH. Repeatability of measurement of fetal nuchal translucency thickness. Ultrsound Obstet Gynecol. 1995;5:334-7
15. Bernardino F, Cardoso R, Montenegro N, Bernardes J, deSa JM. Semiautomated ultrasonographic measurement of fetal nuchal translucency using a computer software tool. Ultrasound Med Biol. 1998; 24:51-4.
16. Scholl J, Iyer C, Heard A, Coletta J, Panda B, Russell M. Thicker nuchal translucency is associated with greater risk of abnormal fetal and neonatal outcomes among fetuses with first trimester cystic hygroma. American Journal of Obstetrics and Gynecology. 2011;204(1, Supplement):S168.
17. Spencer K. Accuracy of Down syndrome risks produced in a first-trimester screening programme incorporating fetal nuchal translucency thickness and maternal serum biochemistry. Prenatal Diagnosis. 2002;22(3):244-6.
18. Ghi T, Huggon I, Zosmer N, Nicolaides K. Incidence of major structural cardiac defects associated with increased nuchal translucency but normal karyotype. Ultrasound in Obstetrics & Gynecology. 2001;18(6):610-4.
19. Goetzl L. Adverse Pregnancy Outcomes After Abnormal First-Trimester Screening for Aneuploidy.Clinics in Laboratory Medicine. 2010;30(3):613-28.
20. Michailidis G, Economides D. Nuchal translucency measurement and pregnancy outcome in karyotypically normal fetuses. Ultrasound in Obstetrics & Gynecology. 2002;17(2):102-5.
21. Sairam S, Carvalho JS. Early fetal echocardiography and anomaly scan in fetuses with increased nuchal translucency. Early Human Development. 2012;88(5):269-72.
22. Hyett J, Moscoso G, Papapanagiotou G, Perdu M, Nicolaides K. Abnormalities of the heart and great arteries in chromosomally normal fetuses with increased nuchal translucency thickness at 11–13 weeks of gestation. Ultrasound in Obstetrics & Gynecology. 1996;7(4):245–50.

23. Muller F, Benattar C, Audibert F, Roussel N, Dreux S, Cuckle H. "First-trimester screening for Down syndrome in France combining fetal nuchal translucency measurement and biochemical markers". Prenat Diagn. 2003;23(10):833-6.
24. Pandya PP, Goldberg H, Walton B, et al.The implementation of first trimester scanning at 10-13 weeks' gestation and the measurement of fetal nuchal translucency thickness in two maternity units. Ultrsound Obstet Gynecol. 1995;5:20-5.
25. Pandya PP. Ultrasound screening for fetal abnormalities in the first trimester. Prenatal Diagnosis. 1997;17:13:1269-8.
26. Comas C, Torrents M, Muñoz A, Antolín E, Figueras F, Echevarría M. Measurement of nuchal translucency as a single strategy in trisomy 21 screening: should we use any other marker? Obstet Gynecol. 2002;100(4):648-54.
27. Monni G, Zoppi MA, Ibba RM, Floris M, Manca F, Axiana C. Nuchal translucency and nasal bone for trisomy 21 screening: single center experience. Croat Med J. 2005;46(5):786-91.
28. del Carmen Saucedo M, DeVigan Vodovar. Measurement of nuchal translucency and the prenatal diagnosis of down syndrome. Obstet & Gynecol. 2009;114(4):829-38.

5

Applications of Three-Dimensional Ultrasound in Obstetrics

Narendra Malhotra, Jaideep Malhotra, Neharika Malhotra Bora

INTRODUCTION

As digital technology advances, patients and health-care professionals benefit from access to modern devices to assist diagnostics and monitor vital signs at the point of care.

Three-dimensional (3D) ultrasound involves imaging of the distribution of ultrasonic echo information in 3D space, while conventional ultrasonography applies to this imaging on a two-dimensional (2D) plane. Now 3D ultrasound is being regarded as the future of ultrasound system after color Doppler system. Voluson 530 D is the only real-time digital 3D system with powerful digital CFM, and it shows what the value of future diagnostic oriented system is all about.

In 1974, Kretztechnik started the first development dedicated in 3D ultrasound. A cylindric-shaped transducer incorporating 25 elements mounted on a drum performed a volume scan consisting of 25 parallel slices.

It was in 1989 in Paris at the French Congress of Radiology, Kretztechnik presented the first commercially available ultrasound system featuring the 3D-Voluson technique (Voluson—volume sonography).

In 1991, Pretorius and Nelson discussed the potential advantages of 3D ultrasound and its usefulness for fetal studies. All the studies mentioned above used systems developed by the authors. The most recent development is real-time 3D ultrasound using a defocusing lens, without computer processing.

With 4D ultrasound, the added dimension is time, so that the 3D images appear to be moving in real time. The 3D/4D image usually appears a golden color on the ultrasound screen, as this color is easy for patients to look at and highlights features on the baby (Figs 5.1A to C).

Although 3D fetal ultrasound can produce more "realistic" and recognizable images than conventional 2D ultrasound, the clinical significance of this remains unclear. The perceived superiority of 3D ultrasound for a number of fetal abnormalities has not been definitively

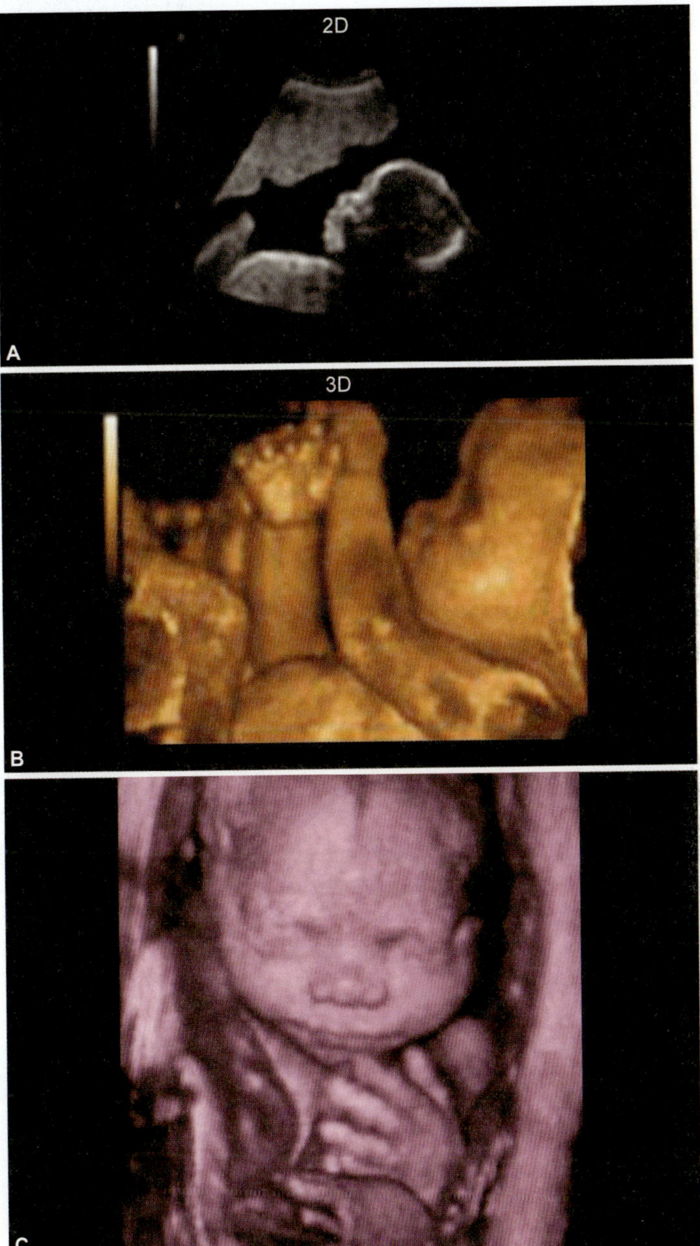

Figs 5.1A to C: (A) 2D fetal profile; (B) 3D fetal profile; and (C) 3D image of a fetus

established, and 2D imaging remains the principal diagnostic modality. (Schellpfeffer MA. Ultrasound imaging in research and clinical medicine. Birth Defects Res C Embryo Today. 2013;99(2):83-92).

THREE-DIMENSIONAL VOLUSON TECHNIQUE

Continuous research and development of this technology led to diagnostic applications in various medical fields. The Voluson system is based on several main components:

Dedicated voluson transducers providing a fully automatic scan of a user-defined region of the patient's body. For different applications various transducers ranging from 3.5—10 MHZ are available.

A special electronic memory to store the ultrasound data as a geometrically correct volume block.

A digital 3D scan converter for lossless and fast image processing.

Immediately after the volume scan is finished (0.5 to 5 sec), the monitor displays three orthogonal planes, longitudinal, transverse and coronal planes. Each of these planes can be moved within the volume block for detailed analyses, either by parallel shifting (tomographic slicing) or by rotation around any of the three spatial axes.

DIGITAL THREE-DIMENSIONAL SONOGRAPHY

Only fully digital technology allows the use of absolutely identical channels. Small deviations in the signal path are enough to produce distortion and noise. Digital technology avoids weakness of this kind and guarantees signal processing which is both distortionless and noiseless. This results in superior image quality, high reliability and the stability of the system.

THREE-DIMENSIONAL ULTRASOUND IN OBSTETRICS

Fetal biometry in the first trimester is often used for the estimation of gestational age. Lasser and co-workers examined 144 first-trimester fetuses by transvaginal ultrasonography and showed that gestational age can be estimated much earlier and more accurately than with the transabdominal approach (Figs 5.2A to C).

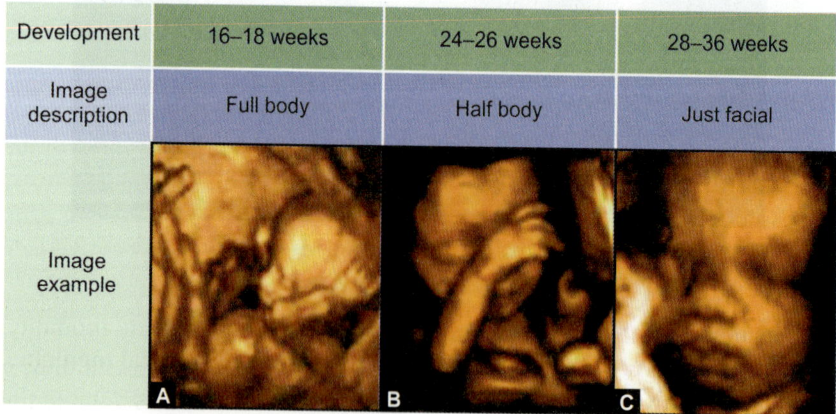

Figs 5.2A to C: Different images obtained at different gestation

However, with the use of conventional transvaginal ultrasonography, it is sometimes difficult to obtain an optimal plane for crown-rump measurement for diagnosis. Three-dimensional ultrasound overcomes this problem and increases the accuracy of fetal biometry.

Transabdominal scanning with conventional 2D ultrasound scan done in/after second trimester, though the general impression of fetal posture can be obtained, it cannot be described precisely. Surface rendering in 3D ultrasound overcomes this problem.

Steiner and colleagues determined gestational sac volume in the first trimester by tracing the contour of the gestational sac using transabdominal 3D ultrasound. In the late second and third trimester, the volume of amniotic fluid decreases relative to fetal size and it becomes increasingly more difficult to obtain 3D images of the whole body of fetus by surface rendering.

Suggested advantages of 3D ultrasound compared to 2D ultrasound in obstetrics include the following:

- Three-dimensional ultrasound appears to be less operator dependent and provides a superior display of structures with complex anatomy compared to conventional ultrasonography.
- Orientations and planes not available with two-dimensional ultrasound, because of anatomic constraints or fetal position are available with three-dimensional ultrasound.
- Volume data may be reviewed millimeter by millimeter after acquisition, simulating real-time scanning.
- Archived volume data with suspected fetal anomalies may be reviewed with other physicians after completion of the ultrasound and data may be transmitted via the internet to other locations.
- Three-dimensional ultrasound has improved accuracy of volume measurements to measure regular and irregular objects.
- Volume-rendered images are easily recognizable by both parents and physicians, which may facilitate decisions by families regarding continuing or terminating the pregnancy and are also said to enable parents to bond more effectively with the fetus. It may also assist them with making lifestyle changes, such as stopping smoking or excessive alcohol intake.

Fetal Head

Blaas and associates obtained 3D images and calculated the volume of the brain cavities at 7–10 weeks of gestation where contours of the brain cavity were interactively drawn in successive 2D slices and displayed as 3D images.

Diagnosis of structural abnormalities such as anencephaly, encephalocele or choroid plexus cyst can be made by 2D ultrasound (Fig. 5.3). However, the defects can be better described by displaying orthogonal triple planes simultaneously.

The corpus callosum, which is difficult to see with 2D ultrasound, may be depicted with 3D ultrasound by constructing a section horizontal to the abdominal wall.

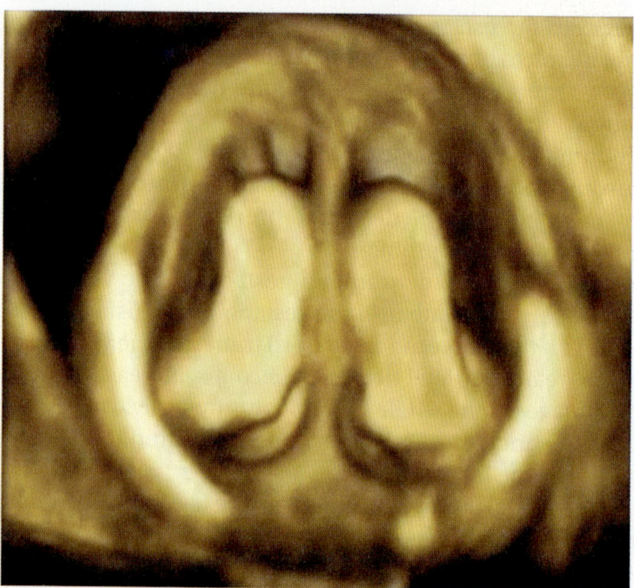

Fig. 5.3: Three-dimensional ultrasound images of fetal choroid plexus

Abnormal development of cranial sutures is seen in many dystrophic syndromes and metabolic disturbance. With 2D ultrasound, curvilinear cranial structures such as cranial sutures and fontanelles cannot be properly evaluated. This is easier with 3D ultrasound using a volume rendering method such as the maximum intensity method or defocusing lens (real-time 3D ultrasound).

Fetal Face (Figs 5.4A to F)

Three-dimensional ultrasound provides clear surface images of the fetal face noninvasively. Images from different directions can also be obtained from 3D data. With 3D ultrasound, the lips, upper gum, nose and eyelids can be observed well and morphological anomalies such as single hostric, flat nose, proboscis, cleft lip, hypotelorism or hypertelorism can be better seen with 3D ultrasound. Even, low set dysplastic ear can be readily diagnosed. The facial origin of a fetal teratoma can be confirmed on a transparent rational display.

Facial defect is one of the markers of chromosomal abnormalities and 3D ultrasound may be useful for increasing the sensitivity of screening.

Fetal Skeleton (Figs 5.5A and B)

The fetal skeleton can be observed by volume rendering, with techniques such as the transparent method and maximum intensity method.

If the vertebral column is pathologically curved laterally, it is impossible to display the whole vertebral column in one tomogram. Anomalies such as scoliosis, kyphosis, lordosis and spina bifida may be overlooked by 2D

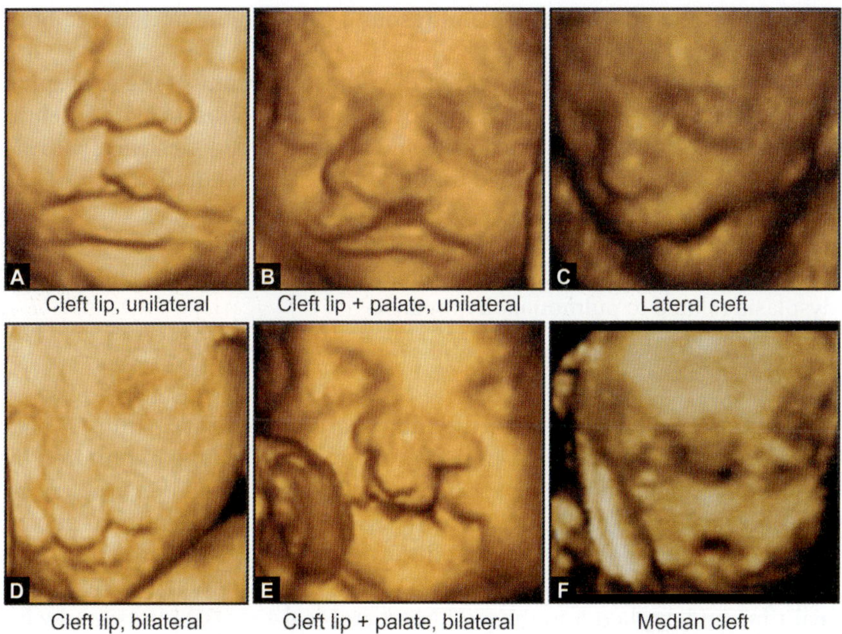

Figs 5.4A to F: Three-dimensional images of fetal facial anomalies

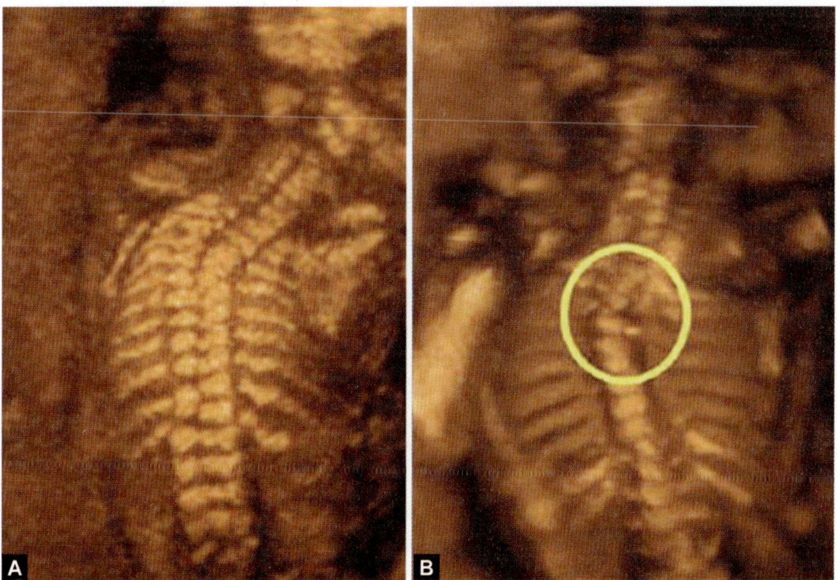

Figs 5.5A and B: (A) 3D maximum mode image of the fetal back; (B) Severe scoliosis with asymmetrical number of ribs (left;12 ribs, right; 9 ribs) is clearly demonstrated

ultrasound. The advantage of 3D ultrasound is the ability to visualize both curvatures at the same time.

Budorick and coworkers reviewed the ultrasonography of the fetal spine and pointed out that the curvature of the spine, continuity of vertebral bodies and costovertebral junctions could be observed more clearly with 3D ultrasound using the depth-cued maximum intensity method, than with 2D ultrasound.

The fetal thorax, ribs, vertebrae, clavicles and sternum are observed with 3D ultrasound, which is useful for diagnosing a small thorax and skeletal dysplasia related to pulmonary hypoplasia.

Fetal Cardiovascular System

In 3D ultrasound examination of the adult heart with regular rhythm, 3D data are generally acquired over a period of many heart beating, monitored by an electrocardiogram (ECG). Nelson and colleagues solved this problem by using the movement of a heart wall/valve instead of the ECG, and constructed 3D images of the fetal heart without distortion due to beating.

Smith and associates developed a 2D array probe for obtaining 3D data in real-time and applied it to the fetal heart and real-time 3D ultrasound with simultaneous multisection display.

Fetal Abdomen

By surface rendering, abnormalities of the abdominal wall such as omphalocele and gastroschisis are well demonstrated. It is now possible to construct any slice nearly parallel to mother's abdominal wall in arbitrary section on orthogonal triple-section display.

Three-dimensional ultrasound confirms suspected, multicystic dysplastic kidney as well as renal agenesis. Also, the pelvic-ureteric junction and ureterovesical junctions are easily observable.

Nagata and coworkers developed a method for 3D reconstruction of the fetal stomach mathematically from one ultrasonogram of a longitutinally transected stomach, using the symmetry of the stomach about the central axis. The inner volume of the stomach can be measured directly from 3D data.

The volume of the bladder is also measurable.

Fetal Limbs

Surface-rendered images in 3D ultrasound give clear displays of distortions of the normal anatomical axis such as club foot (talipes equinovarus) and Rocker-bottom feet as well as limb abnormalies such as phocomelia. Since, with 3D ultrasound, fingers are well visualised, it is useful for detecting overlapping fingers, polydactyly and syndactyly (Figs 5.6A and B).

With 3D ultrasound, two orthogonal sections can be displayed together. The section at the exact midpoint of the limb can be obtained with good reproducibility. Favre and colleagues determined thigh circumference at the

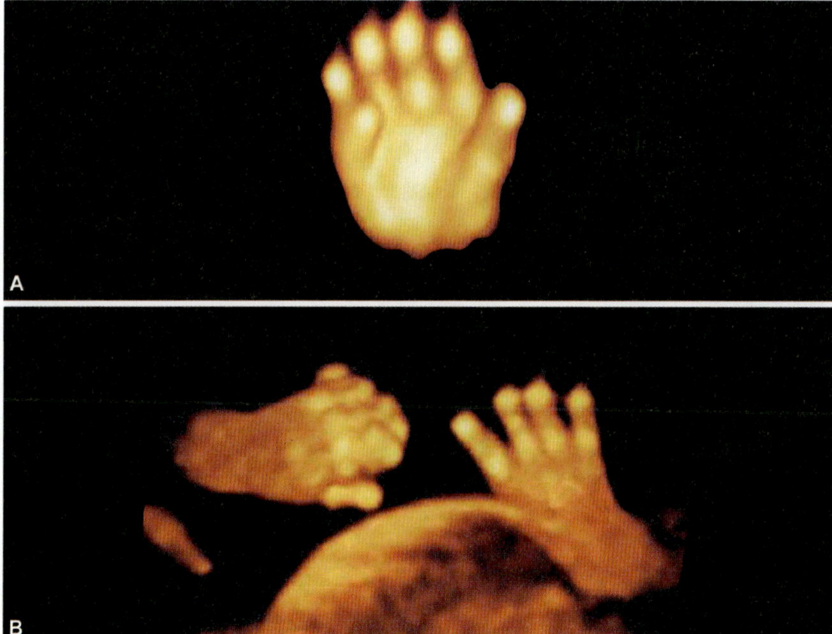

Figs 5.6A and B: Three-dimensional reconstructed ultrasound images clearly depicted bilateral polydactyly (A) and left poly-/syndactyly (B)

midpoint of the femur using 3D ultrasound and proposed a new formula for fetal weight estimation (Fig. 5.7).

Fetal External Genitalia

External genitalia can be observed and malformations of the genitalia such as hermaphroditism and bipartite scrotum can be seen clearly by 3D ultrasound.

Estimation of Fetal Weight and Placental Weight and Amniotic Fluid Volume

If the fetal volume can be measured accurately with 3D ultrasound, more accurate fetal weight estimation may be possible.

Three-dimensional ultrasound not only can measure fetal volume but also placental volume and amniotic fluid.

Fetoplacental Circulation

Three-dimensional ultrasound shows the distributions of blood flow in the placenta. Thus it facilitates the diagnosis of not only morphological abnormalities but also abnormalities of the distribution of blood flow.

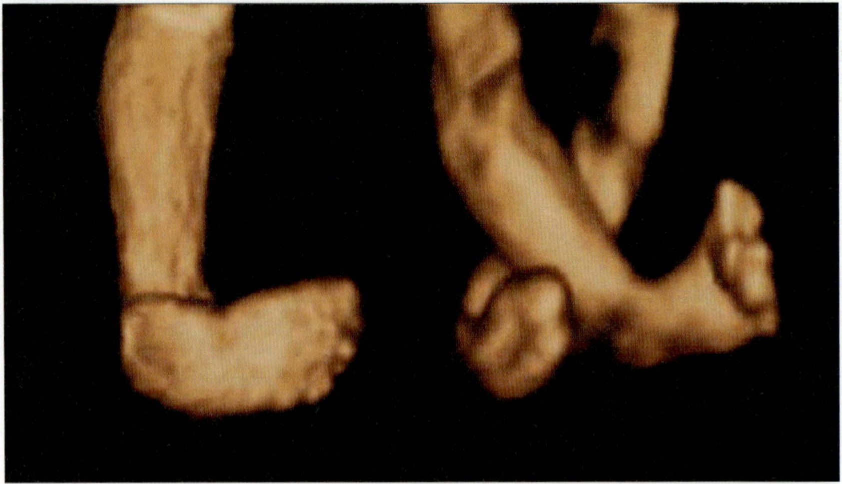

Fig. 5.7: Club foot

LIMITATIONS OF THREE-DIMENSIONAL ULTRASOUND

- *The influence of movement of the object on 3D images:* Distortion of image is caused, if fetus or mother moves during the acquisition of 3D data. So 3D data acquisition should be carried out during periods of fetal rest. Merz and coworkers stated that conventional 2D ultrasound is superior to 3-D ultrasound for the assessment of cardiac anatomy.
- Artifacts and other problems in two-dimensions also exist in three-dimensions.
- The three-dimensional image is not always useful for diagnosis. In cases of severe obesity or in patients with oligohydramnios, fetal imaging with 3D ultrasound is also difficult.
- Preprocessing for three-dimensional image construction is time consuming.
- Scanning range is too narrow, only portions of fetal images can be obtained in the third trimester.

CONCLUSION

Three-dimensional ultrasound is very useful diagnostic method in obstetrics. However, 3D ultrasound is not a substitute for conventional 2D ultrasound and both methods should be used together to get accurate and efficient ultrasonic diagnosis.

Advances in 3D and 4D ultrasound technology now offer capabilities ranging from better visualization of congenital birth defects to dynamic, multiplanar views of the fetal heart.

Intrauterine Growth Restriction: Diagnosis and Management

6

Anupama Rao, Zenab Tambawala

Abstract

Intrauterine growth restriction (IUGR), now also called fetal growth restriction (FGR), is an important cause of perinatal morbidity and mortality. High-risk pregnancies, which can present with IUGR can be identified with history, ultrasound and clinical examination, these pregnancies should be monitored, with ultrasound and Doppler studies and the decision to deliver should be taken, balancing fetal maturity and prognosis of survival.

Doppler findings of absent and reversal of end-diastolic velocity, middle cerebral artery flow and reversal of ducts venosus should help guide the timing of delivery.

INTRODUCTION

Intrauterine growth restriction (IUGR) also called fetal growth restriction (FGR), must be differentiated from small-for-gestation age (SGA). SGA refers to the estimated fetal weight (EFW) below the 10th percentile and severe SGA is below the 3rd percentile. But, 50–70% of the SGA babies are constitutionally small and healthy; and only 10–15% are 'true' IUGR cases and another 5–10% are associated with chromosomal or structural anomalies, or chronic intrauterine infection.[1]

The likelihood of IUGR is higher with severe SGA. The challenge is to identify the pathologically small fetus, monitor and intervene appropriately. The aim also is to avoid iatrogenic harm to the physiologically small but healthy fetus.

IUGR implies fetal compromise, that it is unable to achieve its genetically determined potential, and manifests with abnormal Doppler studies and reduced liquor volumes which is associated with adverse fetal outcomes.

However, a consensus does not exist for the definition of IUGR.

IUGR is of two types:

Symmetrical IUGR is usually early onset, in which all fetal organs are decreased proportionally due to impairment of early fetal cellular hyperplasia, it is nonplacental and due to chromosomal anomaly structural anomaly, viral infection, fetal alcohol syndrome or inborn errors of metabolism.

Asymmetric IUGR is thought to result from the capacity of the fetus to adapt to a hostile environment by redistributing blood flow in favor of vital organs (e.g. brain, heart and placenta) at the expense of non-vital fetal organs (e.g. abdominal viscera, lungs, skin, kidneys) and thus a relative decrease in abdominal size than head circumference. This is seen most commonly seen in maternal conditions involving placental insufficiency (e.g. Pre-eclampsia).

SCREENING FOR INTRAUTERINE GROWTH RESTRICTION

In routine clinical practice, all women should be evaluated for risk factors of IUGR, and women who require more frequent antenatal checks should be identified. The Table 6.1 summarizes the common risk factors of IUGR.

Accurate Determination of the Gestational Age

Knowledge about correct gestational age by last menstrual period (LMP), first trimester examination findings or pregnancy test is of great importance in diagnosis of IUGR. A dating ultrasound in the first trimester provides the most accurate method to determine gestational age.[3] Low first-trimester measurement of crown-rump length in pregnancies is linked with IUGR.[4]

TABLE 6.1 Risk factors for IUGR[2]

Maternal risk factors	*Risk factors in present pregnancy*
Age > 40 years Nullipara	Threatened miscarriage Pregnancy induced hypertension
BMI < 20 IVF	Low maternal weight gain Double marker PAPP-A, 0.4 MoM
Smoking, cocaine, alcohol	Echogenic bowel on ultrasound
Severe malnutrition	Caffeine excessive intake
Hypertension Diabetes	Placental abruption Unexplained APH
Renal disease Antiphospholipid syndrome	
Pregnancy interval, 6 months Previous SGA Previous stillbirth Previous pre-eclampsia	

Abbreviations: APH, antepartum hemorrhage; BMI, body mass index; IVF, in vitro fertilization; SGA, small for gestational age

Symphysio-fundal Measurements

Screening for IUGR in the general population relies on symphysis-fundal height measurements. This is part of routine prenatal care from 20 weeks until term. Although recent studies have questioned the accuracy of fundal height measurements, particularly in obese patients, a discrepancy of greater than 3 cm between observed and expected measurements may prompt a growth evaluation using ultrasound. Lagging fundal height noted during prenatal examination is typically the first indication and should only be used for screening. It is low cost, convenient and readily available, especially in developing countries where more sophisticated assessment is either unavailable or very limited.

Symphysio-fundal height should be plotted on a customized chart based on maternal characteristics rather than a population based chart as this will improve SGA detection and avoid false positives.

Uterine Artery Doppler

The uterine artery Doppler at 20–24 weeks is used to identify severe IUGR. Abnormal uterine artery Doppler (PI > 95th centile) and notching should be referred for further monitoring of IUGR.

The uterine artery is typically measured using color Doppler where it crosses over the external iliac artery. The normal waveform shows high flow throughout diastole. An abnormal waveform is characterized by high resistance and an early diastolic notch. IUGR and pre-eclampsia have been associated with abnormal velocimetry of the uterine arteries. Uterine Doppler evaluation has detection rates of about 75% and 25%, respectively, for a false-positive rate of 5–10%.[5]

Ultrasonography

Ultrasonography should be done for high-risk pregnancies or those with discordant fundal heights. Also women with large fibroids, polyhydramnios, BMI > 35 in whom symphysio-fundal height measurements are difficult should be monitored with serial ultrasounds.

Ultrasound examination of the fetus for serial growth and development should encompass the following measurements:

- *Estimated fetal weight (EFW):* An estimation of the fetal weight lesser than tenth percentile based on standardized percentiles, when combined with assessment of maternal and fetal risk factors and fetal biometric measurements, can provide confirmation of the diagnosis of IUGR.
- *Fetal biometrics:* Serial biometry is the recommended gold standard for assessing pregnancies that are high risk,[6] either on the basis of pasthistory or because of complications that arose during the current pregnancy. In both symmetric and asymmetric growth-restricted fetuses, the AC is the first biometric measure to change due to depleted abdominal adipose tissue and decreased hepatic size. Assessment of the HC: AC ratio (head

circumference: abdominal circumference) assists in the identification of asymmetrically growth-restricted fetuses.

- Comparison of biometric measurements, as well as the estimated fetal weight (EFW) and AC, provide an indication of the fetal growth over time. Serial ultrasounds, with examination of fetal growth and use of standardized growth curves, demonstrate growth velocity. Loss of or decreased growth velocity is the most sensitive indicator of fetal growth.[7]
- *Anatomic survey:* Chromosomal abnormalities and intrauterine infections may present with anatomical defects detected on the 18–20 weeks ultrasonography and usually present with symmetrical IUGR and warrant further evaluation in the form of either fetal karyotyping or TORCH titers if viral infection is suspected.
- *Amniotic fluid:* Assessment for decreased amniotic fluid is not an appropriate screening tool for IUGR as it may or may not be present. However, given that oligohydramnios is one of the sequelae of IUGR, the AFI should still be assessed as low amniotic fluid index (AFI) will identify the fetus at risk for poor perinatal outcome.

Biochemical Markers

In the first trimester, low pregnancy-associated plasma protein A (less than 0.9 MoM), human chorionic gonadotropin (hCG) or elevation of serum alpha-fetoprotein, hCG, or inhibin-A in the second trimester is associated with an increased risk of placental-related IUGR or pre-eclampsia.[8]

CONFIRMATION OF DIAGNOSIS AND FURTHER SURVEILLANCE

Doppler or Velocimetry

Most instances of growth restriction correspond with cases of placental insufficiency.[9] Evaluation of placental function by umbilical artery Doppler is a standard test to distinguish between SGA and IUGR. Umbilical artery Doppler is considered abnormal if diastolic flow is on decreasing trend, greatly reduced, absent, or reversed after 20 weeks gestation. Figure 6.1 demonstrates the appearance of absence and reversal of flows as seen on Doppler an ultrasound. Abnormal Doppler indices have shown to be strong predictor of absent variability, late decelerations, severe variable decelerations, low fetal scalp pH, presence of thick meconium, low Appearance, Pulse, Grimace. Activity and Respiration (APGAR) score and admission to the neonatal intensive care unit. Abnormal umbilical artery Doppler is an indication for enhanced fetal surveillance or delivery.

As the fetus adapts to hypoxemia by redistributing blood flow to the brain and heart thus showing reduced middle cerebral artery resistance (Brain sparing effect) followed by reduced blood flow in the ductus venosus/inferior vena cava or, then in more advanced cases, pulsatile umbilical venous flow

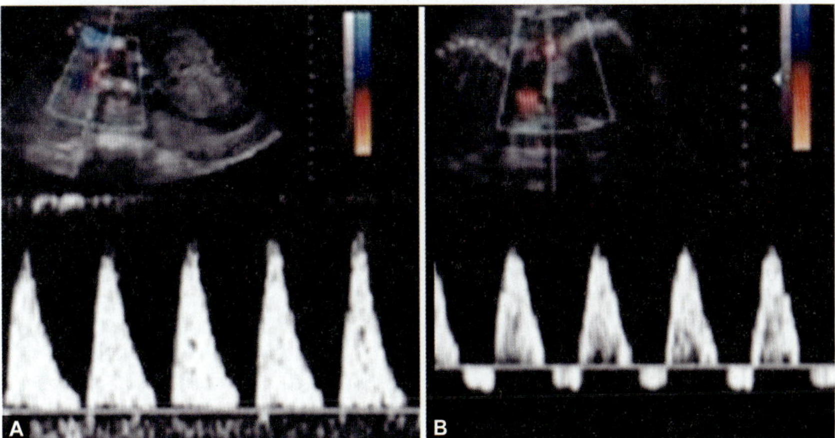

Figs. 6.1A and B: Umbilical artery Doppler: (A) Absent end-diastolic flow; (B) Reversed end diastolic flow

(indicating fetal acidemia and a high risk of intellectual impairment and other postnatal complications). DV flow waveforms become abnormal only in advanced stages of fetal compromise.[10]

Ductus venosus DV Doppler should be used for evaluation in pre term SGA with abnormal umbilical artery Doppler and should be used to time delivery in early onset IUGR.

Amniotic Fluid Index

The assessment of serial AFI forms an important part of the appraisal of the growth restricted fetus, given the strong association between oligohydramnios and a markedly increased risk of perinatal mortality.[11] Conversely, a normal AFI provides a degree of reassurance regarding fetal well-being, but should be interpreted in conjunction with the results of other assessment tools.[12]

NST and Biophysical Profile

Though in most cases, normal non-stress test (NST) is predictive of good perinatal outcome for one week (providing the maternal-fetal condition remains stable), more frequent testing is advocated in definite cases of IUGR.

Biophysical profile (BPP) of the fetus is a non-invasive method used to evaluate five parameters (gross movement, tone, breathing movements, amniotic fluid volume and NST) that may provide useful information in relation to fetal well-being. In the presence of hypoxemia and acidosis, one or more of these five variables may be affected.

It should be noted that BPP itself, should not be used as a single assessment tool in the evaluation of the IUGR fetus as it provides insufficient information related to cardiovascular compromise. BPP should be used in conjunction with umbilical arterial Doppler for more comprehensive fetal assessment.

The BPP is a time consuming test and it is not recommended for routine monitoring in lowrisk/unselected pregnancies or for primary surveillance in SGA fetuses.'[13] Also BPP is not recommended as a surveillance method for preterm SGA.

The loss of short-term FHR variability is considered an acute response to fetal acidosis.[14] Longitudinal series have demonstrated that except for amniotic fluid volume and the fetal heart rate, the other components (tone, breathing, and body movements) of the biophysical profile become abnormal only in advanced stages of fetal compromise. In fact, in about 90% of cases, the biophysical profile becomes abnormal only 48–72 hours after the ductus venosus change.[15]

Staging of IUGR (Mari et al. 2008)

Stage I: Normal NST and umbilical artery Doppler, show no hypoxemia or fetal acidosis.
Stage II: Normal NST and abnormal umbilical artery Doppler found 5% rate of hypoxia or acidosis.
Stage III: Abnormal NST and umbilical artery Doppler found a rate of 60% hypoxia or acidosis.

MANAGEMENT OF IUGR

Because no treatment has been demonstrated to be of benefit for FGR, the assessment of fetal well-being and timely delivery remains as the main strategy for management.
The challenges for healthcare providers are to:

- Identify IUGR fetuses whose health is at risk and intervene appropriately.
- Identify small, yet healthy, fetuses and support these pregnancies appropriately.

The goal is to delay delivery as long as possible to achieve fetal maturation and, hopefully, ensure viability while avoiding the sequelae of fetal acidemia. Frequency of re-evaluation of the IUGR fetus is dependent on many factors. Interval of repeat ultrasound for the assessment of fetal growth can be as frequent as every two weeks depending on the severity of IUGR, gestational age and evidence of fetal compromise. Assessment of fetal well-being through biophysical profile (BPP), with or without Doppler flow assessment, and NST may be done more frequently based on the same factors.

Timing of Delivery

Once IUGR is diagnosed, serial monitoring to assess fetal well-being becomes mandatory. Delivery is indicated when the risk of fetal death or significant morbidity from continued intrauterine existence is greater than the risk of prematurity. This decision making process has been informed by the findings of the growth restriction intervention trial (GRIT) which concluded that, in general, at gestations less than 31 weeks, delivery is best delayed if there is any uncertainty about the need for intervention.[16] The GRIT has not provided evidence to date that early delivery to pre-empt severe hypoxia and acidosis reduces any adverse outcome.

Steroids are given when preterm delivery is anticipated.

Term or Near Term (Beyond 36–37 weeks)

Delivery should be considered for the term fetus with evidence of IUGR. If IUGR is certain, end diastolic flow is present and AFI is normal, delivery may be deferred until the Bishop's score is adequate for induction. If the AFI is reduced, delivery should be expedited. Delivery is considered for no growth over 2–4 weeks, for BPP of 6 or less, and for absent end or reverse diastolic blood flow in the umbilical artery Doppler.

In term SGA fetus with normal umbilical artery Doppler, an abnormal middle cerebral artery Doppler (PI < 5th centile) should be used to time delivery.

The decision on the best mode of delivery is based on the gestation, fetal condition, and cervical status.[17] In cases where there is evidence of fetal acidemia, cesarean section may be appropriate. Fetuses with IUGR have an increased risk of meconium aspiration and intrapartum asphyxia/stillbirth. Therefore, meticulous intrapartum care and monitoring is essential with recourse to obstetric intervention if evidence of additional fetal compromise emerges in labor. Given their oxygen and substrate deprivation during intrauterine life, newborns affected by IUGR may develop hypoxic-ischemic encephalopathy or have meconium aspiration, polycythemia, hypoglycemia or other metabolic abnormalities, as well as hypothermia. Long-term risks faced by survivors of IUGR, include neuro-developmental problems in childhood and degenerative diseases in adulthood. The prognosis is optimized by the appropriate timing of delivery, close intrapartum surveillance, and skilled neonatal care.

Remote from term (Before 36–37 weeks)

Despite numerous approaches to managing IUGR, effective therapies that improve the growth pattern of the fetus have not been identified.[18] Modalities that have been tested with little effect include bed rest, maternal nutritional supplementation, plasma volume expansion, maternal medications (low-dose aspirin), oxygen supplementation and antihypertensives.[19]

Outcome of preterm delivery of IUGR is improved when:

Antenatal steroids have been administered, and delivery occurs at a care center with a neonatal unit that is able to manage the complexities of the IUGR affected preterm newborn.

Individualization is made based on gestational age and fetal status.

Royal College of Obstetricians and Gynaecologists (RCOG) guideline recommends:

In SGA fetus with absence or reversal of end-diastolic velocity detected prior to 32 weeks of gestation, delivery is recommended when ductus venosus becomes abnormal or umbilical vein pulsations appear, provided fetus is viable and steroids have been given.

If Doppler is abnormal delivery is recommended by 32 weeks.

If MCA Doppler is abnormal, delivery is recommended no later than 37 weeks.

When end-diastolic flow is present on UA Doppler, delay delivery until at least 37 weeks, provided other surveillance findings are normal.

SUMMARY

The first step in the management of the IUGR fetus is diagnosis. Fundal height is a useful screening tool, and ultrasound biometry is the best method for detecting the small fetus. Doppler velocimetry is the most important means of diagnosing the IUGR fetus that is at risk for adverse perinatal morbidity and mortality. It is difficult to determine the best time to deliver the IUGR fetus: one must balance the risks of prematurity with the risks of further intrauterine decompensation. For the very preterm fetus, there may be some benefit of delaying delivery until venous evidence of circulatory decompensation is present.

Current best practice would indicate that from the time fetal pulmonary maturity can be inferred, there is little to be gained by allowing a pregnancy to continue if good fetal growth cannot be demonstrated.

REFERENCES

1. Alberry M, Soothill P. Management of growth restriction. Archives Disease and Childhood, Fetal and Neonatal Edition. 2007;72(1):F62–F7.
2. Crowly T. Investigation and management of the small-for-Gestational–Age Fetus. Green-Top Guideline No.31; 2013;29-30.
3. Haram K, Softeland E, Bukowski R. Intrauterine growth restriction. International Journal of Gynecology and Obstetrics. 2006;93:5.
4. Bukowski R, Smith GC, Malone FD, et al. Fetal growth in early pregnancy and risk of delivering low birth weight infant: prospective cohort study. BMJ 2007;334:836.
5. Martin AM, Bindra R, Curcio P, Cicero S, Nicolaides KH. Screening for pre-eclampsia and fetal growth restriction by uterine artery Doppler at 11–14 weeks of gestation. Ultrasound Obstet Gynecol. 2001;18:583.
6. Royal College of Obstetricians and Gynaecologists. The investigation and management of the small-for-gestational age fetus. RCOG Green Top Guideline no. 31. London; Nov 2002. Available at: *www.rcog.org.uk/files/rcogcorp.*
7. Gardosi J, Francis A. Controlled trial of fundal height measurement plotted on customised antenatal growth charts. BJOG. 1999;109:309-17.
8. Killam WP, Miller RC, Seeds JW. Extremely high maternal serum alpha-fetoprotein levels at second-trimester screening. Obstet Gynecol. 1991;78:257-61.
9. Lackman F, Capewell V, Gagnon R, Richardson B. Fetal umbilical cord oxygen values and birth to placental weight ratio in relation to size at birth. Am J Obstet Gynecol. 2001;185:674-82.

10. Ferrazzi E, Bozzo M, Rigano S, et al. Temporal sequence of abnormal Doppler changes in the peripheral and central circulatory systems of the severely growth-restricted fetus. Ultrasound Obstet Gynecol. 2002;19:140-6.
11. Resnik R. Fetal growth restriction: Management. 2005 UpToDate. Available at: *www. uptodate.com.*
12. Divon MY, Ferber A. Fetal growth restriction: Diagnosis-1. 2005 UpToDate.
13. Coomarasamy A, Fisk NM, Gee H, Robson SC. Royal College of Obstetricians and Gynaecologists. Guideline No. 31. The investigation and management of the small for gestational age fetus.
14. Hecher K, Bilardo CM, Stigter RH, et al. Monitoring of fetuses with intrauterine growth restriction: a longitudinal study. Ultrasound Obstet Gynecol. 2001;18:564-70.
15. Baschat A A, Gembruch U, Harman CR. The sequence of changes in Doppler and biophysical parameters as severe fetal growth restriction worsens. Ultrasound Obstet Gynecol. 2001;18:571-7.
16. GRIT study group. A randomised trial of timed delivery for the compromised preterm fetus short term outcomes and Bayesian interpretation. BJOG. 2003;110:27-32.
17. Weiner CP, Baschat AA. Fetal growth restriction: evaluation and management. In: James DK, Sheer PJ, Weiner P, Gonik B, (Eds). High Risk Pregnancy: Management Option. London: WB Saunders, 1999.
18. Gulmezoglu AM, Hofmeyr GJ. Plasma volume expansion for suspected impaired fetal growth. Cochrane Database Syst Rev. 2000: CD000167.
19. Laurin J, Persson PH. The effect of bedrest in hospital on fetal outcome in pregnancies complicated by intra-uterine growth retardation. Acta Obstet Gynecol Scand. 1987;9 66:407.

7

Assessing Fetal Wellbeing in Third Trimester

Ameet Patki, Deepali Kale

Abstract

The goal of antepartum fetal surveillance is prevention of fetal death and avoidance of unnecessary interventions. Most of the current techniques employed to forecast fetal well-being focus on fetal physical activities, including heart rate, movement, breathing, and amniotic fluid production. In most cases, a negative, that is, normal test result is highly reassuring, because fetal deaths within 1 week of a normal test are rare. A successful antenatal fetal testing program would ideally reduce the fetal and neonatal outcomes of asphyxia.

INTRODUCTION

Abnormal fetal surveillance is based on physiologic changes that alter fetal heart rate and fetal activity.[1] Fetal heart rate, fetal movement and tone in particular are impacted by uteroplacental fetal blood flow alterations and are thereby sensitive to fetal hypoxemia and acidemia. While nonreassuring fetal surveillance is associated with fetal hypoxemia and acidemia based on these physiologic adjustments, these indicators can neither predict the degree or duration of the fetal acid base disturbance nor precisely predict neonatal outcome.

Indications fetal surveillance is often warranted in high risk pregnancies, most common being intrauterine growth restrictions (IUGR), pregnancy induced hypertension (PIH) and postdatism, diabetes mellitus and multiple pregnancy. Antenatal fetal testing techniques fall into seven categories and may be used simultaneously or in a hierarchical fashion. They are:

1. Fetal movement counting
2. Nonstress test (NST)
3. Contraction stress test (CST)
4. Biophysical profile
5. Maternal uterine artery Doppler

6. Fetal umbilical artery Doppler
7. Other fetal artery Doppler parameters.

FETAL MOVEMENT COUNTING

The concept of counting fetal movements is attractive, since it requires no technology and is available to all women. A warning sign that a fetus may be at risk of compromise is maternal perception of decrease in fetal movement. If "kick counting" is used by the patient, a nonreassuring count provides the alert for further assessment. A nonreassuring count should prompt notification for further fetal assessment.

Decreased placental perfusion and fetal acidemia and acidosis are associated with decreased fetal movements.This is the basis for maternal monitoring of fetal movements or "the fetal movement count test." A variety of methods have been described, X. The Cardiff method, first reported by Pearson and Weaver suggests a count to 10 movements in a fixed time frame. The original study required counting for 12 hours. Patient is instructed to start counting movements in morning and note the time when she count 10 movements. If 10 movements are counted in 10–12 hours or less, then fetus is likely in good health. Modified protocols include those of Liston (count to 6 hours)[2] and Moore (count to 2 hours).[3] The Sadovsky method suggests a count of movements in a specific time frame (usually 30 minutes to two hours).[4]

Though, simple and effective, literature has produced contradictory results about its clinical utility in preventing late fetal deaths.

NONSTRESS TEST

Nonstress test (NST) assessing fetal heart rate acceleration in response to fetal movement as a sign of fetal health was first introduced by Freeman and Lee and colleagues.[5,6] This test involved the use of Doppler-detected fetal heart rate acceleration coincident with fetal movements perceived by the mother. Nonstress test is primarily a test of fetal condition, and it differs from the contraction stress test, which is a test of uteroplacental function. Currently, nonstress testing is the most widely used primary testing method for assessment of fetal wellbeing. The fetal heart rate is normally increased or decreased by autonomic influences mediated by sympathetic or parasympathetic impulses from brainstem centers.[7] The NST is based on the hypothesis that the heart rate of a nonhypoxic, nonacidotic fetus will temporarily accelerate in response to fetal movement. Heart rate acceleration with movement is a reflex that involves the cerebral cortex and is affected by physiologic or pathologic influences on the fetal brain. The most common physiologic situation suppressing this reflex is fetal sleep, while the most common pathological condition is fetal hypoxia. For this reason, absence of accelerations during a NST must be considered a consequence of fetal hypoxia unless it can be explained otherwise. Technique nonstress test is performed during the antenatal period when the uterus is relaxed, i.e. the fetus is not exposed to the "stress" of uterine contractions. The recording should last for at least 20 minutes. The baseline fetal heart rate should be within the normal range of 110–160 bpm. Moderate variability of 6–25 bpm is expected, but variability assessment was not the original objective of the NST. Results and interpretation historically, a normal (reactive) nonstress test includes at least two accelerations from the baseline within the 20-minute period of testing that reach a peak or acme of at least 15 bpm above the baseline and have a duration from onset to return to baseline of at least 15 seconds.[8] If the fetal heart acceleratory response does not meet the criteria after 20 minutes of testing, the recording should continue for another 20 minutes to account for the average period of non-rapid eye movement sleep when fetal movement and subsequently heart rate variability are reduced. Some authors advocate provoking fetal movement during this period by external manipulation. If there is no acceleration with spontaneous or repeated external stimuli during a 40-minute period, the test is considered nonreactive. The test is unsatisfactory (equivocal) if the quality of the monitor tracing is inadequate for interpretation.

If the fetus lacks accelerations after 40 minutes of testing, the electronic fetal monitoring should be continued. A decision should be made to proceed either to amniotic fluid assessment and or to multiple parameters testing (such as a biophysical profile or contraction stress testing). In most cases a normal NST is predictive of good perinatal outcome for one week (providing the maternal-fetal condition remains stable). More frequent testing is advocated by some investigators for women with post-term pregnancy, multifetal gestation, type 1 diabetes mellitus, fetal-growth restriction, or gestational hypertension.[9,10]

In these circumstances, some investigators perform twice-weekly tests. Others perform nonstress tests daily or even more frequently, for example, with severe pre-eclampsia remote from term. The NST is markedly influenced by the gestational age and approximately 50 and 15% of NSTs done in otherwise healthy fetuses at 24–28 and 28–32 weeks respectively are nonreactive.

Though NST may be performed after 28 weeks onwards, it should be remembered that criteria mentioned above for normal NST are applicable only to fetuses near or at term. Due to immaturity of autonomous nervous system in preterm fetuses, acceleratory response to fetal movement is less causing high possibility of false positive result. Hence, caution should be used in applying the usual acceleratory (reactive) criteria in the interpretation of the nonstress test in the premature fetus. For fetuses less than 32 weeks' gestation, accelerations would be expected to increase 10 bpm for at least 10 secs.[11]

Current clinical practice calls for performing a NST once or twice weekly after 32 0/7 gestational weeks, depending on the indication for testing. If the indication for testing is not persistent, the NST need not be repeated. If the maternal condition is stable and testing is reassuring, the NST is typically repeated weekly. The negative predictive value of NST alone for predicting stillbirths within 1 week of a normal test is 99.8%.[23]

Advantages and disadvantages of NST simple, relatively inexpensive, less time consuming, easy to perform and can be done on OPD basis. Interpretation of trace requires degree of experience, skill and training. To be correlated in context of clinical findings. High degree of false positive rate and may cause unnecessary intervention, leading to high cesarean rate. Fetal sleep pattern or maternal medications can affect result accuracy of test. The false negative rate of test is 3.2 per 1000. Death of fetuses with reactive NST is seen in conditions like postdatism, diabetes, malformation and abruption. The false positive rate is very high, 50% for morbidity and 80% for mortality, indicating that possibility of serious fetal problem is relatively low in nonreactive NST. It also stresses the need of additional testing when test is nonreactive before intervention. Due to very high false positive rate, there is growing concern that wide use of electronic fetal monitoring (EFM) may be responsible for rising incidence of cesarean section.

ACOUSTIC STIMULATION TESTS

Loud external sounds have been used to startle the fetus and thereby provoke heart rate acceleration—an acoustic stimulation nonstress test. Vibroacoustic Manual on Fetal Surveillance 80 stimulation (VAS) also elicits accelerations of the FHR and has been added to the protocol to perform the NST (Zimmer et al 1993).[12] FHR reactivity, spontaneous or obtained with VAS, is a solid indicator of fetal health and absence of acidosis. VAS uses stimulation with an artificial larynx over fetal head during 1-3 seconds. The instrument produces a vibratory acoustic stimulus approximately 80 Hz and 82 db. A healthy fetus will respond with sudden movement (startle response) followed by acceleration of the FHR. VAS was originally designed to decrease the time spent in performance of the NST that is frequently prolonged because of episodes of fetal sleep, and soon the NST with VAS became the predominant method to perform the NST. Maternal perception of fetal movement following VAS is another indicator of fetal well-being. However, if the mother does not perceive fetal movement following VAS, but if there is a clear accelerative response of the FHR, test is considered as normal. An abnormal response to VAS, found in the fetus with chronic asphyxia, consists of no acceleration or declaration of FHR. VAS is safe and no evidence of hearing impairment or other abnormality has been reported in neonates exposed to VAS *in utero*.

CONTRACTION STRESS TEST

The contraction stress test (CST), or oxytocin challenge test, is a test of fetal wellbeing first described by Ray et al. in 1972.[13] It evaluates the response of the FHR to induced contractions and was designed to unmask poor placental function. The CST should not be used in any woman for whom vaginal delivery is contraindicated (i.e. women with placenta previa or previous classical cesarean section).[14] When gestation below 24–28 weeks, at which no intervention would be useful on behalf of the fetus if test is abnormal.[14] This test should be performed in hospital where emergency cesarean section is available, and the woman should be fully informed of the risks and benefits of the test. The objective is to induce three contractions, lasting one minute each, within a ten minute period, and then evaluate the fetal heart response to these contractions. The CST may be performed using maternal nipple stimulation or an oxytocin infusion. Nipple stimulation is associated with no greater risk of uterine hyperstimulation and has a shorter average testing time than oxytocin infusion.[15] Should nipple stimulation fail to induce contractions that meet the test criteria, then oxytocin infusion should be considered. For oxytocin-induced contractions, the woman is place in semirecumbent position with an intravenous line in place.[14] An NST is performed prior to the CST. If then considered appropriate, uterine contractions are induced using exogenous oxytocin, commencing at 0.5 to 1 mU/min, and increasing every 15–30 minutes by 1 mU/min, until optimum contractions are achieved. The tracing is evaluated for baseline rate, baseline variability, and decelerations.[14] A CST is considered positive if late decelerations occur with more than 50% of the induced contractions (even if the goal of three contractions in10-minute).

A negative CST has abnormal baseline fetal heart rate tracing without late decelerations.[13] An equivocal test is defined as repetitive decelerations, not late in timing or pattern. A CST is deemed unsatisfactory if the desired number and length of contractions is not achieved or if the quality of the cardiotocography tracing is poor. The oxytocin stress test requires a lengthy observation period and IV access and has a high rate of equivocal results. With availability of other simpler and reliable tests like BPP and Doppler, CST is rarely used now a days. The advantage of the CST is that it most closely approximates intrapartum surveillance of the fetus at risk.

With the addition of umbilical artery Doppler velocimetry, particularly in the surveillance of fetal growth restriction (FGR), the contraction stress test (CST) is now rarely used to assess for fetal compromise or potential hypoxemia.[16]

BIOPHYSICAL PROFILE

The biophysical profile (BPP) combines data from 2 sources (i.e. ultrasonographic imaging and fetal heart rate [FHR] monitoring). Dynamic realtime B-mode ultrasonography is used to measure the amniotic fluid volume (AFV) and to observe several types of fetal movement. The FHR is obtained using a pulsed Doppler transducer integrated with a high-speed microprocessor, which provides a continuously updated reading.[17] Originally described by Manning and colleagues.[18] The BPP has become a standard tool for providing antepartum fetal surveillance. The BPP integrates 5 parameters to yield a biophysical profile score (BPS) and includes:

1. The nonstress test (NST)
2. Ultrasonographic measurement of the AFV

3. Observation of the presence or absence of fetal breathing movements
4. Gross body movements, and
5. Tone.

Each of the five components of BPP is assigned a numerical value of 2 (if normal) or 0 (if abnormal). A composite score of 8 or 10 indicates that fetal status is reassuring, as long as score of 8 does not include an abnormal AFI, which demands further testing. A score of 6 is equivocal and requires further testing. A score of 4 or less is suggestive of fetal compromise. The modified biophysical profile Vintzileos et al. were first to propose a modification of the biophysical profile. A modified biophysical profile (BPP), consists of a nonstress test with VAST, index of acute fetal problem and an amniotic fluid index (AFI) which is index of chronic fetal heath.[19]

If either the NST or the AFI is abnormal, a complete BPP is performed. Frequency of testing in most high-risk pregnancies, testing plans start with weekly testing, although twice-weekly testing is the standard for pregnancies beyond 42 weeks and for patients with insulin-dependent diabetes. Frequency of testing increases in direct proportion to the severity of the maternal or fetal condition.[20] Reliability of the biophysical profile (BPP) is a reliable method of predicting fetal survival (Table 7.1). Data have been collected on this and other antepartum testing procedures for more than 20 years. Testing methods usually are evaluated by comparing the false-negative mortality rate for each method. The false-negative mortality rate is defined as the number of fetal deaths, corrected for lethal congenital anomalies and unpredictable causes of demise, that occur within 1 week of a normal test result. The BPP has a

TABLE 7.1: Specific criteria for the biophysical profile score

Biophysical variable	Normal (Score = 2)	Abnormal (Score = 0)
Fetal breathing movements	One or more episodes of ≥20 s within 30 min	Absent or no episode of ≥20 s within 30 min
Gross body movements	Two or more discrete body/ limb movements within 30 min (episodes of active continuous movement considered as a single movement	<2 episodes of body/limb movements within 30 min
Fetal tone	One or more episodes of active extension with return to flexion of fetal limb(s) or trunk (opening and closing of hand considered normal tone)	Slow extension with return to partial flexion, movement of limb in full extension, absent fetal movement, or partially open fetal hand
Reactive fetal heart rate	Two or more episodes of acceleration of ≥15 bpm and of >15 s associated with fetal movement within 20 min	One or more episodes of acceleration of fetal heart rate or acceleration of <15 bpm within 20 min
Qualitative amniotic fluid volume	One or more pockets of fluid measuring ≥2 cm in vertical axis	Either no pockets or largest pocket <2 cm in vertical axis

false-negative mortality rate of 0.77 deaths per 1000 tests. Furthermore, the BPS highly correlates with the antepartum fetal umbilical venous cord pH level.

UTERINE ARTERY DOPPLER

In normal pregnancy, the developing placenta implants on maternal decidua, and the trophoblast invades the maternal spiral arteries, destroying the elastic lamina and transforming these vessels into low resistance shunts in order to improve blood supply to the fetoplacental unit. Impaired trophoblastic invasion is associated subsequent development of hypertensive disorders of pregnancy, IUGR, placental abruption, and intrauterine fetal demise. Doppler ultrasound of the uterine arteries is a noninvasive method of assessing the resistance of vessels supplying the placenta. In normal pregnancies, there is an increase in blood flow velocity and a decrease in resistance to flow, reflecting the transformation of the spiral arteries. In pregnancies complicated by hypertensive disorders, Doppler of the uterine artery shows increased flow, early diastolic notching, and decreased diastolic flow. A positive uterine artery Doppler screen consists of mean resistance index of > 0.57, pulsatility index > 95th centile, and/or the presence of uterine artery notching.[21]

UMBILICAL ARTERY DOPPLER

In normal pregnancy, the fetal umbilical circulation is characterized by continuous forward flow, i.e. low resistance, to the placenta, which improves with gestational age. Resistance to forward flow therefore continues to decrease in normal pregnancy all the way to term.[22] Increased resistance to forward flow in the umbilical circulation is characterized by abnormal systolic to diastolic ratio, pulsatility index (PI) or resistance index (RI) greater than the 95th centile and implies decreased functioning vascular units within the placenta. Decreased diastolic flow, absent end-diastolic flow and reversal of diastolic flow is sequence of change in Doppler findings with increasing fetal hypoxia. Umbilical artery Doppler is the only form of fetal surveillance that has been shown to improve perinatal mortality in randomized controlled trials.

OTHER FETAL ARTERY DOPPLER PARAMETERS

Initially, as fetal hypoxemia develops, redistribution of blood flow occurs such that fetal middle cerebral artery (MCA) resistance indices fall as umbilical resistance it arterial resistance increases, leading to the so-called "brain sparing" effect. Changes in the cerebral flow parameters, however, do not correlate well with the final stages of asphyxic compromise and therefore are not helpful in choosing timing for delivery. Increased resistance in the umbilical arteries and descending aorta does lead, however, in an increase in right ventricular end-diastolic pressure (after load), leading to decreased right ventricular compliance and increased venous pressure in the right atrium and systemic veins. Further deterioration of right ventricular contractility will lead to right ventricular dilatation and tricuspid regurgitation (insufficiency), further exacerbating right atrial filling pressure and resistance to venous filling. Resistance to venous filling is reflected best by increased pulsatility in the ductus venosus[23] during atrial contraction, a finding highly correlated with impending asphyxia and acidosis. Further increases in systemic venous pressures lead to maximum dilatation of the ductus venosus and direct transmission of cardiac impulses to the umbilical vein, causing umbilical venous pulsations. This finding is shown to be highly correlated with severe acidosis and impending fetal demise.

SUMMARY

Identification of those at high-or low-risk is essential to offer appropriate surveillance. But, no fetus can be categorized as no risk such that all surveillance can be avoided because despite appropriate surveillance, emergencies can arise that can jeopardize the fetus in a very short time. In such situations one takes action based on clinical judgement, as the hypoxic insult can be severe leading to rapid deterioration if there is delay in delivery.

REFERENCES

1. Bocking AD. Assessment of fetal heart rate and fetal movements indetecting oxygen deprivation in-utero. Eur J Obstet Gynecol Reprod Biol. 2003;110(Suppl 1):S108-S112.
2. Baskett TF, Liston RM. Fetal movement monitoring: clinical application. Clin Perinatol. 1989;16(3):613–25.
3. Moore TR, Piacquadio K. A prospective evaluation of fetal movement screening to reduce the incidence of antepartum fetal death. Am J Obstet Gynecol. 1989; 160(5Pt 1):1075–80.
4. Sadovsky E, Weinstein D, Even Y. Antepartum fetal evaluation by assessment of fetal heart rate and fetal movements. Int J Gynaecol Obstet. 1981;19(1):21–6.
5. Freeman RK: The use of the oxytocin challenge test for antepartum clinical evaluation of uteroplacental respiratory function. Am J Obstet Gynecol. 1975;121:481.
6. Lee CY, DiLoreto PC, O'Lane JM. A study of fetal heart rate acceleration patterns. Obstet Gynecol. 1975;45:142.
7. Matsuura M, Murata Y, Hirano T, et al. The effects of developing autonomous nervous system on FHR variabilities determined by the power spectral analysis. Am J Obstet Gynecol. 1996;174:380.
8. Freeman R, Garite TJ, Nageotte MP. Fetal heart rate monitoring, 3rd edn. Philadelphia: Lippincott Williams and Wilkins; 2003.
9. Devoe LD. Antenatal fetal assessment: Multifetal gestation—an overview. Semin Perinatol. 2008; 32:281.

10. Freeman RK. Antepartum testing in patients with hypertensive disorders in pregnancy. Semin Perinatol. 2008;32:271.
11. Pratt D, Diamond F, Yen H, Bieniarz J, Burd L. Fetal stress and nonstress tests: an analysis and comparison of their ability to identify fetal outcome. Obstet Gynecol. 1979;54(4):419–23.
12. Zimmer EZ, Divon MY. Fetal vibroacoustic stimulation. Obstetl Gynecol. 1993;81: 451–7.
13. Ray M, Freeman R, Pine S, Hesselgesser R. Clinical experience with the oxytocin challenge test. Am J Obstet Gynecol. 1972;114(1):1–9.
14. Lagrew DC. The contraction stress test. Clin Obstet Gynecol. 1995;38(1):11–25.
15. MacMillan JB, Hale RW. Contraction stress testing with mammary self-stimulation. J Reprod Med. 1984;29(4):219–21.
16. American College of Obstetricians and Gynecologists Practice Bulletin number 145: Antenatal Fetal Surveillance. Obstet Gynecol. 2014;124:182–92.
17. Macones GA, et al. The 2008 National Institute of Child Health and Human Development Workshop Report on Electronic Fetal Monitoring Update on Definitions, Interpretation, and Research Guidelines Obstetrics & Gynecology. 2008;112:661-666.
18. Manning FA, Platt LD, Sipos L. Antepartum fetal evaluation: development of a fetal biophysical profile. Am J Obstet Gynecol. 1980;136(6):787–95.
19. Miller DA, Rabello YA, Paul RH. The modified biophysical profile: antepartum testing in the 1990s. Am J Obstet Gynecol. 1996;174(3):812–7.
20. Lalor JG, Fawole B, Alfirevic Z, Devane D. Biophysical profile for fetal assessment in high risk pregnancies. Cochrane Database Syst Rev. 2008;CD000038.
21. Newnham JP, Patterson LL, James IR, Diepeveen DA, Reid SE. An evaluation of the efficacy of Doppler flow velocity waveform analysis as a screening test in pregnancy. Am J Obstet Gynecol. 1990;162(2):403–10.
22. Adamson SL. Arterial pressure, vascular input impedance, and resistance as determinants of pulsatile blood flow in the umbilical artery. Eur J Obstet Gynecol Reprod Biol. 1999;84(2):119–25.
23. Ritter S, Jorn H, Weiss C, Rath W. Importance of ductus venosus Doppler assessment for fetal outcome in cases of intrauterine growth restriction.Fetal Diagn Ther. 2004;19(4):348–55.

8

Imaging Modalities for Adherent Placenta

Vinita Salvi

INTRODUCTION

Adherent placenta is variously known as morbidly adherent placenta or placenta accreta. The chorionic villi of the human placenta are normally attached to the thin layer of uterine decidua. This allows easy detachment of the placenta following delivery of the fetus. In abnormally adherent placentation, the chorionic villi grow through the uterine decidua and can be found attached directly to uterine myometrium (placenta accreta). The villi can invade into the myometrium (placenta increta) or penetrate the uterine serosa or nearby organs (placenta percreta).

Adherent placenta is associated with increased maternal morbidity and mortality due to major obstetric complications such as intractable postpartum hemorrhage often leading to obstetric hysterectomy or maternal mortality. The risk of maternal death in women with abnormal placentation remains as high as 10%.

The incidence of adherent placenta has been rising mainly due to increase in number of cesarean sections, hence various imaging modalities have evolved for the diagnosis. The incidence of abnormal placental invasion is believed to be one per 533 deliveries. The past history of cesarean section or any uterine surgery like myomectomy or curettage, low lying placenta increases the risk of having adherent placenta.

DIAGNOSIS

Ultrasound scanning and magnetic resonance imaging (MRI) are two main imaging modalities for detection of morbidly adherent placenta.

Antenatal imaging techniques that can help to raise the suspicion of a morbidly adherent placenta should be considered in any situation where any part of the placenta lies under the previous cesarean section scar. These techniques include ultrasound and magnetic resonance imaging (MRI). Numerous ultrasound imaging techniques have been reported over the years including gray scale, color and/or three-dimensional power Doppler sonography.

ULTRASONOGRAPHY

Clinically, the most significant feature of placenta accreta is the abundant uteroplacental neovascularization,which can lead to life-threatening hemorrhage. However, its antenatal diagnosis is usually based on characteristic findings on gray-scale ultrasound imaging, such as the loss of subendometrial echolucent zone or the presence of abnormal placental lacunae.

On gray-scale ultrasound imaging, the presence of at least one of the following characteristics is required to indicate placenta accreta: as shown in Figs 8.1A and B.

- Complete loss of the retroplacental sonolucent zone
- Irregular retroplacental sonolucent zone
- Thinning or disruption of the hyperechoic uterine serosa-bladder interface
- The presence of focal exophytic masses invading the urinary bladder and
- The presence of abnormal placental lacunae.

Likewise, the diagnosis of placenta accreta was regarded as positive when any one of these color Doppler criteria was present:

- Diffuse or focal lacunar flow pattern.
- Sonolucent vascular lakes with turbulent flow typified by high velocity (peak systolic velocity >15 cm/s) and low resistance waveform.
- Hypervascularity of the uterine-bladder interface with abnormal blood vessels linking the placenta to the bladder, and
- Markedly dilated vessels over the peripheral subplacental region.

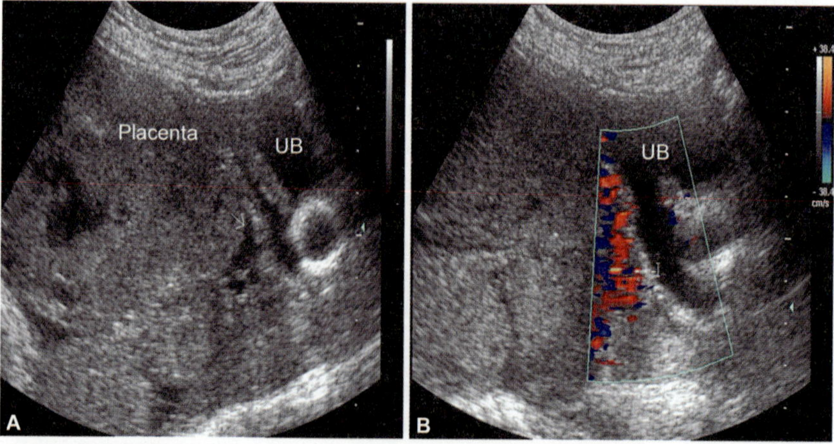

Figs 8.1A and B: Cervix bisected to achieve access to the vesicouterine peritoneum. Slight traction on the bladder with Babcock's forceps brings connecting tissue strands into view for excision and the plane for access.

Source: Sheth SS. Access to vesicouterine and rectouterine pouches. In: Sheth SS (Ed). Vaginal hysterectomy, (2nd edn). New Delhi, India: Jaypee Brothers Medical Publishers (P) Ltd; 2014.pp.31-50

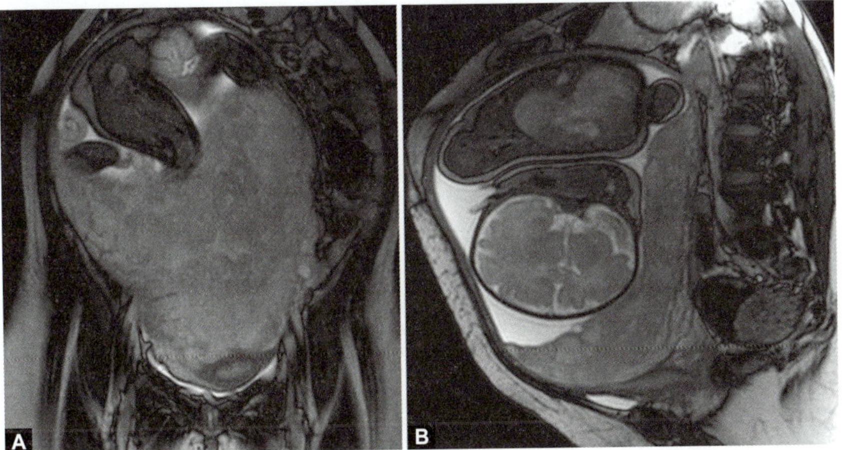

Figs 8.2A and B: MRI images: (A) placenta percreta. (B) placenta previa without invasion

Since the abundant neovascularization of the uteroplacental region is a notable feature of placenta accreta, power Doppler can be used to further analyze the patterns of placental vasculature in an attempt to differentiate between placenta previa totalis and placenta accreta. One of the following criteria is required on three-dimensional power Doppler to make a diagnosis of placenta accreta.

- Numerous coherent vessels involving the whole uterine serosa-bladder junction (basal view)
- Hypervascularity (lateral view)
- Inseparable cotyledonal and intervillous circulations, chaotic branching, detour vessels (lateral view).

MAGNETIC RESONANCE IMAGING

Although ultrasonography remains the primary modality in the evaluation of placental implantation, in recent years there has been interest in the use of magnetic resonance imaging. Some authors have suggested that magnetic resonance imaging is most clearly indicated when there is a posterior placenta or when the US findings are ambiguous.

The role of MRI in diagnosing placenta accreta is still debated. Two recent comparative studies have shown sonography and MRI to be comparable: in the first study 15 of 32 women ended up having accreta (sensitivity 93% versus 80% and specificity 71% versus 65% for ultrasound versus MRI); in the second study 12 of 50 women ended up having accreta and MRI and Doppler showed no difference in detection (P=0.74), although MRI was better at detecting the depth of infiltration in cases of placenta accreta (P<0.001). Many authors have therefore recommended MRI for women in whom ultrasound findings are inconclusive (Figs 8.2A and B).

The main MRI features of placenta accreta include:

- Uterine bulging

- Heterogeneous signal intensity within the placenta
- Dark intraplacental bands on T2-weighted imaging.

CONCLUSION

Single most important factor in management of adherent placenta is antenatal diagnosis. Antenatal diagnosis is possible with ultrasonography especially color Doppler studies and MRI. It provides an opportunity to counsel the patient in advance, plan management and consider interventional radiology as an elective procedure. Hence, these imaging modalities should be routinely advised to patients with placenta previa with risk factors such as scarred uterus.

BIBLIOGRAPHY

1. Cochrane library. Imaging techniques for antenatal detection of morbidly adherent placenta. 2011.
2. Comstock CH, et al. Antenatal diagnosis of placenta accreta: a review. Ultrasound Obstet Gynecol. 2005;26:89-96.
3. SHIH JC, et al. Role of three-dimensional power Doppler in the antenatal diagnosis of placenta accreta: comparison with gray-scale and color Doppler techniques. Ultrasound Obstet Gynecol. 2009;33:193-203.

9

Intrapartum Monitoring of Fetus: What's New?

Vandana Bansal

INTRODUCTION

Continuous electronic fetal heart monitoring in labor was introduced in 1970's to identify events that might result in hypoxic ischemic encephalopathy, cerebral palsy, or fetal death, and was quickly adopted by most obstetricians as a significant improvement in intrapartum fetal care. The purpose of fetal monitoring in labor was to recognize these fetuses which might be at risk of hypoxic injury so that delivery can be expedited and perinatal outcomes improved.

The use of electronic fetal monitoring (EFM) increased exponentially from 1980's. It was used on 45% of laboring women in 1980 to 85% in 2002. In recent year approximately 3.4 million fetuses in the United States were assessed with EFM, making it the most common obstetric procedure.[1] Unfortunately use of EFM has failed to reduce perinatal mortality or incidence of cerebral palsy. In fact, the rate of cerebral palsy has remained the same since World War II despite electronic fetal monitoring, better obstetric and neonatal care. The false positive rate of predicting cerebral palsy with EFM is more than 99%. Only demonstrable benefit of EFM has been a reduction in the incidence of neonatal seizures.[2]

There is evidence that the use of EFM increases the rate of cesarean deliveries and operative vaginal deliveries secondary to erroneous diagnosis of fetal distress in electronically monitored patients (high false positive rate). These limitations are due to high interobserver and intraobserver variability which may play a major role in interpretation.[2] Inspite of all these shortcomings, electronic fetal monitoring provides the obstetricians information with high degree of reliability about both extremes, i.e. presence of fetal well-being (Normal FHR pattern), as well as presence of severe fetal problems (pathological FHR). Most experts and guidelines believe that continuous cardiotocography (CTG) monitoring should be considered in all situations where there is risk of fetal hypoxia.

INTERMITTENT VERSUS ELECTRONIC FETAL MONITORING

Structured intermittent auscultation is a technique that employs the systematic use of a Doppler or Pinard stethoscope assessment of fetal heart rate (FHR) during labor at defined timed intervals. It is equivalent to continuous EFM in screening for fetal compromise in low-risk patients. Safety in using structured intermittent auscultation is based on a nurse-to-patient ratio of 1:1.

The potential benefits and risks of continuous EFM and structured intermittent auscultation should be discussed during prenatal care and labor, and a decision reached by the pregnant woman and her physician, with the understanding that if intrapartum clinical situations warrant, continuous EFM may be recommended.

Intermittent auscultation or continuous electronic monitoring is considered acceptable method of intrapartum surveillance in low-risk pregnancies. Continuous electronic fetal monitoring is recommended in patients with risk factors.

Do not perform cardiotocography for low-risk women in established labor (*NICE 2014 Guideline).*

Auscultation should be commenced immediately after a contraction and continued for at least one minute (*Recent NICE 2014 Guideline).*

Record accelerations and decelerations if heard:

- First stage of labor at least every 15 minutes.
- Second stage at least every 5 minutes.

Palpate maternal pulse if a fetal heart rate abnormality is suspected so as to differentiate between the two heart rates (*2014 NICE Guideline*).

Recommendations ACOG 2009/NICE 2014/Aus NZ Guidelines 2006/SOGC 200.[3-6]

An alternative approach is to provide intermittent CTG monitoring alternating with fetal heart rate auscultation. There is some evidence stating similar neonatal outcomes in low-risk population as compared to continuous CTG.[7]

Admission Cardiotocography

This is a short cardiotocography (CTG) recording made at admission in low risk patients in labor, in order to identify unrecognized 'at risk' fetuses requiring close supervision or immediate delivery. Aim is to categorize patients into low-and high-risk group for effective utilization of resources. However, there is no strong evidence that admission CTG in low-risk pregnancies confer any significant benefit in terms of reduced perinatal loss, neither it appears to be associated with increase in major intervention rates.

Current evidence does not support routine admission test for low risk women as there is no benefit (*SOGC Guidelines).*[6]

Electronic Fetal Monitoring

Electronic fetal monitoring (EFM) is word used synonymously with cardiotocography (CTG). "Cardio" refers to a heart rate, "toco" is derived from the Greek word for birth and refers to uterine activity. The application of a fetal monitor throughout labor with frequent evaluation of the FHR and uterine activity pattern is known as continuous EFM.

Fetal heart rate monitoring may be performed externally or internally. Most external monitors use a Doppler device with computerized logic to interpret and count the Doppler signals. Internal FHR monitoring is accomplished with a fetal electrode, which is a spiral wire placed directly on the fetal scalp or other presenting part. CTG machines should be standardized to enable consistent approach to teaching and interpretation of EFM tracing. Paper tracing of 1cm/ min is adopted universally although few countries still use 2 cm/min and 3 cm/min also.

Continuous EFM should be used when there are abnormalities in structured intermittent auscultation or risk factors arising during labor or for high-risk patients. These include:

- Antenatal risk factors for fetal compromise:
  - Medical disorders like hypertension, diabetes, chronic renal disease.

Cyanotic heart disease, autoimmune disorders, hereditary thrombophilia, antiphospholipid antibody syndrome, poorly controlled hyperthyroidism

- Antepartum hemorrhage
- Previous lowe segment cesarean section (LSCS)
- Prolonged pregnancy
- Oligohydramnios or abnormal umbilical artery Doppler
- Multiple pregnancy
- Prematurity
- Fetal growth restriction
- Intrapartum factors necessitating EFM:
  - Abnormal admission test
  - Significant meconium stained liquor
  - Abnormal fetal heart on auscultation
  - Maternal pyrexia, sepsis, chorioamnionitis
  - Fresh vaginal bleeding in labor
  - Oxytocin use-induction, augmentation
  - Use of epidural for labor analgesia
  - Prolonged rupture of membranes
  - Confirmed delay in the first and second stage of labor.

Guidelines for Nomenclature and Interpretation of Electronic Fetal Heart Rate Monitoring[3]

This chapter will use American College of Obstetricians and Gynecologists (ACOG) 2009, National Institute for Health and Care Excellence (NICE) 2014 and The International Federation of Gynecology and Obstetrics (FIGO) 2015 Guidelines for standardized interpretation and management of electronic fetal heart monitoring for clinicians and students.

To provide a systematic approach to interpreting the electronic fetal monitor tracing, the National Institute of Child Health and Human Development convened a workshop in 2008 to revise the accepted definitions for electronic fetal monitor tracing.[8] The key elements include assessment of baseline heart rate, presence or absence of variability, and interpretation of periodic changes. The workshop introduced a new classification scheme for decision making with regard to tracings. ACOG guidelines issued in 2009 supports the recommendations of the Eunice Kennedy Shriver National Institute of Child and Health Development workshop on electronic fetal monitoring. The objective of the guidelines was to reduce the inconsistent use of common terminology and the wide variability that sometimes occurs in FHR interpretations.[3]

Contractions

It is important to assess the pressure tracing before assessing the fetal tracing to accurately interpret decelerations. The electronic fetal monitor uses an external pressure transducer to measure frequency and duration of contractions. However, the strength of contractions and basal tone cannot always be accurately assessed from an external transducer. Intensity is evaluated subjectively by clinical palpation as mild, moderate and strong. Incorrect placement, reduced tension on the supporting elastic band or abdominal adiposity may result in inadequate registration of contractions.

Intrauterine pressure catheters can provide direct assessment of intrauterine pressures, frequency and duration of contraction. However, they are invasive and expensive and are not routinely used in clinical scenarios.

Uterine contractions are quantified as the number of contractions present in a 10-minute window, averaged over a 30-minute period.

Normal: Five contractions or less in 10 minutes, averaged over a 30-minute window.

Tachysystole: More than five contractions in 10 minutes, averaged over a 30-minute window. Tachysystole should always be qualified with or without associated FHR decelerations.

The term tachysystole applies to both spontaneous and stimulated labor. The clinical response to tachysystole may differ depending on whether contractions are spontaneous or stimulated. The terms hyperstimulation and hypercontractility have been abandoned.[3]

ELECTRONIC FETAL MONITORING: DEFINITIONS[3]

Cardiotocography (CTG) analysis starts with evaluation of five basic features including baseline heart rate, variability, accelerations, decelerations and contractions and then classifying the CTG tracing (Table 9.1).

TABLE 9.1 Cardiotocography: Basic features and definitions

Pattern	*Definition*
Baseline heart rate	• The mean FHR rounded to increments of 5 beats per minute during a 10-minute segment, excluding: Periodic or episodic changes Periods of marked FHR variability • The baseline must be for a minimum of 2 minutes in any 10-minute segment, or the baseline for that time period is indeterminate. In this case, one may refer to the prior 10-minute window for determination of baseline. • *Normal FHR baseline*: 110–160 beats per minute • *Tachycardia*: FHR baseline is greater than 160 beats per minute • *Bradycardia*: FHR baseline is less than 110 beats per minute
Baseline variability	• Fluctuations in the baseline FHR that are irregular in amplitude and frequency • Variability is visually quantitated as the amplitude of peak-to-trough in beats per minute. —Absent—amplitude range undetectable —Minimal—amplitude range detectable but 5 beats per minute or fewer —Moderate (normal)—amplitude range 6–25 beats per minute —Marked—amplitude range greater than 25 beats per minute
Acceleration	• A visually apparent abrupt increase (onset to peak in less than 30 seconds) in the FHR • At 32 weeks of gestation and beyond, an acceleration has a peak of 15 beats per minute or more above baseline, with a duration of 15 seconds or more but less than 2 minutes from onset to return • Before 32 weeks of gestation, an acceleration has a peak of 10 beats per minute or more above baseline, with a duration of 10 seconds or more but less than 2 minutes from onset to return • Prolonged acceleration lasts 2 minutes or more but less than 10 minutes in duration • If an acceleration lasts 10 minutes or longer, it is a baseline change
Early deceleration	• Visually apparent usually symmetrical gradual decrease and return of the FHR associated with a uterine contraction • A gradual FHR decrease is defined as from the onset to the FHR nadir of 30 seconds or more • The nadir of the deceleration occurs at the same time as the peak of the contraction • In most cases the onset, nadir, and recovery of the deceleration are coincident with the beginning, peak, and ending of the contraction, respectively

Contd...

Contd...

Pattern	*Definition*
Late deceleration	• Visually apparent usually symmetrical gradual decrease and return of the FHR associated with a uterine contraction • The deceleration is delayed in timing, with the nadir of the deceleration occurring after the peak of the contraction • In most cases, the onset, nadir, and recovery of the deceleration occur after the beginning, peak, and ending of the contraction, respectively
Variable deceleration	• Visually apparent abrupt decrease in FHR • An abrupt FHR decrease is defined as from the onset of the deceleration to the beginning of the FHR nadir of less than 30 seconds • The decrease in FHR is 15 beats per minute or greater, lasting 15 seconds or greater, and less than 2 minutes in duration • When variable decelerations are associated with uterine contractions, their onset, depth, and duration commonly vary with successive uterine contractions
Prolonged deceleration	• Visually apparent decrease in the FHR below the baseline • Decrease in FHR from the baseline that is 15 beats per minute or more, lasting 2 minutes or more but less than 10 minutes in duration • If a deceleration last 10 minutes or longer, it is a baseline change
Sinusoidal pattern	• Visually apparent, smooth, sine wave-like undulating pattern in FHR baseline with a cycle frequency of 3–5 per minute which persists for 20 minutes or more

Abbreviation: FHR, fetal heart rate

Baseline Heart Rate

The mean fetal heart rate, when stable during a 10-minute segment, excluding accelerations and decelerations is defined as baseline fetal heart and normally ranges between 110 and 160 bpm (Fig. 9.1). Mild bradycardia (100–110 bpm) is associated with post-term infants and occipitoposterior position. Rates of less than 100 bpm may be seen in fetuses with congenital heart disease, myocardial conduction defects, drugs like beta-blockers and narcotics or maternal hypothermia. A baseline > 160 bpm is defined as tachycardia. This is associated with certain maternal and fetal conditions, such as chorioamnionitis, fever, dehydration, drugs like beta-mimetics and fetal tachyarrhythmias. Preterm fetuses tend to have heart rate toward upper end of the range and post-term fetuses towards the lower end.

As per the new NICE guidelines a baseline fetal heart rate between 100 and 109 bpm with normal baseline variability and no variable or late decelerations is normal and shoud not prompt further action (provided it is confirmed to be not maternal heart rate). A stable baseline heart rate between 90 and 99

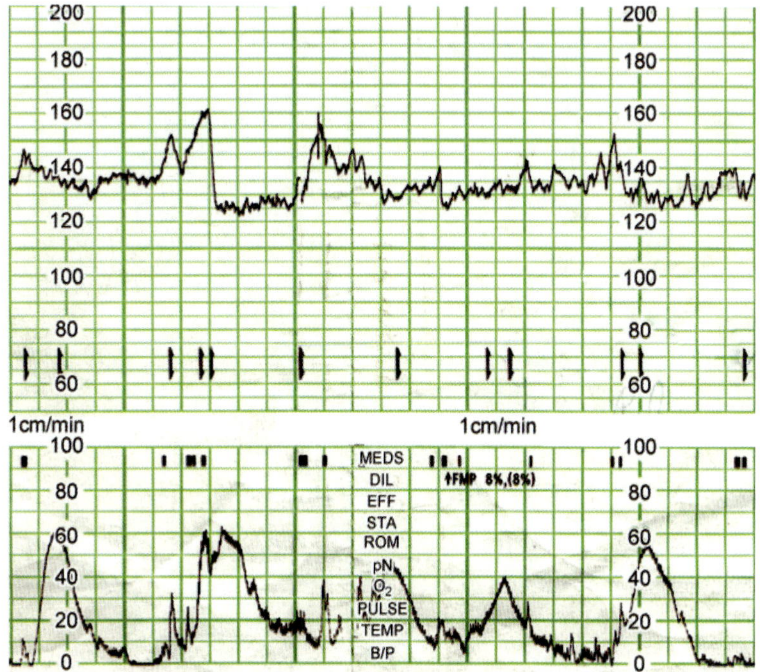

Fig. 9.1: Cardiotocography showing normal fetal heart rate, normal baseline variability with accelerations

bpm with normal baseline variability may be a normal variation and needs a senior obstetricians opinion.[9]

A baseline fetal heart rate between 161–180 bpm with no other nonreassuring or abnormal features on CTG, think of the possibility of underlying causes like infection and perform appropriate investigations. Check woman's temperature and pulse and offer fluids and paracetamol if either is raised (Fig. 9.2). If the woman's pulse and temperature are normal, continue CTG and manage as normal labor, since the risk of fetal acidosis is low (New NICE guidelines).[9]

If baseline heart rate is between 100 bpm and 109 bpm or above 160 bpm and there is 1 other nonreassuring feature on CTG, start conservative measures to improve fetal wellbeing.[9]

If there is bradycardia or a single prolonged deceleration with fetal heart rate below 100 bpm for 3 minutes or more, start conservative measures, seek urgent help, make preparation for urgent delivery, expedite birth if bradycardia persists for 9 minutes.[9]

Variability

It is the amplitude of fluctuations in the fetal heart rate baseline measured in beats per minute. The fetal heart rate (FHR) normally exhibits variability, with an average change of 6–25 bpm of the baseline rate, and is linked to the fetal central nervous system. Therefore, it is a vital clue in determining the

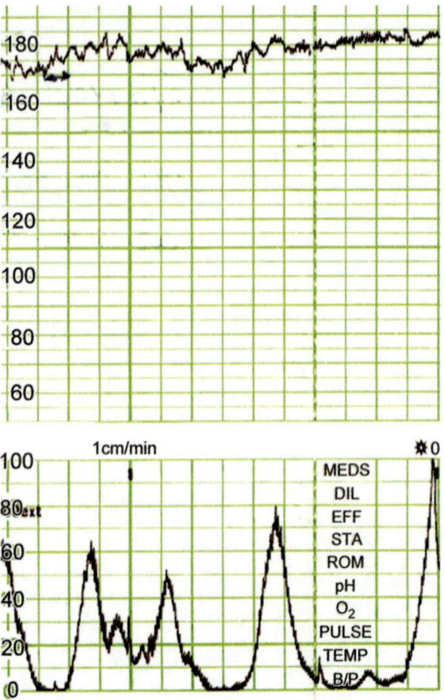

Fig. 9.2: Cardiotocography of a patient with fever showing fetal tachycardia with a baseline heart rate of 180 bpm

overall fetal condition. The National intensive of Child Health and Human Development (NICHD) has stated that it is no longer useful to distinguish between short-term and long-term variability and has categorized variability into absent, minimal, moderate and marked. Sleep cycles of 20–40 minutes or longer may cause a normal decrease in FHR variability, as can certain medications, including analgesics, anesthetics, barbiturates, and magnesium sulfate. Loss of variability, accompanied by late or variable decelerations, increases the possibility of fetal acidosis if uncorrected.

Intermittent periods of reduced baseline variability <5 bpm are normal during the quiescent sleep state. Minor pseudosinusoidal pattern (oscillations of amplitude 5–15 bpm) are of no significance.

If there is reduced baseline variability (<5 bpm) with a normal baseline fetal heart and no variable or late decelerations persisting for over 30 minutes, start conservative measures (Fig. 9.3). However, if it persists for more than 90 minutes, offer fetal blood sampling to measure lactate or pH. If the reduced variability for more than 30 minutes is accompanied with one or more of tachycardia (>160 bpm), bradycardia (<100 bpm) or variable or late decelerations, start conservative measures and offer fetal blood sampling.[9]

Sinusoidal pattern is a smooth, undulating sine wave pattern defined by an amplitude of 10 bpm with three to five cycles per minute, lasting at least 20 minutes. This uncommon pattern is associated with severe fetal anemia and hydrops, and it usually requires rapid intervention in these settings. Similar

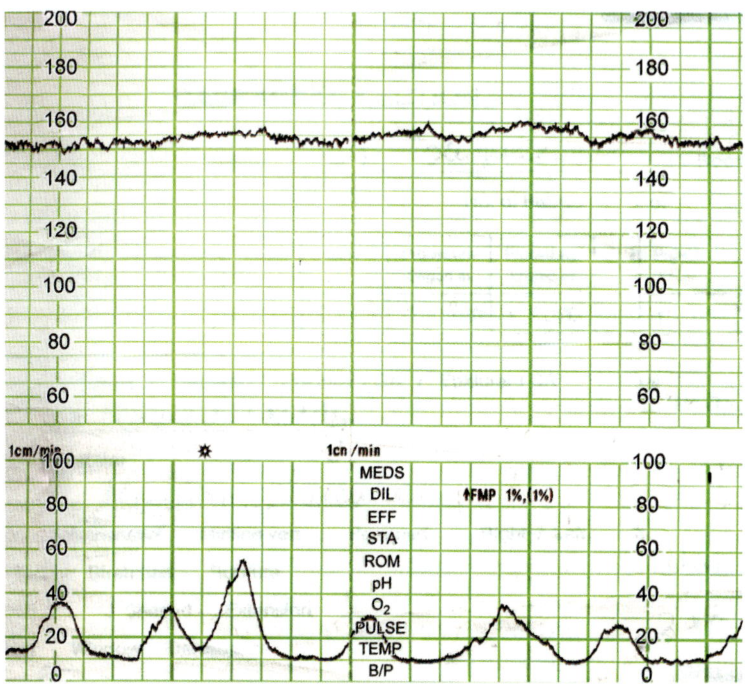

Fig. 9.3: Cardiotocography strip showing reduced variability in a women in labor

appearing benign tracings occasionally occur because of "fetal thumb sucking" or maternal narcotic administration, and generally these will persist for less than 10 minutes.

Accelerations

Abrupt increases in the FHR (15 beats for 15 seconds) are associated with fetal movement or stimulation and are indicative of neurologically responsive non-hypoxic healthy fetus. Preterm fetuses below 32 weeks have acceleration with an amplitude of 10 bpm for 10 seconds. The absence of acceleration in an otherwise normal CTG does not indicate acidosis.

Decelerations

Transient decrease in fetal heart rate of 15 beats for 15 seconds is defined as decelerations. These periodic changes in FHR relate to uterine contractions are classified as recurrent if they occur with 50% or more of contractions in a 20-minute period, and intermittent if they occur with less than 50% of contractions. The decrease in FHR is calculated from the onset to the nadir of the deceleration.

When describing a deceleration following need to be specified:[9]

- The depth and duration
- Timing in relation to the peak of contractions

- Whether or not the fetal heart rate return to baseline
- How long they have been present?
- Whether they occur with over 50% of contractions.

Early deceleration are transient, shallow, gradual decreases in FHR that are visually apparent and usually symmetric. The time from onset to nadir is >30 seconds (gradual). They occur with and mirror the uterine contraction and seldom go below 100 bpm. The nadir of the deceleration occurs at the same time as the peak of the contraction. Early decelerations are nearly always benign and probably indicate head compression and reflex vagal stimulation, which is a normal part of labor. Early decelerations with no non-reassuring or abnormal features need no action (Fig. 9.4).

Variable decelerations, as the name implies, vary in terms of shape, depth, duration and timing in relationship to uterine contractions, but they are visually apparent, abrupt decreases in FHR (onset to nadir <30 seconds) (Fig. 9.5). Characteristics of a typical variable decelerations include rapid descent and recovery, good baseline variability, and accelerations at the onset and at the end of the deceleration (i.e. "shoulders"/"overshoots"). When they are associated with uterine contractions, their onset, depth, and duration commonly vary with successive uterine contractions. Overall, typical variable decelerations are usually benign, and their physiologic basis is usually related to cord compression, with subsequent changes in peripheral vascular resistance or oxygenation. They occur especially in the second stage of labor, when cord compression is most common.

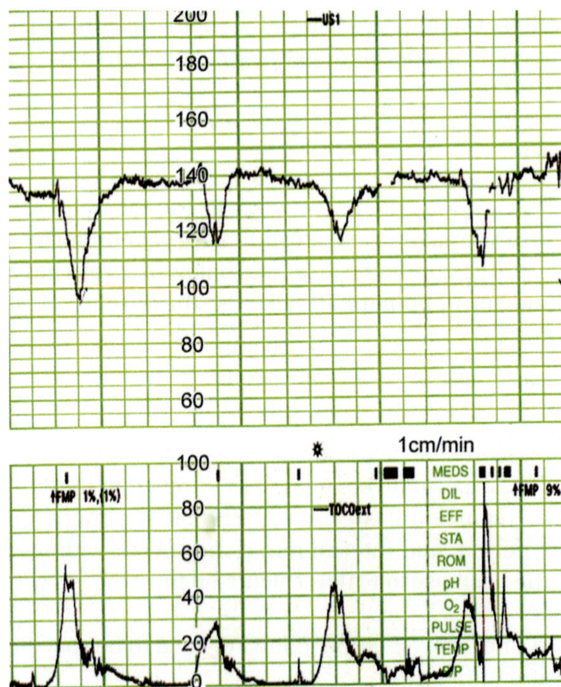

Fig. 9.4: Early decelerations in active labour – delivered vaginally after 3 hours

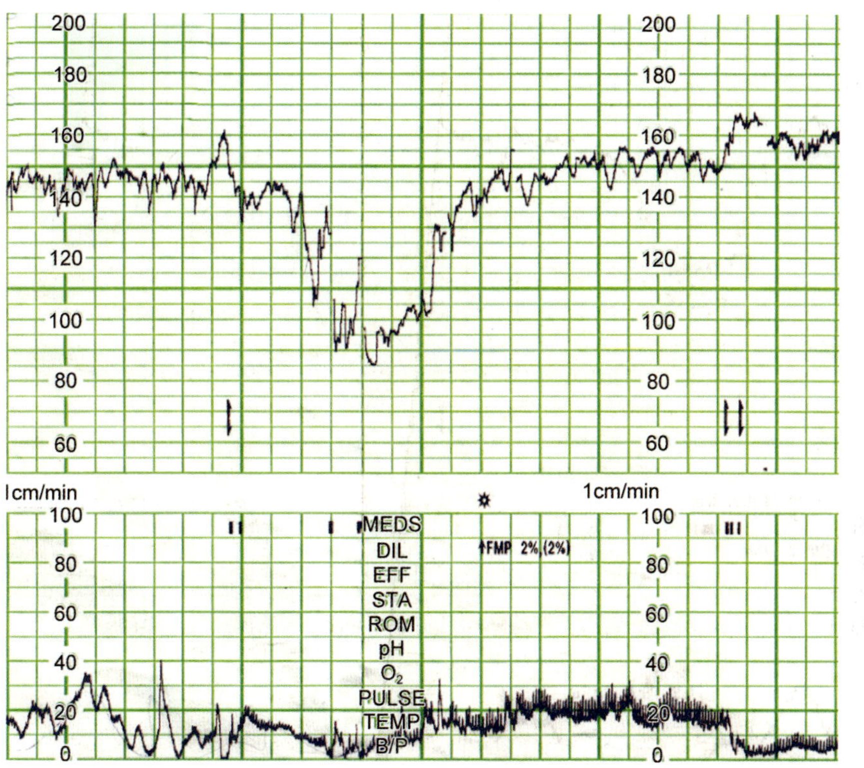

Fig. 9.5: Single unprovoked variable deceleration with normal baseline heart rate, variability and accelerations

Atypical variable decelerations may indicate fetal hypoxemia. Variable decelerations with any of the following additional characteristics are called atypical variable decelerations (Fig. 9.6). These include:

- Loss of primary and secondary rise in baseline rate—loss of shouldering
- Slow return to baseline FHR after the end of contraction
- Prolonged secondary rise in baseline rate
- Biphasic decelerations—M pattern
- Loss of variability during the decelerations
- Continuation of baseline rate at lower level.

If variable decelerations are present with normal baseline heart rate, normal baseline variability with a drop of 60 beats/minute or less and taking 60 seconds or less to recover, present for 90 minutes and occurring in 50% of contractions start with conservative measures.

If variable decelerations are present with normal baseline heart rate, normal baseline variability with a drop of more than 60 beats/minute or taking more than 60 seconds to recover, present for 30 minutes and occurring in 50% of contractions start with conservative measures (Fig. 9.7).

Offer fetal blood sampling if variable deceleration persists after 30 minutes of starting conservative treatment or accompanied by tachycardia or reduced baseline variability.[9]

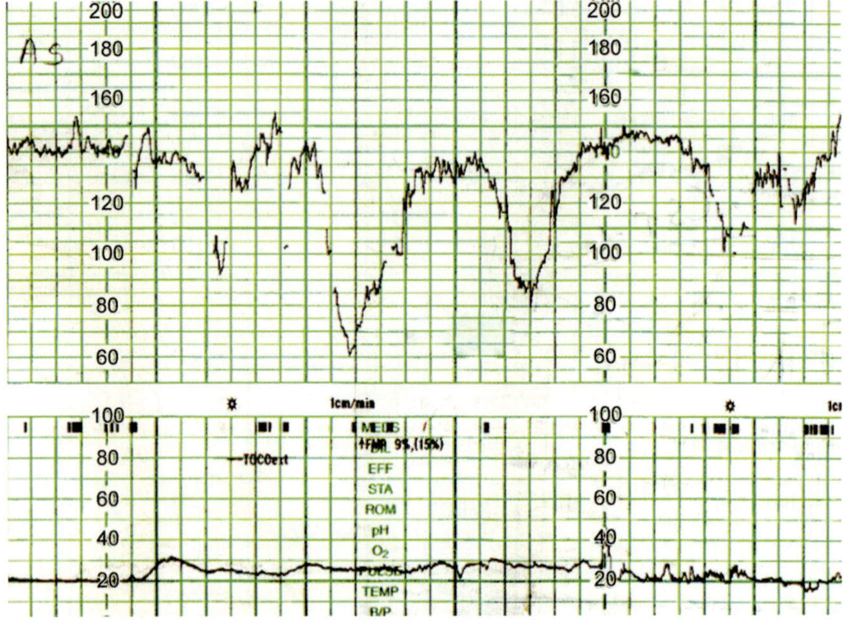

Fig. 9.6: Atypical variable deceleration—biphasic pattern

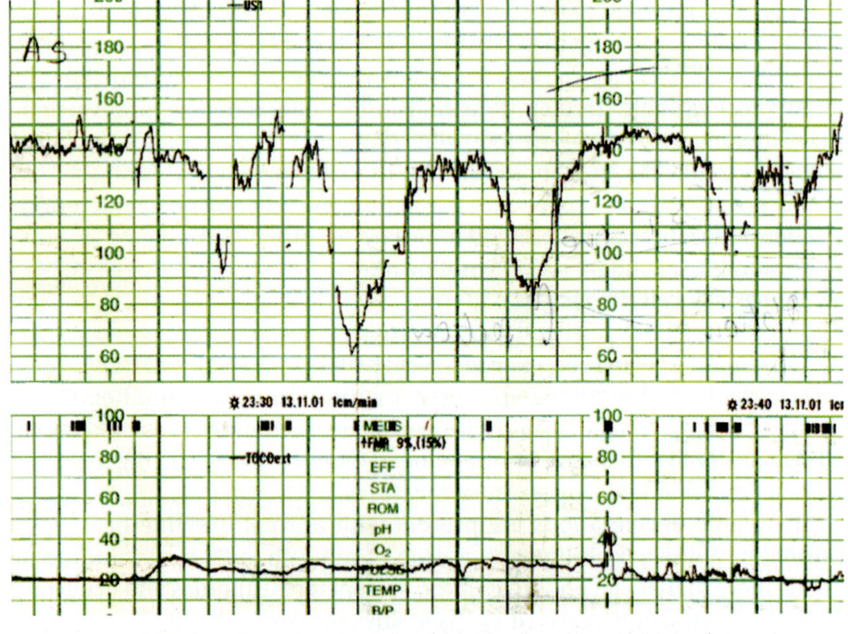

Fig. 9.7: Typical persistent variable deceleration with normal baseline heart rate, variability

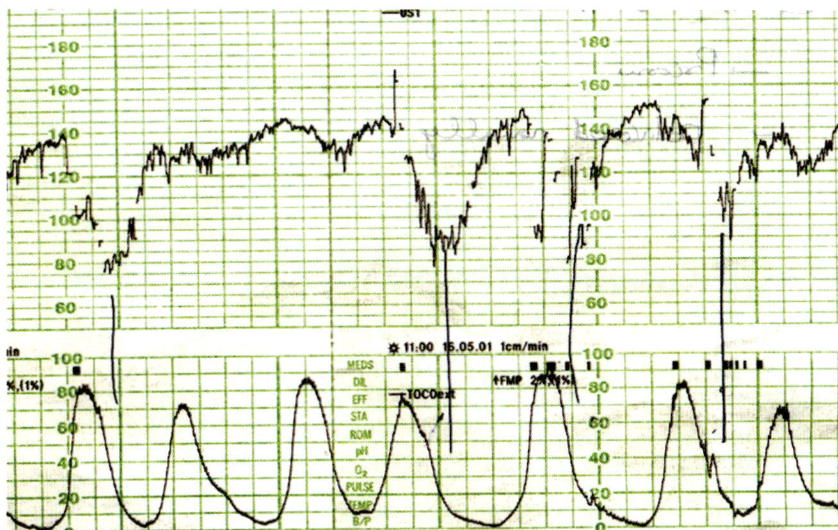

Fig. 9.8: Late decelerations with > 50% of contractions

Late decelerations are visually apparent, usually symmetric, gradual (onset to nadir >30 seconds) and have the characteristic feature of onset of the deceleration after the onset of the uterine contraction. The timing of the deceleration is delayed, with the nadir of the deceleration occurring after the peak of the contraction (Fig. 9.8). The physiology behind late deceleration is uteroplacental insufficiency and is indicative of chemoreceptor mediated response to fetal hypoxemia. Transient late deceleration patterns may be seen with maternal hypotension or uterine hyperstimulation and abruption.

If late decelerations occur with over 50% of contractions, start conservative measures. Offer fetal blood sampling and / or expedite delivery if late decelerations persist for over 30 minutes and occur for over 50% of contractions or late decelerations accompanied with abnormal baseline heart rate and / or reduced variability.[9]

Prolonged decelerations last longer than two minutes, but less than 10 minutes. They may be caused by a number of factors, including head compression (rapid fetal descent), cord compression, or uteroplacental insufficiency. Management depends on the clinical picture and presence of other FHR characteristics. A deceleration that lasts more than 10 minutes is a baseline change.

Overall assessment: The recommendations for the overall management of FHR tracings by NICHD, the International Federation of Gynecology and Obstetrics and ACOG agree that interpretation is reproducible at the extreme ends of the fetal monitor strip spectrum. For example, the presence of a normal baseline rate with FHR accelerations or moderate variability predicts the absence of fetal acidemia. Bradycardia, absence of variability with decelerations, and presence of recurrent late or variable decelerations may predict current or impending fetal asphyxia. However, more than 50% of fetal strips fall between these two extremes, in which overall recommendations cannot be made reliably. In the 2008 revision of the NICHD, a three-tiered system for the categorization of FHR patterns was recommended and adopted by ACOG: normal (category I), indeterminate (category II), and abnormal (category III). Category III tracings need intervention to resolve the abnormal tracing or to move toward expeditious delivery.

CLASSIFICATION OF FETAL HEART RATE TRACINGS[3]

It is important to recognize that FHR tracing patterns provide information only on the current acid-base status of the fetus. Categorization of the FHR tracing evaluates the fetus at that point in time. A FHR tracing may move back and forth between the categories depending on the clinical situation and management strategies used.

Category I: *FHR tracings are normal.* Category I FHR tracings are strongly predictive of normal fetal acid-base status at the time of observation. Category I FHR tracings may be monitored in a routine manner and no specific action is required.

Category II: *FHR tracings are indeterminate.* Category II FHR tracings are not predictive of abnormal fetal acid-base status, yet presently there is not adequate evidence to classify these as category I or category III. Category II FHR tracings require evaluation and continued close surveillance and re-evaluation, taking into account the entire associated clinical circumstances. In some circumstances, either ancillary tests to ensure fetal wellbeing or intrauterine resuscitative measures may be used with category II tracings.

Category III: *FHR tracings are abnormal.* Category III tracings are associated with possible decreased fetal oxygenation and/or abnormal fetal acid-base status at the time of observation. category III FHR tracings require prompt evaluation. Depending on the clinical situation, efforts to expeditiously resolve the abnormal FHR pattern may include but are not limited to provision of maternal oxygen, change in maternal position, discontinuation of labor stimulation, treatment of maternal hypotension, and treatment of tachysystole with FHR changes. If a category III tracing does not resolve with these measures, prompt delivery should be undertaken.

Three-tiered Fetal Heart Rate Interpretation System[8]

Category I

Category I FHR tracings include all of the following:
- *Baseline rate*: 110–160 beats per minute
- *Baseline FHR variability*: Moderate
- *Late or variable decelerations*: Absent
- *Early decelerations*: Present or absent
- *Accelerations*: Present or absent.

Category II

Category II FHR tracings includes all FHR tracings not categorized as Category I or Category III. Category II tracings may represent an appreciable fraction of those encountered in clinical care. Examples of Category II FHR tracings include any of the following:

Baseline rate
- Bradycardia not accompanied by absent baseline variability
- Tachycardia.

Baseline FHR variability
- Minimal baseline variability
- Absent baseline variability with no recurrent decelerations
- Marked baseline variability.

Accelerations
- Absence of induced accelerations after fetal stimulation.

Periodic or episodic decelerations
- Recurrent variable decelerations accompanied by minimal or moderate baseline variability.
- Prolonged deceleration more than 2 minutes but less than10 minutes.
- Recurrent late decelerations with moderate baseline variability.
- Variable decelerations with other characteristics such as slow return to baseline, overshoots, or "shoulders".

Category III

Category III FHR tracings include either:
- Absent baseline FHR variability and any of the following:
  - Recurrent late decelerations
  - Recurrent variable decelerations
  - Bradycardia
- Sinusoidal pattern.

Medications that can Influence the Fetal Heart Rate

Fetal heart rate patterns can be influenced by the medications administered in the intrapartum period. Most often, these changes are transient, although they sometimes lead to obstetric interventions.

Epidural analgesia with local anesthetic agents (i.e. lidocaine, bupivacaine) can lead to sympathetic blockade, maternal hypotension, transient uteroplacental insufficiency, and alterations in the FHR.

Use of magnesium sulfate show small changes in baseline, significant decrease in short-term variability but no decelerations. Caution should be used in ascribing unfavorable findings on EFM to the use of magnesium only.

The use of betamethasone transiently decreased the FHR variability, which returned to pretreatment status by the fourth to seventh day. There also may be a decrease in the rate of accelerations with the use of betamethasone. These effects are seen primarily with betamethasone and not with dexamethasone.

Narcotics (75 mg meperidine, 10 mg morphine, 0.1 mg fentanyl, 10 mg nalbuphine, cocaine) use decreases variability and cause a decrease in the frequency of accelerations.

Terbutaline: Increase in baseline FHR and incidence of fetal tachycardia.

Zidovudine: No difference in the FHR baseline, variability, number of accelerations.

METHODS OF INTRAUTERINE RESUSCITATION USED FOR CATEGORY II OR CATEGORY III TRACINGS[3] CONSERVATIVE MEASURE (NICE 2014)[9]

Category II or Category III FHR tracing requires evaluation of the possible causes. Initial evaluation and treatment may include the following:

- Discontinuation of any labor stimulating agent
- IV fluid bolus of Ringers Lactate solution.
- Cervical examination to determine umbilical cord prolapse, rapid cervical dilation, or descent of the fetal head, fresh vaginal bleeding.
- Changing maternal position to left or right lateral recumbent position, specially avoiding supine position and reducing compression of the vena cava and improving uteroplacental blood flow.
- Monitoring maternal blood pressure level for evidence of hypotension, especially in those with regional anesthesia (if present, treatment with volume expansion or with ephedrine or both, or phenylephrine may be warranted).
- Assessment of patient for uterine tachysystole by evaluating uterine contraction frequency and duration. Discontinue oxytocin if in use. In cases, not secondary to oxytocin infusion, the use of tocolytic agents may be considered to stop uterine contractions and perhaps avoid umbilical cord compression. A suggested regimen is subcutaneous terbutaline 0.25 mg.
- Prolonged use of maternal facial oxygen therapy may be harmful to the baby and should be avoided. There is no research evidence evaluating the benefits or risks associated with the short-term use of maternal facial oxygen therapy in cases of suspected fetal compromise.
- When the FHR tracing includes recurrent variable decelerations, amnioinfusion to relieve umbilical cord compression may be considered. However, the new NICE guideline recommends no amnioinfusion for intrauterine fetal resuscitation.

ADJUNCTS TO THE USE OF CONTINUOUS ELECTRONIC FETAL MONITORING INCLUDING FETAL BLOOD SAMPLE

Ancillary tests available that help to ensure fetal wellbeing in the face of a Category II or Category III FHR tracing, thereby reducing the high false-positive rate of EFM include:

- Fetal scalp sampling
- Fetal scalp stimulation
- Vibroacoustic stimulation
- Digital scalp stimulation.

Because vibroacoustic stimulation and digital scalp stimulation are less invasive than the other two methods, they are the preferred methods. When there is an acceleration following stimulation, acidemia is unlikely and labor can continue.

When a Category III FHR tracing is persistent, a scalp blood sample for the determination of pH or lactate may be considered. However, the use of scalp pH assessment has decreased. There are likely many reasons for this decrease, including physician experience, difficulty in obtaining and processing an adequate sample in a short amount of time, and the need for routine maintenance and calibration of laboratory equipment that may be used infrequently and patients choice. More importantly, scalp stimulation, which is less invasive, provides similar information about the likelihood of fetal acidemia as does scalp pH. The sensitivity and positive predictive value of a low scalp pH to identify a newborn with hypoxic-ischemic encephalopathy was 50% and 3%, respectively. However, the greater utility of scalp pH is in its high negative predictive value (97–99%) (Table 9.2).

Fetal blood sampling should be done in left lateral position to measure either lactate or pH levels.

Interpret fetal blood sampling taking into account previous lactate or pH values, the rate of progress of labor and the clinical circumstances.

TABLE 9.2 Classification of fetal blood sample results (New NICE Guidelines)[9]

Lactate (mmol/L)	*pH*	*Interpretation*	*Response*
≥4.1	≥7.25	Normal	Repeat in 1 hour if FHR trace remains pathological
4.2–4.8	7.21–7.24	Borderline	Repeat in 30 minutes if FHR trace remains pathological
≤4.9	≤7.20	Abnormal	Deliver

Abbreviation: FHR, Fetal heart rate

Where there is clear evidence of acute fetal compromise (for example, prolonged deceleration greater than 3 minutes), FBS should not be undertaken and urgent preparations to expedite birth should be made.

Contraindications to FBS

- Maternal infection (for example, HIV, hepatitis viruses and herpes simplex virus)
- Fetal bleeding disorders (for example, haemophilia)
- Prematurity (less than 34 weeks).

When a fetal blood sampling is indicated but cannot be obtained either because it is contraindicated or technically not possible or unsuccessful, fetal heart rate response to scalp stimulation may be used for fetal wellbeing. Decision to continue labor or expedite delivery should be taken in the light of the clinical situation and in discussion with the obstetrician and woman.[9]

INTERPRETATION OF FHR TRACES/ CARDIOTOCOGRAPHS (NICE GUIDELINES)[4,9]

The recommended definitions and classifications of the FHR trace/ cardiotocograph as per the NICE guideline 2007 were accepted by The Royal College of Obstetrics and Gynecology (UK). These were somewhat similar to the ACOG guidelines with Category I,II,III synonymous with normal, suspicious, pathological trace respectively (Tables 9.3 to 9.6).

- If repeated accelerations are present with reduced variability, the FHR trace should be regarded as reassuring.
- True early uniform decelerations are rare and benign, and therefore they are insignificant.
- Most decelerations in labor are variable.
- If a bradycardia occurs in the baby for more than 3 minutes, urgent medical aid should be sought and preparations should be made to urgently expedite the birth of the baby, classified as a Category I birth. This could include moving the woman to theater if the fetal heart has not recovered by 9 minutes. If the fetal heart recovers within 9 minutes the decision to deliver should be reconsidered in conjunction with the woman if reasonable.

TABLE 9.3 Definition of Normal, Suspicious and Pathological FHR Traces[4] (NICE guideline 2007)

Definition	*Traces*
Normal	An FHR trace in which all four features are classified as reassuring.
Suspicious	An FHR trace with one feature classified as non-reassuring and the remaining features classified as reassuring.
Pathological	An FHR trace with two or more features classified as non-reassuring or one or more classified as abnormal.

TABLE 9.4 Category Definition (Old NICE Guideline 2007)[4]

Features	*Baseline (bpm)*	*Variability (bpm)*	*Deceleration*	*Acceleration*
Reassuring	110–160	≥ 5	None	Present
Non-reassuring	100–109 161–180	< 5 for 40–90 minutes	Typical variable Decelerations with over 50% of contractions, occurring for over 90 minutes Single prolonged deceleration for up to 3 minutes	The absence of accelerations with otherwise normal trace is of uncertain significance
Abnormal	< 100 > 180 Sinusoidal pattern ≥ 10 minutes	< 5 for 90 minutes	Either atypical variable decelerations with over 50% of contractions or late decelerations, both for over 30 minutes Single prolonged deceleration for more than 3 minutes	

TABLE 9.5 Category Definition (NICE Guidelines 2015)[9]

Description	*Features Baseline (bpm)*	*Baseline variability(bpm)*	*Deceleration*
Reassuring/ Normal	100–160	5 or more	None or early
Non-reassuring	161–180	Less than 5 for 30–90 minutes	Variable decelerations: • Dropping from baseline by 60 bpm or less and taking 60 seconds or less to recover • Present for over 90 minutes • Occurring with over 50% of contractions OR Variable decelerations : • Dropping from baseline by more than 60 bpm or taking over 60 seconds to recover • Present for up to 30 minutes • Occurring with over 50% of contractions OR Late deceleration • Present for up to 30 minutes • Occurring with over 50% of contractions

Contd…

Contd...

Description	*Features Baseline (bpm)*	*Baseline variability(bpm)*	*Deceleration*
Abnormal	Above 180 or below 100	Less than 5 for over 90 minutes	Non- reassuring variable decelerations • Still observed 30 minutes after starting conservative measures • occurring with over 50% of contractions OR Late decelerations • Present for over 30 minutes • Do not improve with conservative measures • Occurring with over 50% of contractions OR Bradycardia or a single prolonged Deceleration lasting 3 minutes or more

TABLE 9.6 Management based on interpretation of cardiotocography traces (New NICE guidelines CG190, 2014).[9]

Category	*Definition*	*Interpretation*	*Management*
CTG normal / reassuring	All three features are normal / reassuring	Healthy fetus	• Continue CTG and normal care • If CTG was started because of concern arising from intermittent auscultation, remove CTG after 20 minutes if no nonreassuring or abnormal features and no ongoing risk factors
CTG non-reassuring and suggests need for conservative measures	1. Non-reassuring feature and 2. Normal / reassuring features	Combination of features that may be associated with increased risk of fetal acidosis; If acceleration present acidosis is unlikely	• Think about possible underlying causes • If baseline fetal heart rate is over 160 bpm, check the women's temperature and pulse. If either is raised, offer fluids and paracetamol. • Start 1 or more conservative measures: - Encourage women to mobilize or adopt left lateral position, avoid supine position - Offer oral or IV fluids - Reduce contraction frequency by stopping oxytocin and/or offering tocolysis

Contd...

Contd...

Category	*Definition*	*Interpretation*	*Management*
CTG abnormal and indicates need for conservative measures and further testing	1. Abnormal feature OR 2. Non-reassuring feature	Combination of features that is more likely to be associated with fetal acidosis	• Think about possible underlying causes • If baseline fetal heart rate is over 160 bpm, check the women's temperature and pulse. If either is raised, offer fluids and paracetamol. • Start 1 or more conservative measures • Offer to take a FBS (for lactate or pH) after implementing conservative measures, or expedite birth if an FBS cannot be obtained and no acceleration are seen as a result of scalp stimulation • Take action sooner than 30 minutes if late decelerations are accompanied by tachycardia and/or reduced baseline variability
Category	*Definition*	*Interpretation*	*Management*
CTG abnormal and indicates need for urgent intervention	Bradycardia or a single prolonged deceleration with baseline below 100 bpm persisting for 3 minutes or more	An abnormal feature that is very likely to be associated with current fetal acidosis or imminent rapid development of fetal acidosis	• Start 1 or more conservative measures • Make preparation for urgent birth • Expedite birth if persists for 9 minutes • If heart rate recovers before 9 minutes, reassess decision to expedite birth in discussion with the woman

Abbreviation: CTG, Cardiotocography

- A tachycardia in the baby of 160–180 bpm, where accelerations are present and no other adverse features appear, should not be regarded as suspicious. However, an increase in the baseline heart rate, even within the normal range, with other non-reassuring or abnormal features should increase concern.

As per the new NICE guidelines 2014 these terminology has been replaced with categories based on management strategy, i.e. normal/reassuring, non-reassuring needing conservative measures, abnormal with need for conservative measures and further testing and abnormal and need for urgent delivery. Parameters used for assessment includes only three features rather than four as per old guidelines. However, the 4th feature—presence of acceleration, is taken into account in management decisions.[9]

Overall Care

- Do not make any decisions about a woman's care in labor on the basis of CTG findings alone.
- Take into account any antenatal and intrapartum risk factors, the current wellbeing of the woman and the unborn baby and the progress of labor when interpreting the CTG trace.
- Remain with the women at all times in order to continue providing one to one support.
- Ensure that the focus of care remains with the woman rather than the CTG trace.
- Make a documented systemic assessment of the condition of the woman and the unborn baby (including the CTG) hourly or more frequently if there are concerns.

PRINCIPLES OF INTRAPARTUM CTG TRACE INTERPRETATION

- When reviewing the CTG, assess and document all 4 features (baseline fetal heart rate, baseline variability, presence or absence of decelerations, presence of accelerations)
- It is not possible to categorize or interpret every CTG trace. Senior obstetric input is important in these cases.

Accelerations

- The presence of fetal heart rate accelerations is generally a sign that the fetus is healthy.
- If a fetal blood sample is indicated and the sample cannot be obtained, but the associated scalp stimulation results in fetal heart rate acceleration, decide whether to continue labor or expedite the birth in the light of the clinical circumstances and in discussion with the woman.

ELECTRONIC FETAL MONITORING AND RECORD-KEEPING[4]

In order to ensure accurate record-keeping regarding EFM:

- The date and time clocks on the EFM machine should be correctly set.
- Traces should be labelled with the mother's name, date, hospital number and maternal pulse at the beginning of the monitoring.
- Any intrapartum events that may affect the FHR should be noted at the time on the FHR trace, which should be signed and the date and time noted (for example, vaginal examination, FBS or sitting of an epidural).
- Any member of staff who is asked to provide an opinion on a trace should note their findings on both the trace and the woman's medical records along with the date, time and signature.

- Following birth, the health care professional should sign and note the date, time and mode of birth on the FHR trace.
- The FHR trace should be stored securely with the woman's medical records at the end of the monitoring process.

CONCLUSION

Electronic fetal monitoring can be effective and useful only when the test is performed correctly, the results are interpreted satisfactorily as per standardized guidelines and finally the interpretation must provoke an appropriate response. Inspite of its limitations of high false positive result for predicting adverse outcome, it has a potential to be extremely useful if the entire obstetric team providing care to the women in labor use standardized terminology and communicate data correctly and manage patient appropriately. Decisions about patient management must be made in the light of total clinical situation.

REFERENCES

1. Martin JA, Hamilton BE, Sutton PD, Ventura SJ, Menacker F, Munson ML. Births: final data for 2002. Natl Vital Stat Rep. 2003;52(10):1-113.
2. Alfirevic Z, Devane D, Gyte GML. Continuous cardiotocography (CTG) as a form of electronic fetal monitoring (EFM) for fetal assessment during labour. Cochrane Database of Systematic Reviews 2006;3. Art. No.:CD006066. DOI: 10.1002/14651858.CD006066. (Metaanalysis)
3. ACOG Practice Bulletin No. 106: Intrapartum fetal heart rate monitoring: nomenclature, interpretation, and general management principles. Obstet Gynecol. 2009;114(1):192-202.
4. National Institute for Health and Clinical Excellence. Intrapartum care: management and delivery of care to women in labour. September 2007. *http:// guidance. nice.org.uk/CG55. Accessed July 6, 2009.*
5. RANZCOG Intrapartum Fetal Surveillance Clinical Guidelines (second edition), 2006.
6. Fetal Health Surveillance: Antepartum and Intrapartum Consensus Guideline No. 197 (Replaces No. 90 and No. 112). Journal of Obstetrics and Gynaecology Canada; 2007;29(9).
7. Diogo AC, Catherine YS, Edwin C. FIGO consensus guidelines on intrapartum fetal monitoring: Cardiotocography. International Journal of Gynecology and Obstetrics. 2015;131:13-24.
8. Macones GA, Hankins GD, Spong CY, Hauth J, Moore T. The 2008 National Institute of Child Health and Human Development workshop report on electronic fetal monitoring: update on definitions, interpretation, and research guidelines. Obstet Gynecol. 2008;112:661-6.
9. National Institute for Health and Clinical Excellence. Intrapartum care for healthy women and babies. December 2014. *http://guidance. nice.org.uk/guidance/* CG190.

Vaginal Hysterectomy in Case of Previous Lower Segment Cesarean Section

10

Shirish S Sheth

Today in most countries, over 20–50% of births are carried out by cesarean section, and this figure may rise disproportionately. It is therefore conceivable that the surgeon of tomorrow will be confronted by the need to carry out hysterectomies in women who have had one or multiple previous cesarean sections. Women who have not delivered vaginally and have had previous cesarean sections are 'vaginally nulliparous' and 'abdominally parous'.

The decision to carry out vaginal hysterectomy in women who have had previous cesarean sections should be guided by two questions: 'with the same pelvic findings, in the absence of cesarean section in past, would I attempt vaginal hysterectomy?' If the response is yes, then the second question is 'will I be able to access the vesicouterine peritoneum (VUP)?' Gynecologists need to remember that previous cesarean sections *per se* does not contraindicate vaginal hysterectomy but improves our operative skill, gives relief to patients and promotes vaginal surgery. Anxiety is to get an access to anterior or vesicouterine peritoneum (VUP).[1-3]

ACCESS TO THE VESICOUTERINE PERITONEUM: ANTERIOR POUCH

The intraoperative identification of correct planes and space depends on the gynecologist's knowledge of surgical anatomy and especially the surgical landmarks as seen in the operative fields. The gynecologist takes separate anterior and posterior incisions or has a circumferential incision around the cervix below the line of the bladder.

A central approach should be the routine to get an access to VUP but in those with a past history of cesarean section(s), the approach should always be from the lateral space by putting Allis laterally on cut vaginal edge. Thus access to VUP should be ideally via uterocervical broad ligament space or the lateral space or window. Anatomically, the free space laterally between bladder and uterocervical surface, namely uterocervical broad ligament space was first described by the author in the year 1993 and 1995 as space for the vaginal approach to hysterectomy in uteri with C-section(s) in past.[3-6]

Important is to have familiarity with friendliness in the area with cervico vesical strands, bladder, bladder pillars and vesicouterine space.[2,6]

Approach to access VUP from the lateral part of the cervix is safer as in lateral one fifth there are no adhesions and bladder lies at distance and not directly on the uterocervical surface. Figure 10.1 distinctly shows extra or more space between the bladder and cervix laterally than in the 3/5 centrally.[3-6] Hence, adhesions between the bladder and the lower uterine segment after C-section in past, if present, are usually in the middle three fifths and therefore accessing the peritoneal fold can become difficult and risky from the central area.

Uterocervical Broad Ligament Space

Presence of anterior adhesions between the bladder and lower uterine surface in the central 3/5 following C-section in past can prevent access to the vesicouterine peritoneum but it can still be gained by the lateral window approach.

Anatomically 2 × 1.5 cm + space is bound anteriorly by the under surface of the bladder and the anterior leaf of the broad ligament. It is bound posteriorly by the uterocervical surface as it slopes towards uterocervical border and the posterior leaf of the broad ligament. Medially the space ends where the bladder comes in close contact with the uterocervical surface (Fig. 10.1). Space continues laterally between the two leaves of the board ligament. The contents are the loose areolar tissue, lateral uterocervical margin and may have descending cervical vessels. It must be noted that the space does not contain uterine vessels and the ureter is well away from it.[2,6]

This anatomical space has been demonstrated by magnetic resonance imaging (MRI) that at the isthmic level through different planes shows

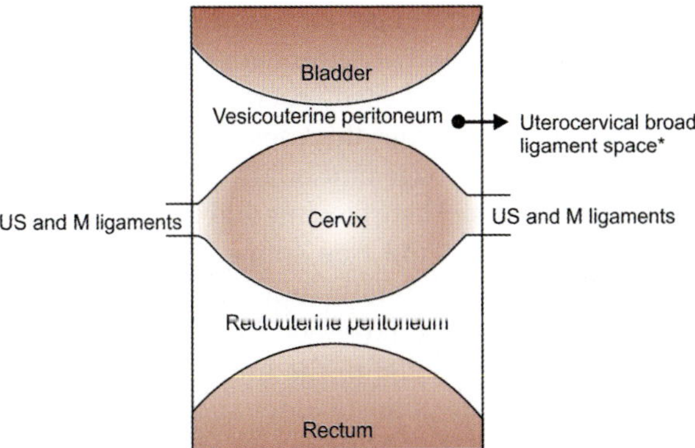

Fig. 10.1: The space between bladder and cervix or cervicouterine surface*, which is much more under lateral one fifth of bladder when compared with central three fifths of bladder

Source: Sheth SS. Access to vesicouterine and rectouterine pouches. In: Sheth SS (Ed). Vaginal hysterectomy, 2nd edition. New Delhi, India: Jaypee Brothers Medical Publishers (P) Ltd; 2014.pp.31-50.

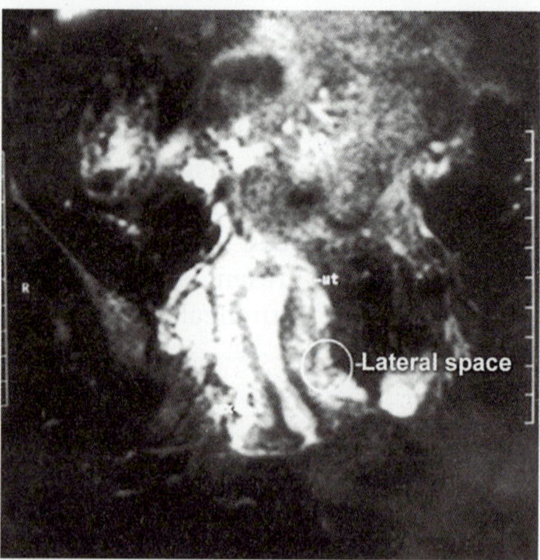

Fig. 10.2: Coronal section MRI shows a distinct vacant space medial to the line joining the maximally bulging uterus above and the cervix below with its continuity laterally

Source: Sheth SS. An approach to vesicouterine peritoneum through a new surgical space. J Gynecol Surg. 1996;12:135-40. Sheth SS. Vaginal hysterectomy. Best Practice & Research – Clinical Obstetrics & Gynaecology. S Arulkumaran (Ed). 2005;19(3):307-32.

a distinct vacant space medial to the line joining the maximally bulging uterus above and the cervix below with its continuity medially between the uterocervical surface and the bladder until they come intimately close to each other in the midline (Figs 10.2 and 10.3).

After making transverse incision on vaginal mucosa below the bladder bulge, Allis forceps was put laterally, close to the lateral uterocervical border of the incised upper vaginal mucosa (Fig. 10.4). An upward pull through Allis guides to the site to get an access to the uterocervical broad ligament space (UCBLS). Usually underneath the bladder, entry to space is easily seen. If the space is not easily seen even by the push of scissor's tip, one needs to gauge the bladder thickness of approx. 1.5 cm + from the cut upper vaginal or mucosal edge and boldly push the closed scissor's tip (Fig. 10.5), on the uterocervical surface medial to the lateral uterocervical border and open it to widen the free space below the gauged bladder thickness. Dissection is made laterally little beyond lateral cervicouterine border to enter between the two layers of broad ligament. Space provides bare cervicouterine surface medial to the uterocervical border permitting to put bladder retractor and keep the bladder and ureter away. This makes it easy to severe the uterosacral and Mackenrodt's complexes and descending cervical vessels. Uterine vessels are easily seen. Small ooze from tiny vessel (s) may need cauterization. Important is to obtain bare cervical-uterine surface on both sides of the centrally adherent bladder. Gentle traction with Babcock on separated free lateral bladder border facilitates the separation of the bladder medially and upwards. This gives an access to the uterine serosa

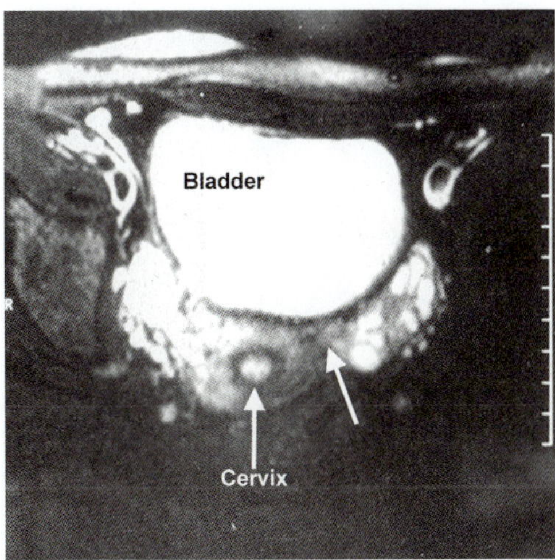

Fig. 10.3: Transverse section MRI at the isthmic level shows clear space between the bladder in front and the uterocervical surface behind, with continuity laterally between the two leaves of the broad ligament

Source: Sheth SS. An approach to vesicouterine peritoneum through a new surgical space. J Gynecol Surg. 1996;12:135-40. Sheth SS. Vaginal hysterectomy. Best Practice & Research – Clinical Obstetrics & Gynaecology. S Arulkumaran (Ed). 2005;19(3):307-32.

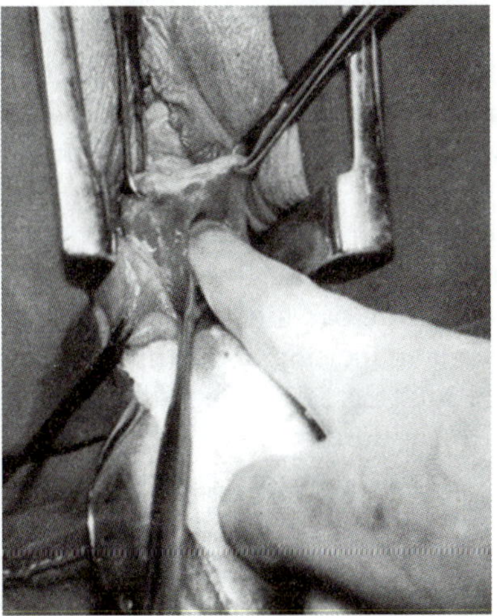

Fig. 10.4: At vaginal hysterectomy, the finger is on the uterocervical surface, with the bladder anteromedially, as it insinuates further between the two leaves of the broad ligament laterally

Source: Sheth SS. An approach to vesicouterine peritoneum through a new surgical space. J Gynecol Surg. 1996;12:135-40. Sheth SS. Vaginal hysterectomy. Best Practice & Research – Clinical Obstetrics & Gynaecology. S Arulkumaran (Ed). 2005;19(3):307-32.

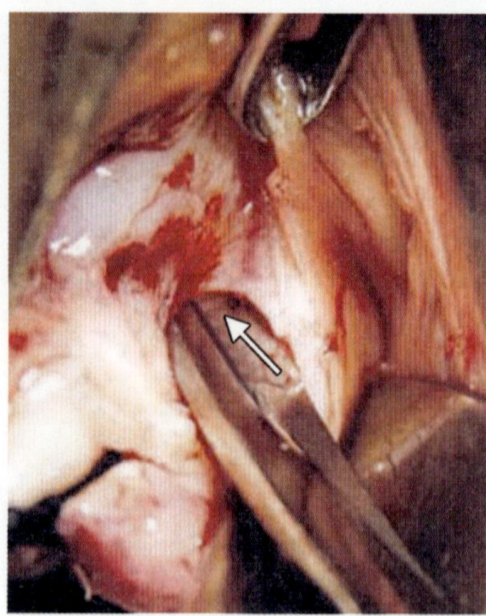

Fig. 10.5: Entry and access to the uterocervical-broad ligament space. The uterocervical-broad ligament space is widened using scissors while the edge of the anterior vaginal mucosa is held with Allis' forceps and the cervix is pulled with black silk traction suture

Source: Sheth SS. Vaginal hysterectomy in women with a history of 2 or more cesarean deliveries. Int J Obstet Gynecol. 2013;121:92-3.

from one side and thus to the peritoneum higher up. Tactile sensation plus backup of experience are useful for further dissection, if required.

If the case of a patient with two or more previous cesarean sections, often a similar dissection is required from the other end and either to meet in the center or to go completely around from one to other end. This surgically created space aids and will provide access to the vesicouterine fold of the peritoneum.

If an anterior access is difficult after uterines are secured and fundus is at close distance, the index and middle fingers of the left hand can be inserted through the posterior cul-de-sac and brought to the front or uterovesical reflection so as to permit an incision of the thin peritoneum as it rests on the fingers under direct vision (Fig. 10.6). This is followed by severance of upper pedicles to complete the hysterectomy.

During early parts of the learning curve or in case of the occasional difficulty, bladder sound or metal catheter or instilling a few milliliters of methylene blue in the bladder can act as a guide to get the plane of dissection.

Same space is also utilized for the bladder separation at laparoscopic hysterectomy by Sizzi and Rossetti[7] and at abdominal hysterectomy in women with history of C-section(s) in the past,[8] where in the separation is reversed and is from above downwards. John M. Monaghan, an eminent gynec-oncologist from UK[9] finds this space useful for accessing the vesicouterine peritoneum and labels it as Sheth's space. Khung[10] writes, that nonadherent portion of the bladder can be easily approached for separation through Sheth's uterocervical broad ligament space or a surgical window. Surgeons

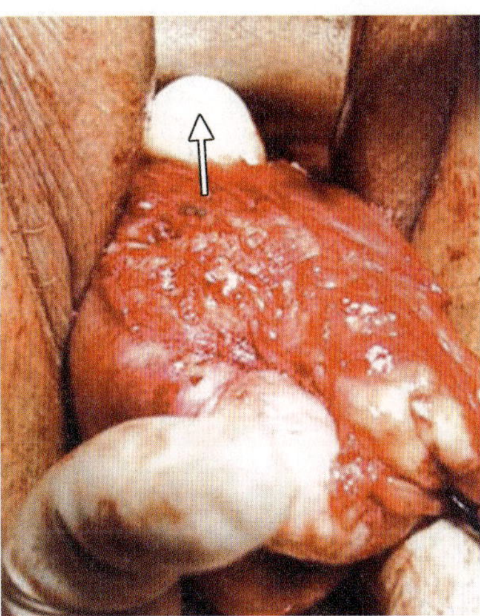

Fig. 10.6: Access to the vesicouterine peritoneum via step 3B. After a finger pushes some of the thin peritoneum anteriorly out of the pouch of Douglas, the peritoneum is incised and the finger emerges. This causes the separation of the bladder from the uterine surface, allowing placement of the bladder retractor

Source: Sheth SS. Vaginal hysterectomy in women with a history of 2 or more cesarean deliveries. Int J Obstet Gynecol. 2013;121:92-3.

who want to learn and progress may choose to practice access to VUP with help of uterocervical broad ligament space in 5 to 10 vaginal hysterectomies in parous women who have not had cesarean section in past.

Unger and Meeks[11] reported 2.8% bladder injury in vaginal hysterectomy (VH) with previous versus 1.6% without C-section in the past. Fear of injury to the urinary bladder causes many surgeons to resort to LAVH or total laparoscopic hysterectomy (TLH), which is heavily propagated via workshops or via laparotomy even though hysterectomy by the vaginal route is the least invasive and the choicest one.

The author is "as a rule" utilizing described space with great safety to the bladder for almost last 25 years to obtain access to VUP[3-6] in all women scheduled for VH with a history of C-section(s) in the past. This includes more than 300 women who underwent VH with history of two or more C-sections in past.[12]

SURGICAL TECHNIQUE IN WOMEN WITH HISTORY OF TWO OR MORE C-SECTIONS IN PAST

Surgical technique may be usual like after one C delivery in past or more depending on the adhesions, uterine size etc. If more is required, technique is described in four steps. It is very likely that step 4 will not be required and only up to step 2 or 3 is required in some to complete the hysterectomy vaginally.[12]

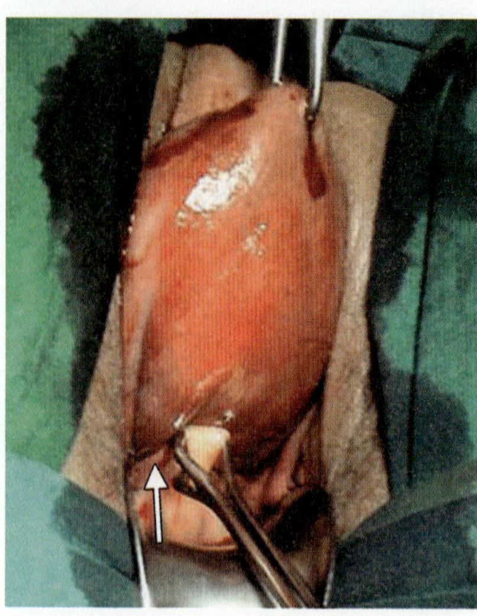

Fig. 10.7: Access to the vesicouterine peritoneum via step 3A. After the uterine fundus is brought out of the pouch of Douglas (POD) and pulled as anteriorly as possible, the bladder is seen drooping in the POD. With the bladder held with Babcock's forceps from the POD, its separation is performed by incising the vesicouterine peritoneum from laterally—from near cornual area; thus, easier access is made to the anterior POD from this site

Source: Sheth SS. Vaginal hysterectomy in women with a history of 2 or more cesarean deliveries. Int J Obstet Gynecol. 2013;121:92-3.

Four operative steps in reaching the VUP, when required in women with 2 or more C-sections in past are: (1) entering the cervicouterine surface from the uterocervical-broad ligament space; (2) creating a large bare cervicouterine surface and reaching the lateral uterine serosal surface; (3) freeing the bladder, either via POD through one of two techniques or by separating the centrally adherent bladder, which is already made free laterally. If required debulking can facilitate. If possible, after uterines are secured, uterine fundus was brought out through the POD using Allis forceps and held sufficiently anteriorly for the bladder to droop through the space in the POD and appear behind the uterus (3A) (Fig. 10.7). The bladder with nonadherent VUP (preferably from an area close to a cornual area laterally) was easily separated from the bladder which enabled the surgeon to free the bladder completely from lateral to medial and gain access to the peritoneal cavity or anterior pouch. For the second technique (3B) a finger was passed laterally from the POD into one of the proximal cornual areas and guided by tactile sensation, emerged anteriorly covered with only VUP. The VUP was then incised to let the finger through, which caused separation of the bladder laterally from the uterine surface (Fig. 10.6).[12] The opening produced by the finger was widened and the bladder retractor inserted to keep the bladder away. For this technique, guidance comes from the distance to the fundus—which is judged by palpation via POD—and from earlier clinical and sonographic findings. (4) Occasionally bisecting the cervix, to split the cervix

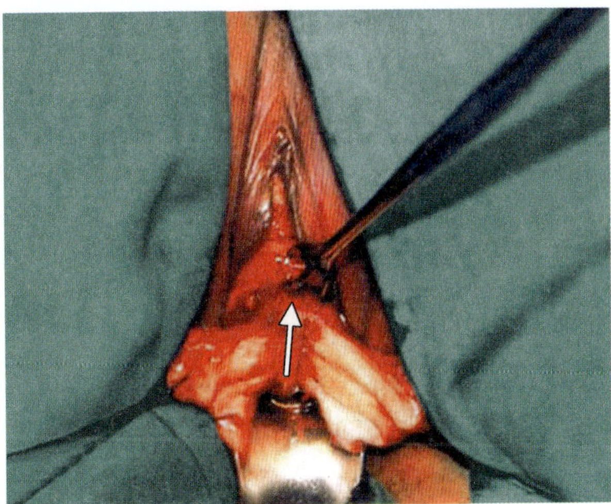

Fig. 10.8: Cervix bisected to achieve access to the vesicouterine peritoneum. Slight traction on the bladder with Babcock's forceps brings connecting tissue strands into view for excision and the plane for access

Source: Sheth SS. Access to vesicouterine and rectouterine pouches. In: Sheth SS (Ed). Vaginal hysterectomy, 2nd edition. New Delhi, India: Jaypee Brothers Medical Publishers (P) Ltd; 2014.pp.31-50.

upwards gives an access to the peritoneum. Adherent bladder is carefully kept a way by Babcock forceps (Fig. 10.8).

If in doubt as to the appropriate route, operating surgeon can perform investigatory laparoscopic examination and/or take her as 'Trial VH' case. At any stage, if he or she is concerned about causing trauma to the bladder and/or cannot complete the VH procedure, one should not hesitate to take laparoscopic assistance or perform laparotomy.[12]

REFERENCES

1. Sheth SS, Paghdiwalla KP, Hajari AR. Vaginal route: A gynaecological route for much more than hysterectomy. In: S Arulkumaran (Ed). Best Practice & Research - Clinical Obstetrics & Gynaecology. Elsevier, UK. 2011;25(2):115-32.
2. Sheth SS. Access to vesicouterine and rectouterine pouches. In: Sheth SS (Ed). Vaginal hysterectomy, 2nd edition. New Delhi, India: Jaypee Brothers Medical Publishers (P) Ltd. 2014.pp.31-50.
3. Sheth SS. Vaginal hysterectomy. In: Studd J (Ed). Progress in obstetrics and Gynecology, 10th edition. London: Churchill Livingston. 1993.pp.317-40.
4. Sheth SS, Malpani AN. Vaginal hysterectomy following previous cesarean section. Int J Gynecol Obstet. 1995;50:165-9.
5. Sheth SS. An approach to vesicouterine peritoneum through a new surgical space. J Gynecol Surg. 1996;12:135-40.
6. Sheth SS. Vaginal hysterectomy. Best Practice & Research - Clinical Obstetrics & Gynaecology. S Arulkumaran (Ed). 2005;19(3):307-32.

7. Sizzi O, Rossetti A. Overcoming technical limits to laparoscopic hysterectomy. J Gynecol Surg Endoscopy. 2006; http://*thetrocar.net/viewNew.asp?ID=7&IDArticolo=39.*
8. Sheth SS. Bladder separation at abdominal hysterectomy. Int J Gynaecol Obstet. 2013;122:157-8.
9. Monaghan J. Personal communication.
10. Khung TTG. Use of Sheth's uterocervical broad ligament space for vaginal hysterectomy in a patient with history of cesarean section. Malaysian J Obstet and Gynaecol. 1995;4:39-42.
11. Unger JB, Meeks GR. Vaginal hysterectomy in women with history of previous cesarean delivery. Am J Obstet Gynecol. 1998;179:1473-8.
12. Sheth SS. Vaginal hysterectomy in women with a history of 2 or more cesarean deliveries. Int J Obstet Gynecol. 2013;121:92-3.

11

Management of Third and Fourth-Degree Perineal Tears

Bipin Pandit

DEFINITION

A third-degree perineal tear is defined as a partial or complete disruption of the anal sphincter muscles, which may involve either or both the external (EAS) and internal anal sphincter (IAS) muscles.

A fourth-degree tear is defined as a disruption of the anal sphincter muscles with a breach of the rectal mucosa.

The overall risk of obstetric anal sphincter injury is 1% of all vaginal deliveries. With increased awareness and training, there appears to be an increase in detection of anal sphincter injury. Obstetricians who are appropriately trained are more likely to provide a consistent, high standard of anal sphincter repair and contribute to reducing the extent of morbidity and litigation associated with anal sphincter injury.

Obstetric anal sphincter injury encompasses both third- and fourth-degree perineal tears (Fig. 11.1).

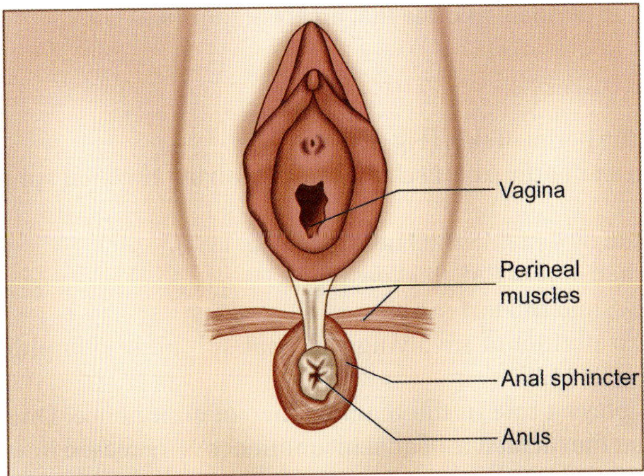

Fig. 11.1: Anatomy of the perineum

PREDICTION AND PREVENTION OF OBSTETRIC ANAL SPHINCTER INJURY

Clinicians need to be aware of the risk factors for obstetric anal sphincter injury but also recognize that known risk factors do not readily allow its prediction or prevention.

Where episiotomy is indicated, the mediolateral technique is recommended, with careful attention to the angle cut away from the midline.

The following factors are associated with an increased risk of a third degree tear:

- Birth weight over 4 kg (up to 2%)
- Persistent occipitoposterior position (up to 3%)
- Nulliparity (up to 4%)
- Induction of labor (up to 2%)
- Epidural analgesia (up to 2%)
- Second stage longer than 1 hour (up to 4%)
- Shoulder dystocia (up to 4%)
- Midline episiotomy (up to 3%)
- Forceps delivery (up to 7%).

Most of the risk factors identified cannot readily be used to prevent or predict the occurrence of a third- and fourth-degree tear. Severe perineal tears that involve the anal sphincter complex and/or the anal epithelium (obstetric anal sphincter injury) are identified in 0.6–9.0% of vaginal deliveries where mediolateral episiotomy is performed. However, since the introduction of endoanal ultrasound, sonographic abnormalities of the anal sphincter anatomy has been identified in up to 36% of women after vaginal delivery, in prospective studies.

A lower risk of third-degree tear is associated with a larger angle of episiotomy. In a prospective case-control study there was a 50% relative reduction in risk of sustaining third-degree tear observed for every six degree away from the perineal midline that an episiotomy was cut.

Classification and Terminology

I: Injury to the perineal skin (Fig. 11.2).
II: Injury to the perineal muscle but not involving the anal sphincter (Fig. 11.3).
IIIa: Less than 50% of EAS thickness torn (Fig. 11.4).
IIIb: More than 50% of EAS thickness torn.
IIIc: Both EAS and IAS torn.
IV: Injury to perineum involving the anal sphincter complex and anal epithelium (Fig. 11.5).

The IAS plays a role in the maintenance of continence. One study has reported that the incidence of anal incontinence is increased in women who had both IAS and EAS damage compared with those who had EAS damage alone.

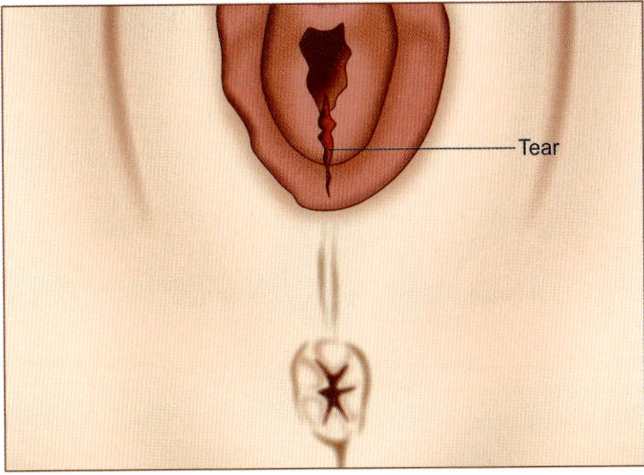

Fig. 11.2: First-degree injury to perineal skin only

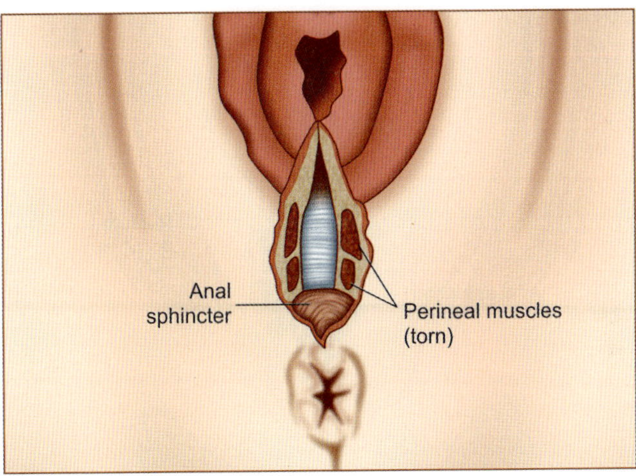

Fig. 11.3: Second-degree injury to perineum involving perineal muscles but not involving the anal sphincter

Inclusion of the IAS in the classification below would allow differentiation between future incontinence related to IAS injury rather than EAS alone. It is, however, recognized that in acute obstetric trauma, identification of the IAS may not be possible but a record of the degree of EAS damage (more or less than 50%) should be possible in all cases. If the tear involves only anal mucosa with intact anal sphincter complex (buttonhole tear) this has to be documented as a separate entity. If not recognized and repaired this type of a tear may cause anovaginal fistulae.

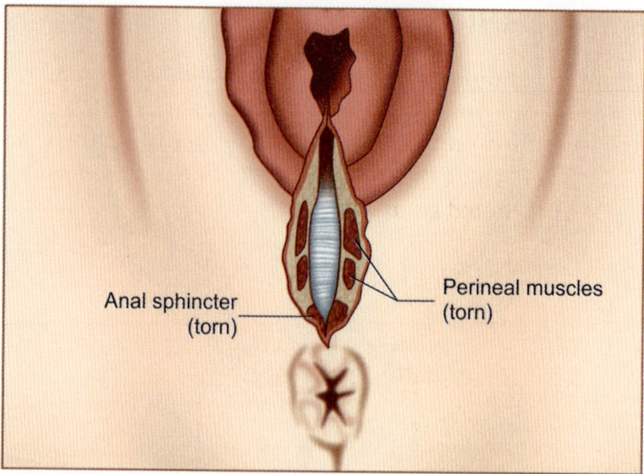

Fig. 11.4: Third-degree injury to perineum involving the anal sphincter complex

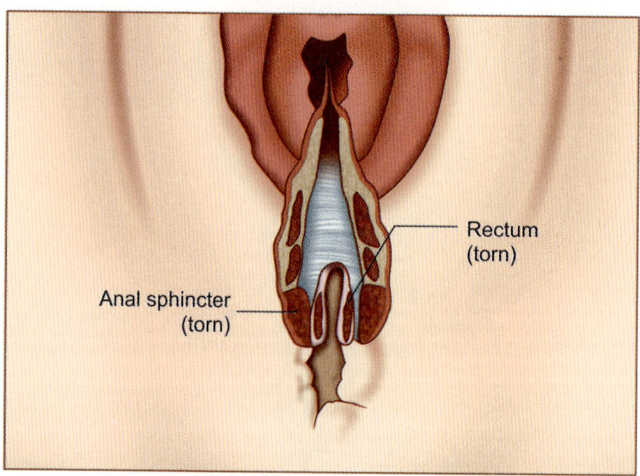

Fig. 11.5: Fourth-degree injury to perineum involving the anal sphincter complex (EAS and IAS) and anal epithelium

Identification of Obstetric Anal Sphincter Injuries

All women having vaginal delivery with evidence of genital tract trauma, or operative vaginal delivery or who have experienced perineal injury should be examined by an experienced practitioner trained in the recognition and management of perineal tears.

One observational study showed that increased vigilance about anal sphincter injury can double the detection rate. In another study where endoanal ultrasound was used immediately following delivery, the detection rate of anal sphincter injury was not significantly increased compared to clinical examination alone.

SURGICAL TECHNIQUES

Which techniques should be used to accomplish the repair of obstetric anal sphincter injury? For repair of the external anal sphincter, either an overlapping or end-to-end (approximation) method can be used, with equivalent outcome. Where the IAS can be identified, it is advisable to repair separately with interrupted sutures.

OVERLAPPING (FIG. 11.6)

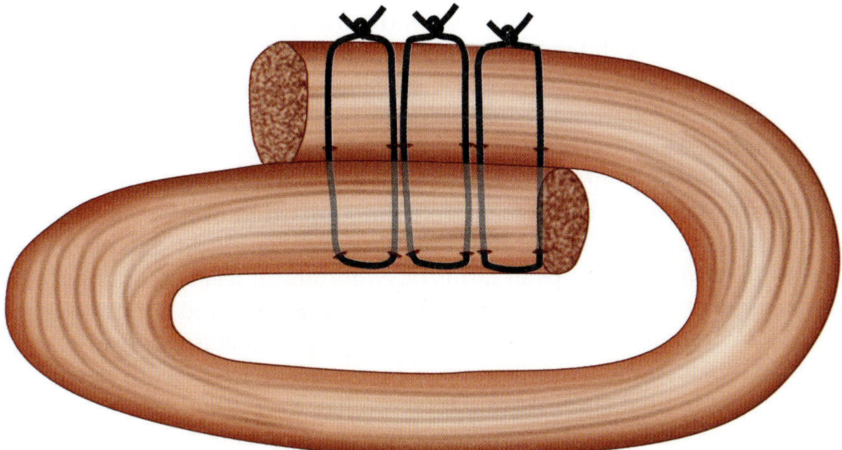

Fig. 11.6: Repair of EAS—Overlapping technique

END-TO-END (APPROXIMATION) (FIG. 11.7)

Repair of third- and fourth-degree tears should be conducted in an operating theater, under regional or general anesthesia.

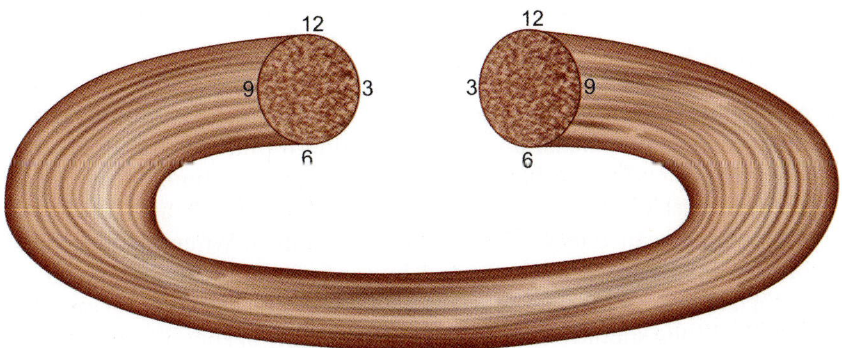

Fig. 11.7: Repair of EAS—end-to-end approximation

A systematic review on the method of repair for third-degree tears examined three trials involving 279 women. This review showed that there was no significant difference in perineal pain, dyspareunia, flatus incontinence and fecal incontinence, between the two repair techniques at 12 months but showed a significantly lower incidence in fecal urgency in one trial, 52 women and lower anal incontinence score in the overlap group. Overlap technique was also associated with a significant lower risk of deterioration of anal incontinence symptoms over 12 months. There was no significant difference in quality of life. The reviewers concluded that the limited data available show that compared with immediate primary end-to-end repair of obstetric anal sphincter injuries, early primary overlap repair appears to be associated with lower risks for fecal urgency and anal incontinence symptoms. As the experience of the surgeon is not addressed in the three studies reviewed, it would be inappropriate to recommend one type of repair over another. However, most of these conclusion were based on one study.

A separate randomized controlled trial of 41 women with complete third- and fourth-degree perineal tears were randomized to overlap and end-to-end groups and followed up for 3 months. No significant difference was found between the groups in terms of symptoms of fecal incontinence or transperineal ultrasound findings. In another randomized controlled trial of secondary repair, 24 women were randomized to either end-to-end or overlap repair. At median follow-up of 26 months, there were no significant differences in anal continence. Other studies have evaluated secondary sphincter repair for anal incontinence in colorectal patients and showed a significant increase in continence rate with overlap repair.

One study, however, has shown a deterioration of anal continence 5 years following secondary repair for obstetric anal sphincter injuries.

Repair in an operating theater will allow the repair to be performed under aseptic conditions with appropriate instruments, adequate light and an assistant. Regional or general anesthesia will allow the anal sphincter to relax, which is essential to retrieve the retracted torn ends of the anal sphincter. This also allows the ends of the sphincter to be brought together without any tension.

Choice of Suture Materials

When repair of the EAS muscle is being performed, either monofilament sutures such as polydioxanone (PDS) or modern braided sutures such as polyglactin (Vicryl®) can be used with equivalent outcome. When repair of the IAS muscle is being performed, fine suture size such as 3-0 PDS and 2-0 Vicryl may cause less irritation and discomfort. When obstetric anal sphincter repairs are being performed, burying of surgical knots beneath the superficial perineal muscles is recommended to prevent knot migration to the skin. Women should be warned of the possibility of knot migration to the perineal surface, with long-acting and non-absorbable suture materials.

There are no systematic reviews to assess the best suture material for repair of the external anal spincter. Use of fine suture size such as 3-0 PDS and 2-0 Vicryl may cause less irritation and discomfort. The only randomized controlled trial comparing Vicryl and PDS reported no significant difference in morbidity from anal incontinence, perineal pain or suture migration with 12 months follow-up. There are no systematic reviews or randomized studies to evaluate the type of suture materials use for the repair of IAS. Similar to EAS, use of fine suture size, such as 3-0 PDS and 2-0 Vicryl may cause less irritation and discomfort.

Surgical Competence

Obstetric anal sphincter repair should be performed by appropriately trained practitioners. Formal training in anal sphincter repair techniques is recommended as an essential component of obstetric training. Inexperienced attempts at anal sphincter repair may contribute to maternal morbidity, especially subsequent anal incontinence. A survey of UK consultant obstetricians and trainee obstetricians in two regions highlighted the deficiency and their dissatisfaction with their training in the management of third-degree tears. Many regions now conduct training workshops and different approaches to teaching these skills should be evaluated. Training may be improved by the implementation of surgical skills workshops with the use of models and audiovisual material. A report on the effect of hands-on training workshops on repair of third- and fourth-degree perineal tears showed that there is increased awareness of perineal anatomy and recognition of anal sphincter injury following attendance at hands-on training workshops.

POSTOPERATIVE MANAGEMENT

The use of broad-spectrum antibiotics is recommended following obstetric anal sphincter repair to reduce the incidence of postoperative infections and wound dehiscence. The use of postoperative laxatives is recommended to reduce the incidence of postoperative wound dehiscence. Local protocols should be implemented regarding the use of antibiotics, laxatives, examination and follow-up of women with obstetric anal sphincter repair. All women should be offered physiotherapy and pelvic-floor exercises for 6–12 weeks after obstetric anal sphincter repair.

All women who have had obstetric anal sphincter repair should be reviewed 6–12 weeks postpartum by a consultant obstetrician and gynecologist. If a woman is experiencing incontinence or pain at follow-up, referral to a specialist gynecologist or colorectal surgeon for endoanal ultrasonography and anorectal manometry should be considered. A small number of women may require referral to a colorectal surgeon for consideration of secondary sphincter repair. Intraoperative and postoperative broad-spectrum antibiotics are recommended because the development of infection will pose a high-risk of anal incontinence and fistula formation in the event of breakdown of the anal sphincter repair.

Inclusion of metronidazole is advisable to cover the possible anaerobic contamination from fecal matter. No systematic reviews were identified which evaluated the use of postoperative laxatives and stool softeners. Laxatives are recommended during the postoperative period as passage of a hard stool can disrupt the repair.

Use of stool softener such as Lactulose® and a bulking agent such as Fybogel® is recommended for about 10 days after the repair. One randomized control study compared laxatives and constipating agents in the postoperative period following primary obstetric anal sphincter repair. In this study, women in the laxative group had a significantly earlier and less painful bowel motion and earlier postnatal discharge. There was no difference in the symptomatic or functional outcome of repair between the two regimens.

There were no systematic reviews or randomized controlled trials to suggest the best method of follow-up after obstetric anal sphincter repair. It is helpful to review women in the postnatal period to discuss injury sustained during childbirth, assess for symptoms and offer advice on how to seek help if symptoms develop, offer treatment and/or referral if indicated and advice on future mode of delivery. If facilities are available, follow-up of women with obstetric anal sphincter injury should be in a dedicated perineal clinic with access to endoanal ultrasonography and anal manometry, as this can aid decision on future delivery.

PROGNOSIS

Women should be advised that the prognosis following EAS repair is good, with 60–80% asymptomatic at 12 months. Most women who remain symptomatic describe incontinence of flatus or fecal urgency.

Several prospective case-control and retrospective, studies have looked at the outcome of primary repair in terms of reported symptoms and results of anal sphincter investigations. All of these studies describe end-to-end suturing of the EAS, using either interrupted or figure-of-eight sutures, but suturing of the IAS is reported in only some of these studies. Initial studies report anal incontinence symptoms in 20–67% of women who have undergone primary third-degree tear repair. In these studies, the type of incontinence is mainly flatus (up to 59%) with leakage of liquid and solid stool in up to 11%, while fecal urgency occurred in 26% of these women. In one study, there was a marked increase in anal incontinence symptoms after four years of follow-up (17–42%). These studies used different questionnaires to assess anal incontinence symptoms and it is therefore difficult to compare study outcomes directly. However, several recent randomized controlled studies carried out since 2000 comparing overlap and end-to-end techniques of EAS repair have reported low incidence of anal incontinence symptoms in both arms, with 60–80% of women described as asymptomatic at 12 months.

Studies using endoanal ultrasound as part of follow-up demonstrated persistent defects in 54–88% of women after primary repair of recognized third-degree tears. More recently, the published randomized controlled trials have reported fewer residual defects, about 19–36% overall. The clinical relevance of asymptomatic defects demonstrated by ultrasound is currently unclear.

FUTURE DELIVERIES

All women who sustained an obstetric anal sphincter injury in a previous pregnancy should be counselled about the risk of developing anal incontinence or worsening symptoms with subsequent vaginal delivery. All women who sustained an obstetric anal sphincter injury in a previous pregnancy should be advised that there is no evidence to support the role of prophylactic episiotomy in subsequent pregnancies. All women who have sustained an obstetric anal sphincter injury in a previous pregnancy and who are symptomatic or have abnormal endoanal ultrasonography and/or manometry should have the option of elective cesarean birth. There were no systematic reviews or randomized controlled trials to suggest the best method of delivery following obstetric anal sphincter injury. The risks of a subsequent vaginal delivery after third-degree tear were examined in four studies, which showed between 17% and 24% of women developed worsening fecal symptoms after a second vaginal delivery. This sseemed to occur particularly if there had been transient incontinence after the index delivery. All women who have suffered an obstetric anal sphincter injury should be counselled at the booking visit regarding the mode of delivery and this should be clearly documented in the notes. If the woman is symptomatic or shows abnormal anorectal manometric or endoanal ultrasonographic features, it may be advisable to offer an elective cesarean section. This is an area that should be assessed within the confines of a randomized controlled trial.

RISK MANAGEMENT

When third-and fourth-degree repairs are performed, it is essential to ensure that the anatomical structures involved, method of repair and suture materials used are clearly documented and that instruments, sharps and swabs are accounted for. The woman should be fully informed about the nature of her injury and the benefits to her of follow-up. This should include written information where possible. There is a steady increase in litigation related to obstetric anal sphincter injury. The majority are related to failure to identify the injury after delivery, leading to subsequent anal incontinence and rectovaginal fistulae. At present, the occurrence of obstetric anal sphincter injury is not considered substandard care because it is a known complication of vaginal delivery. However, failure to recognize anal sphincter damage and to carry out a repair may be considered substandard care. Poor technique, poor materials or poor healing may cause a repair to fail. Clear documentation and patient counselling are of utmost importance. A patient information leaflet is recommended. Future research recommendations. There is a clear deficit in the evidence for the short- and long-term management of obstetric anal sphincter injury. This needs to be addressed by encouraging multicenter randomized controlled trials involving a large number of women.

BIBLIOGRAPHY

1. Anthony S, Buitendijk SE, Zondervan KT, van Rijssel EJ, Verkerk PH. Episiotomies and the occurrence of severe perineal lacerations. BJOG. 1994;101:1064–7.
2. Bodner-Adler B, Bodner K, Kaider A, Wagenbichler P, Leodolter S, Husslein P, et al. Risk factors for third degree perineal tears in a vaginal delivery with an analysis of episiotomy types. J Reprod Med. 2001;46:752–6.
3. Buekens P, Lagasse R, Dramaix M, Wollast E. Episiotomy and third degree tears. BJOG. 1985;92:820–3.
4. Christiansen LM, Bovbjerg VE, McDavitt EC, Hullfish KL. Risk factors for perineal injury during delivery. Am J Obstet Gynecol. 2003;189:255–60.
5. de Leeuw JW, Sruijk PC, Vierhout ME, Wallenburg HC. Risk factors for third degree perineal ruptures during delivery. BJOG. 2001;108:383–7.
6. Donnelly V, Fynes M, Campbell D, Johnson H, O'Connell R, O'Herlihy C. Obstetric events leading to anal sphincter damage. Obstet Gynecol. 1998;92:955–61.
7. Eason E, Labrecque M, Wells G, Feldman P. Preventing perineal trauma during childbirth: A systematic review. Obstet Gynecol. 2000;95:464–71.
8. Fitzpatrick M, Harkin R, McQuillan K, O'Brien C, O'Connell PR, O'Herlihy C. A randomised controlled trial comparing the effects of delayed versus immediate pushing with epidural on mode of delivery and faecal continence. BJOG. 2002;109:1359–65.
9. Fitzpatrick M, McQuillan K, O'Herlihy C. Influence of persistent occiput posterior position on delivery outcome. Obstet Gynecol. 2001;98:1027–31.
10. Gjessing H, Backe B, Sahlin Y. Third degree obstetric tears: outcome after primary repair. Acta Obstet Gynecol Scand. 1998;77:736–40.
11. Handa VL, Danielsen BH, Gilbert WM. Obstetric anal sphincter lacerations. Obstet Gynecol. 2001;98:225–30.
12. Jander C, Lyrenas S. Third and fourth degree perineal tears: predictor factors in a referral hospital. Acta Obstet Gynecol Scand. 2001;80:229–34.
13. McLeod NL, Gilmour DT, Joseph KS, Farrell SA, Luther ER. Trends in major risk factors for anal sphincter lacerations: a 10 year study. J Obstet Gynecol Can. 2003;25:586–93.
14. Poen AC, Felt-Bersma RJ, Dekker GA, Deville W, Cuesta MA, Meuwissen SG. Third degree obstetric perineal tears: risk factors and the preventative role of mediolateral episiotomy. BJOG. 1997;104:563–6.
15. Poen AC, Felt-Bersma RJF, Strijers RL, Dekker GA, Cuesta MA, Meuwissen SG. Third degree obstetric perineal tear: long-term clinical and functional results after primary repair. Br J Surg. 1998;85:1433–8.
16. Richter HE, Brumfield CG, Cliver SP, Burgio KL, Neely CL, Varner RE. Risk factors associated with anal sphincter tear: a comparison of primiparous vaginal births after caesarean deliveries, and patients with previous vaginal delivery. Am J Obstet Gynecol. 2002;187:1194–8.
17. Samuelsson E, Ladfors L, Wennerholm UB, Gareberg B, Nyberg K, Hagberg H. Anal sphincter tears: prospective study of obstetric risk factors. BJOG. 2000;107:926–31.
18. Sultan AH, Monga AK, Kumar D, Stanton SL. Primary repair of obstetric anal sphincter rupture using the overlap technique. BJOG. 1999;106:318–23.
19. Williams A, Tincello DG, White S, Adams EJ, Alfirevic Z, Richmond DH. Risk scoring system for prediction of obstetric anal sphincter injury. BJOG. 2005; 112:1066–9.
20. Wood J, Amos L, Rieger N. Third degree anal sphincter tears: risk factors and outcome. Aust NZ J Obstet Gynaecol. 1998;38:414–7.

12

Human Papillomavirus Vaccination

Neerja Bhatla, Deepali Kale

Abstract

Human papillomavirus (HPV) is associated with the development of anogenital cancer (including cervical, vaginal, vulvar, penile, and anal), oropharyngeal cancer, and genital warts. Human papillomavirus vaccination can significantly reduce the incidence of anogenital cancer and genital warts. Despite the benefits of HPV vaccines, only approximately one-third of girls in the recommended age group have received the vaccines. The Centers for Disease Control and Prevention and the American College of Obstetricians and Gynecologists recommend routine vaccination with HPV vaccine for girls and boys. The 9-valent HPV vaccine is recommended by the Advisory Committee on Immunization Practices and was licensed by the US Food and Drug Administration in December 2014 for girls and boys aged 11–12 years.

INTRODUCTION

Cervical cancer continues to be the most common cancer among women in India, with an estimated 134, 420 new cases and 72, 825 deaths annually, which is nearly one-fourth of the global burden.[1] Secondary prevention is possible to a large extent by screening for pre-cancers and treatment of lesions. However, screening by cytology is mostly opportunistic and there is a lack of awareness and commitment even in urban areas. Thus <5% of women receive adequate cervical screening. Although alternative low resource methods like visual inspection with acetic acid (VIA) and visual inspection with Lugol's iodine (VILI) have been recommended by the National Cancer Control Programme of the Ministry of Health & Family Welfare, they have still not been implemented widely. New techniques like HPV testing have shown excellent promise with better sensitivity than Pap smear, but are not yet widely available. Thus primary prevention by prophylactic HPV vaccines is an excellent complementary method for cervical cancer prevention.

Out of more than 100 subtypes, HPV 16 and 18 account for up to 72% of cervical cancers, whereas HPV 6 and 11 cause 90% of the anogenital warts. Results from trials indicate that the vaccine is safe, well tolerated and highly efficacious in HPV naive women. The optimal target age is in pre-pubertal women before coitarche, while it will remain an individual decision for older women. Vaccination and screening are complementary strategies and synergy in a cost-effective manner will be required for the next few decades.

TYPES OF VACCINE AND VACCINATION SCHEDULE

Two prophylactic HPV vaccines are available in India. Both target HPV 16/18, the two genotypes responsible for 70% of cervical cancers worldwide and 82.5% of cancers in India.[2]

The bivalent vaccine (bHPV)has HPV 16/18 virus-like particles (VLPs) with ASO4 adjuvant and is targeted against cervical cancer.

The quadrivalent vaccine (qHPV) has HPV 16/18 VLPs as well as HPV 6/11 VLPs for protection against genital warts, 90% of which are caused by these two genotypes. Both the vaccines have shown excellent protection against new infection, persistent infection and CIN 2/3 lesions caused by HPV 16/18, and some degree of cross-protection against related genotypes.[3] Further, protection against VIN and VAIN has also been demonstrated in trials.

The 9-valent Human Papillomavirus Vaccine

The 9-valent HPV vaccine is recommended by ACIP and was licensed by the FDA in December 2014 for girls and boys aged 11–12 years. Catch-up vaccination for females and males through age 26 years is recommended for those not vaccinated at the target age of 11–12 years. In a phase III efficacy trial comparing the 9-valent HPV vaccine with the quadrivalent HPV vaccine among approximately 14,000 females aged 16–26 years, the 9-valent HPV vaccine had high efficacy for prevention of greater than or equal to CIN 2, vulvar intraepithelial neoplasia (VIN) 2 or 3, and vaginal intraepithelial neoplasia 2 or 3 due to HPV genotypes 31, 33, 45, 52, and 58.[4] The antibody titer against HPV genotypes 6, 11, 16, and 18 was not reduced with the addition of the other five HPV genotypes. Revaccination with the 9-valent HPV vaccine in individuals who previously completed the three-dose series with the quadrivalent HPV vaccine or the bivalent HPV vaccine currently is not a routine recommendation.

The US Food and Drug Administration (FDA) has approved three vaccines shown to be effective at preventing HPV infection. All three vaccines are given in a three-dose series with a schedule of 0, 1–2, and 6 months. The durability of the immune response (i.e. how long protection lasts) is being monitored in various long-term studies, and there currently is no indication for a booster vaccine. The series does not need to be restarted if there is a delay in administration of the second or third dose.

Safety

Safety data for all three HPV vaccines are reassuring. According to the vaccine adverse events reporting system, more than 60 million doses of HPV vaccine have been distributed, and there are no data to suggest that there are any severe adverse effects or adverse reactions linked to vaccination.[5]

The 9-valent and quadrivalent vaccines had similar safety profiles, except that the 9-valent HPV vaccine had a higher rate of injection site swelling and erythema than the quadrivalent HPV vaccine, and the rate increased after each successive dose of the 9-valent HPV vaccine.[4]

Obstetrician-gynecologists or other providers should counsel patients to expect discomfort after vaccination and that such discomfort is not a cause for concern. Available data demonstrate no safety concerns in individuals who were vaccinated with the 9-valent HPV vaccine after having been vaccinated with the quadrivalent HPV vaccine. Anyone who has ever had a life-threatening allergic reaction to any component of the HPV vaccine, or to a previous dose of the HPV vaccine, should not get the vaccine. Obstetrician-gynecologists or other providers should assess patients for severe allergies, including an allergy to yeast. Individuals with a moderate or severe illness should wait until their illness improves before receiving a vaccine.

An immune bridging study of the safety and immunogenicity of the bHPV vaccine carried out at several centers in India showed excellent acceptability, 100% seroconversion with comparable titers to previous major trials and no major side effects.[6] In fact, there are very few contraindications to these vaccines. Demonstration projects have shown positive acceptance of HPV vaccination with the understanding provided to parents that they protect against cervical cancer and the majority (92.9%) of girls completing all three doses.[7]

The Major Barriers to Implementation of HPV Vaccination in India

These include lack of awareness of this eminently preventable condition, misinformation on safety and efficacy of the vaccine, and cost. The EPI Programme has paved the way for adequate infrastructure to maintain the logistics of the cold chain as well as deal with the challenges of compliance with a multiple-dose regime. However, preliminary results of on going 2-dose vs 3-dose trials are very promising with comparable immunogenicity, but efficacy data are awaited. This will help to decrease costs and improve logistics. Recently, very encouraging results have emerged from population based data from Australia, the country that first introduced free HPV vaccination for all girls aged 10–13 years in their National Programme, with catch-up vaccination to 26 years in the initial phase. Data from the sexual health clinics have shown a decline in genital warts among girls who received qHPV vaccination in the National Programme. In addition, there is evidence of herd immunity from the reduction in genital warts among heterosexual men as well. There is also a decline in the incidence of high grade cervical intraepithelial neoplasia among young women who received vaccination.

Summary of Recommendations

- It is crucial that obstetrician-gynecologists and other providers educate parents and patients on the benefits and safety of human papillomavirus (HPV) vaccination.
- The Centers for Disease Control and Prevention (CDC) and the American College of Obstetricians and Gynecologists (the College) recommend routine vaccination with HPV vaccine for girls and boys.
- The 9-valent HPV vaccine has been added to the Advisory Committee on Immunization Practices (ACIP) recommendations for girls and boys at the target age of 11–12 years with catch-up for females and males through age 26 years if not vaccinated in the target age.
- Testing for HPV DNA is not recommended before vaccination in any group and if the patient is tested for HPV DNA and the results are positive, vaccination is still recommended.

THE FUTURE PERSPECTIVE

Since the discovery that HPV is causally associated with cervical cancer, there has been a development of several tests and biomarkers. Several studies are investigating how these may improve and personalize the management of women with abnormal findings at screening. The introduction of prophylactic vaccination is the latest important landmark in the history of prevention of cervical cancer. If it is applied nation-wide, in the pre-pubertal population with complete coverage, it is estimated that it may lead to a 40% reduction in low grade CIN, 50–60% in high grade CIN, and 90% in AIS within about 5–7 years. In the next 3 decades, it is expected that there might be an almost 75–80% reduction in the incidence of cervical cancers. Further research to assess screening strategies in vaccinated cohorts is needed. The introduction of vaccination is especially important in the developing countries, like India but affordability remains a major issue.

CONCLUSION

HPV vaccination is a safe and effective method for primary prevention of HPV related diseases. In the future, there will be vaccines that will cover more HPV types and perhaps alternate dose schemes and routes will develop. New vaccines may develop that do not require a cold chain. Meanwhile, the present vaccines have shown good efficacy for prevention of genital warts and cervical cancer and should be offered to all girls as a part of preventive health care. They should also be told the importance of screening even after vaccination. Comprehensive cervical cancer prevention can happen if we can adopt the slogan of "Every woman screened by 40, every girl vaccinated by 14".

REFERENCES

1. Ferlay J, Shin HR, Bray F, et al. GLOBOCAN 2008 v2.0, Cancer Incidence and Mortality Worldwide: IARC Cancer Base No. 10 [Internet]. Lyon, France: International Agency for Research on Cancer; 2010. Available from: *http://globocan.iarc.fr, accessed on* 10/11/2012.
2. WHO ICO. *http://apps.who.int/hpvcentre/statistics/dynamic/ico/country_pdf/IND, p 28.* Accessed on Sep 30, 2012.
3. The WHO Position Paper on Vaccines against Human Papillomavirus (HPV). *Weekly Epidemiological Record. 2009;15:118-32. http://www.who.int/wer/2009/wer8415.pdf.*
4. Petrosky E, Bocchini JA Jr, Hariri S, Chesson H, Curtis CR, Saraiya M, et al. Use of 9-valent human papillomavirus (HPV) vaccine: updated HPV vaccination recommendations of the advisory committee on immunization practices. Centers for Disease Control and Prevention (CDC). MMWR Morb Mortal Wkly Rep 2015;64:300–4.
5. Centers for Disease Control and Prevention. Vaccine safety: human papillomavirus (HPV) vaccine. Available at: *http://www.cdc.gov/vaccinesafety/vaccines/HPV/index.html. Retrieved June 8, 2015.*
6. Bhatla N, Suri V,Basu P, et al. Immunogenicity and safety of human papillomavirus-16/18 AS04-adjuvanted cervical cancer vaccine in healthy Indian women. J ObstetGynaecol Res. 2010;36(1):123–32.
7. LaMontagne DS, Barge S, Nga TL, et al. Human papillomavirus vaccine delivery strategies that achieved high coverage in low- and middle-income countries. Bull World Health Organ 2011;89:821-30B.

13

Treatment of Cervical Intraepithelial Neoplasia

Nikhil Purandare, Deepali Kale

Abstract

Cervical cancer is both preventable and curable. Its long natural history with a prolonged precancerous phase makes it amenable for easy detection and treatment. Exfoliative cytology being the mainstay for screening of cervical intraepithelial neoplasia (CIN). Assessment of women presenting with abnormal cervical cytology and the selection of those requiring treatment relied mainly on colposcopic interpretations of the cervical transformation zone and the histological appraisal of directed punch biopsies. The necessity to maximize clinical resources, achieve rapid and more effective management of patients, limit postoperative complications and preserve reproductive function has led to the popularity of local excisional methods for cervical premalignancy.

INTRODUCTION

Cervical dysplasia is diagnosed by histopathology assessment of the biopsy or excised sample. Cervical intraepithelial neoplasia (CIN) is diagnosed depending on how much of the cervical epithelium is involved by dysplastic cells. CIN is graded into I, II and III.

The published literature would suggest that 11% of CIN I lesions will progress to higher-grade disease and there is some role in the use of human papilloma virus (HPV) detection in the management of CIN I (Duggan MA, 1998). But there is general consensus that CIN I does not need to be biopsied every time and can be safely managed conservatively (NHSCSP Guideline) though it would be ideal to be able to predict which lesion is likely to progress. There is lesser consensus though on how CIN II needs to be treated. There is a suggestion that up to 68% of CIN II lesions diagnosed in adolescents (i.e. the under 24) will spontaneously regress but require close follow-up (Moscicki AB, 2010 and Discacciati MG, 2011). Infection with HPV 16/18 or infection with multiple HPV types decreases the likelihood of spontaneous regression of the lesion (Ho GY, 2011). Strong evidence suggests that CIN III is a true precursor of cancer and needs to be treated (Petry KU, 2011). Electrosurgical excision is the most common treatment for high-grade lesions (Volsante R, 2006). Clinics operating according to 'See and Treat' policy must ensure that women who are offered treatment at their first visit have been given adequate and appropriate information (100%). Anxiety is greater in women attending 'See and Treat' clinics if they are not adequately informed of the potential for treatment at their first visit (NHSCSP Guideline 20, 2010).

TREATMENTS OF CERVICAL INTRAEPITHELIAL NEOPLASIA

The treatments should be efficient in eradicating the intraepithelial lesions, but it should also have minimum morbidity and adverse effects on future fertility and reproductive outcomes. The conservative methods of CIN are easy to perform, of low cost and are usually performed under local anesthesia, in an outpatient setting.

These are divided into ablative and excisional techniques:

EXCISION AND ABLATIVE TECHNIQUES

Excisional Treatments

Excisional methods of treatment are indicated particularly in cases of repeat conization, suspected invasion, glandular epithelium involvement, in cases of unsatisfactory colposcopy and in cases of discrepancy between cytology, colposcopy and biopsy. The specimen should ideally be removed as a single sample. The advantages of excisional procedures such as the large loop excision of the transformation zone (LLETZ) are its low cost, high success rate, ease of use, it can be used within on office setting and it is possible to get comprehensive histology. René Cartier invented the small low-voltage high dielectric loops to biopsy and excise the transformation zone (Cartier R, 1994). In 1989, Walter Prendiville used large loops, thereby removing the transformation zone with better histological evaluation (Prendiville W, 1989).

Large Loop Excision of the Transformation Zone (LLETZ)/Loop Electrosurgical Excision Procedure (LEEP)

The LLETZ/LEEP using low voltage apparatus is now the most widely practiced technique. It is performed under local anesthetic. There are different available sizes of loops. There should be minimal artefactual damage to the specimen and cervix and roller ball can be used for hemostasis. Women should avoid intercourse and insertion of menstrual tampons for 4 weeks post-treatment.

Various loops are demonstrated in Figure 13.1.

Local anesthetic drug is injected into the cervix circumferential before the LLETZ for adequate pain relief (Fig. 13.2). The solution usually contains octapressin or adrenaline to reduce the bleeding. A 'Top Hat' lesion excision may be done in cases where it is suspected that the appropriate depth

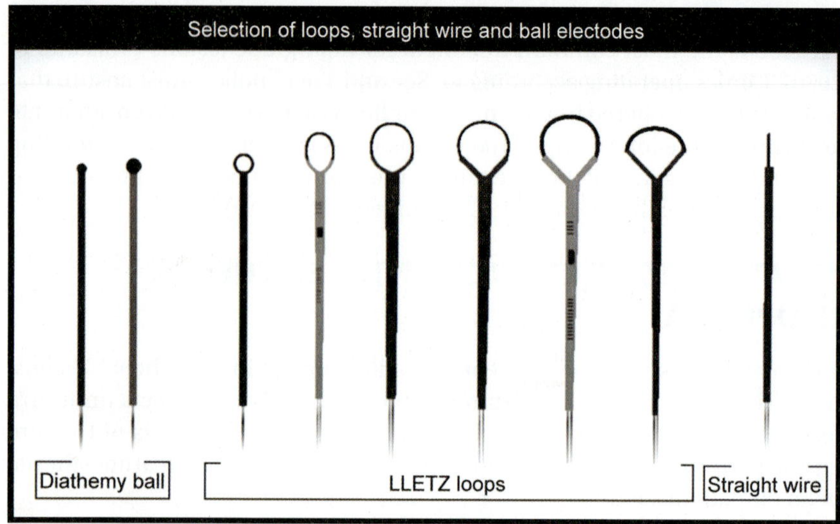

Fig. 13.1: Loops for excision, roller balls for diathermy and the straight wire for excision are demonstrated

of excision has not been achieved. The safety profile of LLETZ has been confirmed by a number of studies (Prendiville WJ, 1989 and Bigrigg MA, 1990) but it needs to be used cautiously. LLETZ procedures may be associated with bleeding, infection and even preterm labor in the future. The risk of preterm labor depends on the size of the loop and the depth of excision (Khalid S, 2012).

Needle Excision of Transformation Zone (NETZ) /Straight Wire Excision of Transformation Zone (SWETZ)

It is a recent modification that uses a straight wire rather than a loop. This technique allows individualization of the procedure and aims to eradicate the lesion without removing redundant healthy cervical tissue.

Laser Conization

It follows the same principle of LLETZ and needle excision of transformation zone (NETZ). It is technically more demanding, requires longer treatment time and more expensive equipment to buy and maintain.

Cold Knife Conization

It is used relatively rarely today as it has been superseded by more conservative techniques. It requires general anesthesia and hospitalization. This technique is particularly useful in cases of suspected invasion and glandular disease; the lack of diathermy minimizes the thermal artefact and allows accurate assessment of the excision margins. There is comparatively increased risk of hemorrhage, fertility and pregnancy morbidity with knife conization as compared to the other techniques.

Hysterectomy

It still retains a place in the management of CIN in women who have other gynecological conditions such as fibroids, menorrhagia or prolapse. It may also be used in cases of glandular lesions where fertility does not need to be spared, especially in cases of treatment failure or incomplete excision. It is important to ensure complete excision of the cervix, the transformation zone (TZ) and any vaginal lesion; the preferential route is vaginal hysterectomy preceded by a colposcopic assessment.

Ablative Techniques

Ablative techniques destroy the cervical epithelium and preclude the histological assessment of the TZ; accurate pretreatment biopsy samples are required at a separate initial visit, which increases the risk of noncompliance. Furthermore, the accuracy of punch biopsies is questionable; it is estimated that punch biopsies under-diagnose the severity of the lesion in 20% of the cases when these were compared to the histology of subsequent large loop excisions. All treatment techniques should remove tissue to a depth of more than 7 mm to ensure eradication of CIN that may involve the gland crypt. Ablative treatment may be an option in selected cases when the TZ and the lesion are fully visible, the colposcopy satisfactory and there is no discrepancy between cytology, colposcopy and histology. Before using any form of ablative therapy, histological assessment with colposcopically directed biopsies is necessary to rule out invasion. These techniques are contraindicated in women with glandular lesions, suspicion of invasion or history of a previous cone.

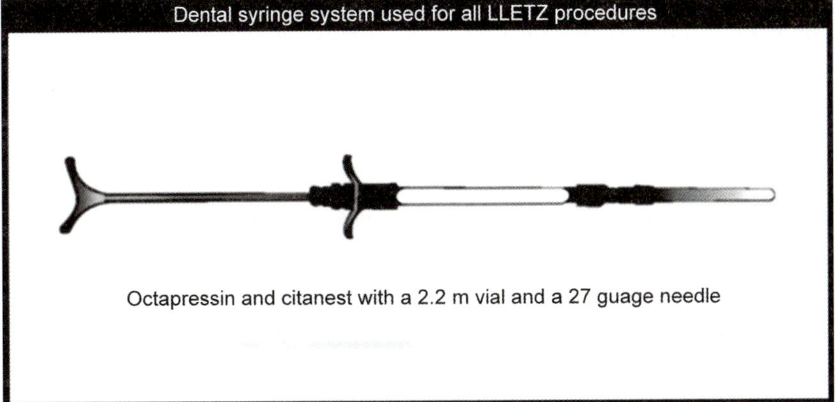

Fig. 13.2: Syringe and needle used for anesthetic infiltration

- Cryocautery destroys tissue by freezing using probes of various shapes and sizes, and is probably best reserved for small, low-grade lesions as the rates of clearance of CIN III are poor in comparison to other techniques. The duration of the freeze is 2 minutes from the appearance of the ice ball. A freeze/thaw/freeze technique is advocated as this increases the cure rate.
- Electrodiathermy requires general, regional or local anesthesia. Under colposcopic control it is possible to destroy up to 1 cm depth using a combination of needle and ball electrodes. The apparatus required is cheap and easy to maintain but the thermal necrosis may be considerable more than anticipated and more difficult to control.
- *Cold coagulation*: In the cold coagulation technique, heat at 100–120°C is applied to tissue using a Teflon-coated thermosound for 30 seconds. The procedure is easy and does not usually require analgesia.
- *Laser ablation*: A micromanipulator attached to the colposcope is used to manipulate the laser and treatment is conducted under direct vision. As the technique is precise, it gives good control over depth of destruction, good hemostasis and excellent healing, with minimal damage to the adjacent tissue. The technique is particularly useful in lesions that extend to and involve the vagina. The vaginal epithelium does not have gland crypts and, as a result, a depth of destruction of about 2–3 mm is usually sufficient. Despite these benefits, the cost of the equipment and maintenance is high and not easily available.

Summary of treatment methods for CIN

Ablative	*Excisional*
Cryocautery	Large loop excision of the TZ (LLETZ-Europe)/Loop electrosurgical excisional procedure (LEEP-North America)
Radical	Needle excision of the TZ (NETZ)/straight wire excision of the TZ (SWETZ)
Cold coagulation	Laser conization
CO_2 laser	Cold knife conization
Ablation	Hysterectomy

Complications of Treatment

The complications of CIN treatment are rare. These are divided into:

Early complications	*Late complications*
Perioperative pain, primary hemorrhage, secondary hemorrhage, adverse obstetric outcome	Cervical stenosis inadequate or unsatisfactory colposcopy (common with cold knife conization)

Although the cure rates for all local ablative and excisional methods are more than 90% after one treatment, the excisional methods provide a more reliable histopathological diagnosis and the patient can be treated at the initial visit. The recognition that persistent infection with oncogenic human papilloma virus (HPV) causes cervical cancer has led to the development of new HPV tests/biomarkers and prophylactic vaccines against HPV. The HPV DNA test that targets the viral DNA has been introduced as a test of cure after CIN treatment and as a triage tool in women presenting with borderline or low grade findings at cytology. HPV DNA test will be introduced in primary screening in the future.

GLANDULAR DISEASE

Atypical glandular cytology may be suggestive of invasive cervical adenocarcinoma or cervical glandular intraepithelial neoplasia (CGIN). It may be associated with other conditions like CIN and endometrial pathology. If endometrial cells are seen on the cytology report in a postmenopausal woman not taking hormone replacement therapy, this may indicate endometrial disease and warrants investigations. If borderline glandular changes are present, colposcopic assessment with appropriate cervical biopsies and selective endometrial biopsy are indicated. Colposcopic findings are usually non-specific (for example, stain acetowhiteness in fused villi) but colposcopy is always essential, as a high percentage of these women have concomitant CIN. Punch biopsy in the setting of atypical glandular cytology is unreliable, as the lesions are often small and may occur in the base of gland crypts. Excisional conization for diagnosis and perhaps treatment is recommended.

Women with CGIN can be managed conservatively with local excision provided adequate close surveillance is possible. The excision margins should be free from disease; if involved, further excision is recommended. If the family is complete, the option of hysterectomy should also be considered.

FOLLOW-UP AFTER TREATMENT

The risk of future invasive cancer remains 4–5% greater than that of the general population following treatment.The majority (90%) of treatment failures (residual and recurrent disease) will be detected within 24 months of treatment. Previously, women postconization for high-grade disease were followed up closely with cytology with or without colposcopy for 10 years after treatment. More recently, HPV DNA test has been introduced as a 'test of cure'. Data from a series of clinical trials and meta-analyses report that HPV DNA testing.

Glandular Intraepithelial Lesions

Women with previously treated cGIN are at higher risk of recurrent disease. Postexcision cytology is less accurate and the ability to detect residual/recurrent disease may be compromised. The use of HPV DNA test in the surveillance after treatment for glandular lesions has been recently introduced.

Recent Advances

The most recent development in treatment of CIN is the "Test of Cure" following the treatment, whether ablative or excisional, after 6 months of treatment of CIN I, II, III, these women need to be asked to follow-up for a cervical cytology and HPV DNA test. If cytology is low grade dyskaryosis and HPV is positive she needs a colposcopy. If low grade dyskaryosis is seen with HPV negative then she needs a 3 year recall. Previously all these women used to be called for yearly recalls, the introduction of HPV test of cure decreases the anxiety and frequency of follow-up with out compromising on patient care. If the cytology at 6 months is high grade dyskaryosis, she needs to be referred to colposcopy immediately. (NHS Cancer screening Programmes, April 2014)

Women who test negative for high-risk oncogenic HPV types may return back to routine recall. The management of confirmed CIN I lesions varies and depends on their families are usually managed conservatively with surveillance. Older women with persistent disease may undergo treatment depending upon the woman's age, the length of persistence of the disease and her fertility wishes. Large proportion of women with CIN are of reproductive age with a mean age around thirties.

BIBLIOGRAPHY

1. *http://globocan.iarc.fr/old/FactSheets/cancers/cervix-new.asp.*
2. *http://www.cancerscreening.nhs.uk/cervical/.*
3. Jordan JA, Singer A, Jones III H, Shafi MI. The cervix. Oxford: Blackwell Publishing, 2006.
4. Luesley DM, Leeson S. Colposcopy and programme management: guidelines for the NHS cervical screening programme. NHSCSP Publication no. 20, Sheffield; 2004.
5. Obstetrics, Gynecology and Reproductive Medicine Review, 2014.
6. Shafi MI, Nazeer S. Colposcopy e a practical guide. 2nd edn. Cambridge University Press, 2012.
7. Shafi MI, Nazeer S. Grading system for abnormal colposcopic findings, EAGC course book on colposcopy. Bosze and Luesley, 2003. pp. 33- 6.

Electrosurgery and Energy Use at Endoscopy

14

CV Hegde

Electrosurgery use is seldom learned as a special subject by most of those who embark on the journey of endoscopic surgery and is often learned 'on the job' during the duration of apprenticeship. As a consequence 'knowledge' imbibed is very often hearsay, secondhand and often wrong which may ultimately result in a catastrophe during surgery and seeking of true knowledge later on wiser and suitably chastened.

Historically though electrical energy was used in the nineteenth century—Bottini used galvanocautery in 1875 during prostatectomy, it was its use during neurosurgery in the 1920s by Cushing and Bowie that really popularized its use subsequently. They were the first to describe the three main effects of electrical energy—desiccation, cutting and coagulation.

There are three effects of electricity on living tissues namely electrolytic—produced by current of low frequency, faradic—stimulation of nerve and muscles and thermal—which is the effect desired for clinical use. Tissue gets heated by electrical energy and one of the three effects of electrical energy as outlined occur depending on current density, duration of application and tissue resistance. Spread of heat in surrounding areas can result in collateral damage.

Electrical energy is due to the flow of current. Ampere (A) is the rate of flow of electrons, volt (V) is the force driving the electrons and ohm is tissue resistance. Watt is the work amount produced. Wattage is equal to volt multiplied by ampere. Therefore, the same wattage (work) may be produced by higher voltage and lesser ampere—more force as in monopolar coagulation current or by low voltage and high current—precise cut as in pure monopolar current or bipolar desiccation. Alternating current (AC) is used at electrosurgery. Three forms can be used—1. Continuous/cut—uninterrupted flow of electrons. 2. Coagulation—interrupted, modulated, dampened. 3. Blend—energy delivered at variable intervals producing a cutting and coagulation effect.

The electrosurgical unit must be carefully researched before purchase. The machine should be user programmable, should have autofunctions, should have separate and noninterchangeable monopolar and bipolar connections, there should also be safety alarms and error detection and machine shutoffs functions. There should also be underwater coagulation and a bipolar 'cut' function if possible. Fourth generation digital technology has now given way to microprocessor controlled diathermy.

The biological effects of electrical current on tissue depend on the kind of current used— monopolar 'pure' cutting current, monopolar coagulating current or a bipolar desiccating current, the shape and size of the electrode, the intensity and duration of use, the tissue being coagulated/cut and the finesse of its use.

Monopolar energy flows from the electrosurgical unit through the applicant device through the patient and out via the patient plate which is attached to the patient. It is therefore, a mandatory precaution to personally ensure prior to every surgery that an appropriate sized, preferably disposable patient plate be attached either to an electrically conductive area like large muscle mass— the lateral aspect of the thigh or the gluteal region is appropriate. The patient plate is the negative pole through which the electrical energy returns to the electrosurgical generator. A large size plate ensures that electrical energy does not get concentrated at one point and is dissipated appropriately. Metal plates are not in use anymore. The consequences of forgetting to attach the patient plate or the use of a poorly functioning plate are horrendous and resulting electrical injuries can be fatal. There can be no medicolegal defense when injuries of this nature occur. For absolute safety it is better that a plate is in position even when one is almost certain that only bipolar energy would be used. In some old model generators monopolar energy electrodes can be activated by error when bipolar energy is being sought to be used.

Monopolar energy is unidirectional. It can be of three modes—pure cut, coagulation and blend. All modern electrosurgical units allow a personalized setting for use at surgery. Pure cut mode setting can be from 60 to 100 W. This mode is high current and low voltage; therefore there is minimal force in this energy. A pure cut mode use is best served and most effective when a point or right angled electrode is used. This energy acts like a sharp knife. The effect obtained is a clean-cut incision. This energy does not coagulate tissue and does not spread. Therefore, it can be used to cut tissue near sensitive areas without fear of spread. At laparoscopy this type of energy is used to perform colpotomy at total laparoscopic hysterectomy, for incising the fibroid capsule at laparoscopic myomectomy, for dissection of tissue in severe endometriosis, for incision of an ovarian cyst capsule at laparoscopic cystectomy. Hysteroscopic uses include resection of submucous fibroids, septum resection and endometrial resection. At hysteroscopic surgery the distension medium used must be nonelectrolytic like glycine when this energy is being used.

Monopolar coagulation energy setting is usually between 40 and 60 W. This energy is low current and high voltage. As a result this energy has a great degree of force. At laparoscopy the electrode most suitable for the use of this energy is a spatula. This energy can coagulate and due to the high voltage can achieve a 'cutting' effect by blasting through tissue. This energy results in tissue around the target area getting damaged due to spread of heat. Therefore, its use in areas near the ureter can result in ureteric injury.

Monopolar blend energy has a large voltage and therefore, great force and the effects can be most destructive. Its use is limited.

Bipolar energy passes from one pole of the instrument to another through the tissue held. The setting is between 30 and 60 W. It is a high current low voltage setting. The force is minimal but the heat generated in the coagulated/desiccated tissue spreads laterally and can result in surrounding tissues getting affected. This must be recognized especially when the uterine vessels are coagulated at laparoscopic hysterectomy and ureteric injury is a possibility when the vessels are coagulated laterally. Bipolar energy is a desiccating energy. The effect is best when a small amount of tissue is held. Tissue is gradually heated, the water driven out, cell plasma coagulates, vessels shrink and bleeding stops. Most modern electrosurgical devices shut off or signal when tissue desiccation is complete. Desiccation takes place at 90–100°C. Charring indicates that a temperature of 200°C and is undesirable. During surgery the tips of the bipolar electrode must be cleansed of char intermittently for obtaining an optimum effect. There is no need for the use of a patient plate when this is the only energy being used. Bipolar energy is the most common energy used for multiple indications at laparoscopic surgery. Vessel sealing systems also use this form of energy and act by a combination of pressure and energy to create vessel fusion. Vessels up to 7 mm can be fused and feedback system ensures that energy is cut off when the effect is achieved. A facility to cut coagulated tissue in some such systems can aid in the performance of surgery by freeing up an extra- port for use since with the use of conventional bipolar energy use another port is used to introduce a scissor for cutting coagulated tissue.

The use of ultrasonic sound waves at a vibrating capacity of 55,500 times per second of the movable blade of the harmonic device enables denaturation of protein to form a sticky coagulum. Pressure exerted on tissue with the blade surface collapses blood vessels and allows the coagulum to form a hemostatic seal. The surgeon controls cutting and coagulation by adjusting the power level, blade edge, tissue tension and blade pressure. By using only mechanical longitudinal vibration at the distal end, no electrical current is passed to or through the patient, and damage to surrounding tissue and nerves is minimized.

There is no question of using a patient plate since no electrical energy is used. Usually however, since surgery at some stage, e.g. when dealing with uterine vessel coagulation/colpotomy at total laparoscopic hysterectomy may require the use of concurrent monopolar/bipolar energy it may be sound surgical practice to have a patient plate in position prior to surgery. Ultrasonic energy does not spread, does not heat surrounding tissue, does not char and can be thus used safely near sensitive areas, it does not produce smoke and can coagulate and cut simultaneously and therefore, frees up a port for other use. The only fly in the ointment is the humangous cost of the handset and the strict instructions of the manufacturer that the handset is meant for a single use only. A rule which is flouted more often than it is followed. Which in turn leads to ethical questions about informing the patient about the reuse of an essentially one time use instrument, informing the cost levied for the instrument under the circumstances and also whether the instrument would perform optimally under the conditions of being reused. The harmonic device requires a learning curve and is not a magic wand by any stretch of imagination.

Any energy source used without precision, knowledge and technique can lead to disastrous consequences including skin burns, bowel injury which could be discovered days after the surgery as peritonitis, ureteral and bladder injury, conductance capacitance-related injuries, etc. all of which if not dealt with professionally can be fatal.

A must know list therefore, would include amongst others—a knowledge of electrosurgical energy. Preoperative check of electrosurgical units, cord connections, electrodes, insulation of monopolar electrodes. A correct placement of adequate size patient plate when monopolar energy is used. Activation of all devices—monopolar or bipolar undervision. Avoid using electrodes for retraction of bowels. Recognize and appropriately treat viscus or vessel injury. Energy use during endoscopy is to be used well and wisely.

15

The Art of Laparoscopic Suturing

Rajendra Sankpal

INTRODUCTION

Laparoscopic surgery has become the part of the day-to-day gynecological practice. In recent years, the need for advanced laparoscopic surgeries has increased manifolds. More number of the practicing gynecologists are venturing into the practice of gynecological endoscopy. Suturing is the essential part of any surgery. Similar to the principles of laparotomy surgery one must know and master the technique of laparoscopic suturing before embarking on the advanced endoscopic surgeries. Tissue approximation by suturing remains the most reliable, cost effective and professionally satisfying method for repair of defects and achieving hemostasis. This applies as equally to endoscopic surgical interventions as it dose to open conventional surgery.

Considering the advancement of today's electrosurgical generators the following laparoscopic surgeries in gynecology require laparoscopic suturing:

- Laparoscopic myomectomy
- Laparoscopic closure of vaginal vault in total laparoscopic hysterectomy
- Laparoscopic tubo-tubal anastomosis
- Laparoscopic closure of bladder and intestinal trauma
- Closure of ureteric injuries
- Uncommonly reconstruction of ovary after removal of large ovarian cyst and laparoscopic surgery for uterine or vault prolapse surgery.

Although approximation by clips and stapling techniques expedites the process of surgical reconstruction in general, the two approaches are complimentary and indeed the safe execution of stapling anastomotic techniques necessitates intracorporeal suturing and knot tying. Situations are often encountered when stapling or use of clips cannot be used. Failure of stapling devices is infrequent due to mechanical malfunction or human error. So, surgeon must deal with the problem by laparoscopic suturing techniques.

This article will give you the step-by-step approach to perform effective laparoscopic suturing. Author states that the following points are the guidelines to perform laparoscopic suturing and are not the rules of the suturing.

Laparoscopic suturing requires a good needle holder, assistant grasper and suture material.

NEEDLE HOLDER

The design of the needle driver is now standardized. You must be able to grasp the curved needle securely. The handle of the instrument should be in line with the long-axis of the barrel of the instrument in order allow physiological position of function to prevent excessive hand fatigue (Fig. 15.1).

Needle holder must have minimum ratchets. When needle holder is holding the needle, it should also allow the manipulation of the needle in order to achieve the upright position of the needle. More ratchets cause a violent set of movements at the tip of the needle holder reducing suturing efficiency. The release mechanism should be simple, requiring only one click to release the needle.

ASSISTING NEEDLE GRASPER

As in laparotomy the nondominant hand can have a simple tooth grasper with a design of 2×4 teeth. A nontraumatic fenestrated simple grasper is also sufficient to assist the suturing. Remember this instrument should not have a ratchet.

CHOICE OF NEEDLES

Straight needles have very limited application in laparoscopic surgery, just as they have in open surgery. The tip of the straight needle has tendency to remain buried in the tissue, making the tip difficult to grasp. Curved needles are preferred in laparoscopic surgery.

CHOICE OF LAPAROSCOPE

The 30° laparoscope is preferred to 0° laparoscope. It has a look down capacity and allows to adequately visualize the operative sites (Fig. 15.2).

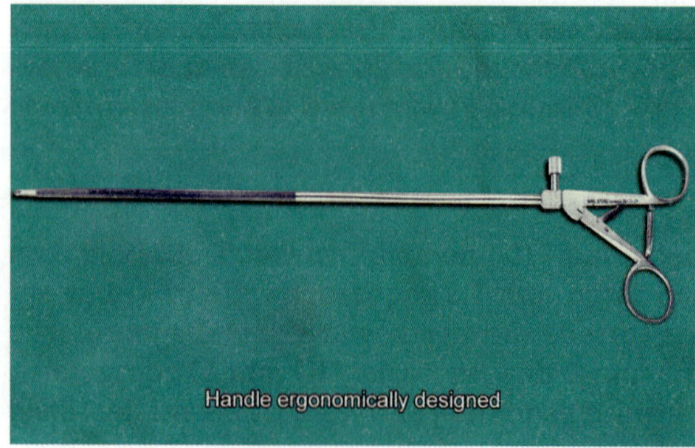

Fig. 15.1: Needle holder

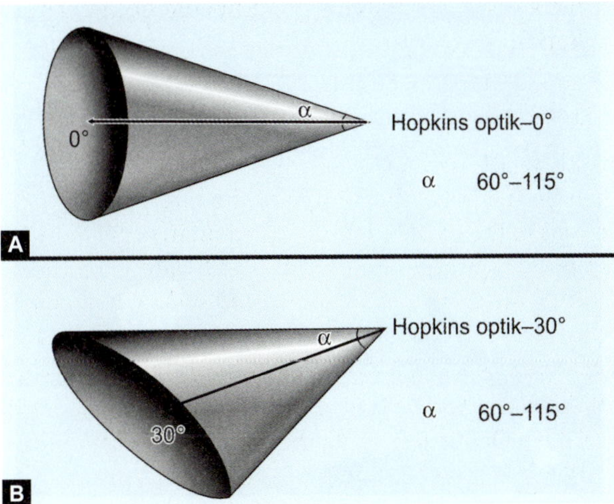

Figs 15.2A and B: Choice of laparoscope

CHOICE OF SUTURE MATERIAL

Author prefers to use no. 1 delayed absorbable braided suture on 40 mm half circle round body needle (Code No. 2347) for gynecological surgeries such as myomectomy, vaginal vault closure, sacrocervicopexy and vault prolaspe surgery. In the beginning of the suturing experience it is preferable to use suture length of 10 cm for simple interrupted sutures and 20 cm suture length for continuous suturing. Once the surgeon is familiar with the technique of laparoscopic suturing he or she may choose a longer length of the suture material. In case of long sutures such as more than 30 cm the suturing becomes cumbersome in the limited magnified abdomen.

CAMERA PORT

Placement of camera port is now standardized. Author prefers to place the camera port intraumbilical or supraumbilical area (Fig. 15.3).

ANCILLARY PORTS

Laparoscopic surgery requires minimum two ancillary ports. Author prefers to put two ports on the right side of the midline. First ancillary port is placed at the spinoumbilical line two fingers medial to the anterior superior iliac spine and the second port is placed in the midclavicular line at the level or just above the level of the umbilicus. The distance between the two ancillary ports should be minimum of 12–15 cm in a distended abdomen (Fig. 15.4). If the two ports are placed close to each other then the needle driver and tooth grasper in these ports will not converge at the tissue site and will be parallel to each other making the suturing experience more difficult. If these two ports are too widely separated then it will lead to unphysiological situation leading to pain at the arms and the shoulder even after minimal operative time.

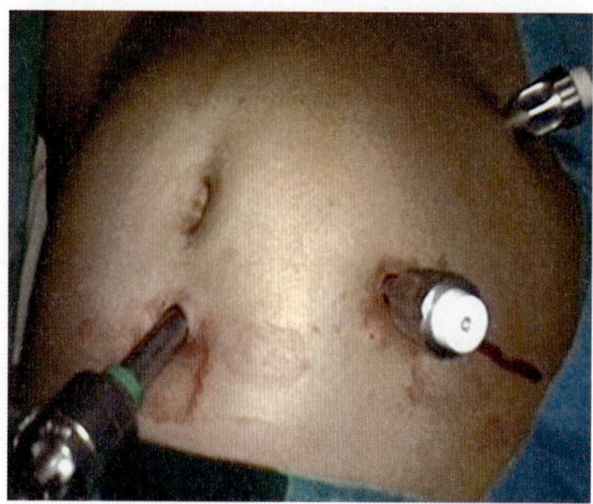

Fig. 15.3: Port placement

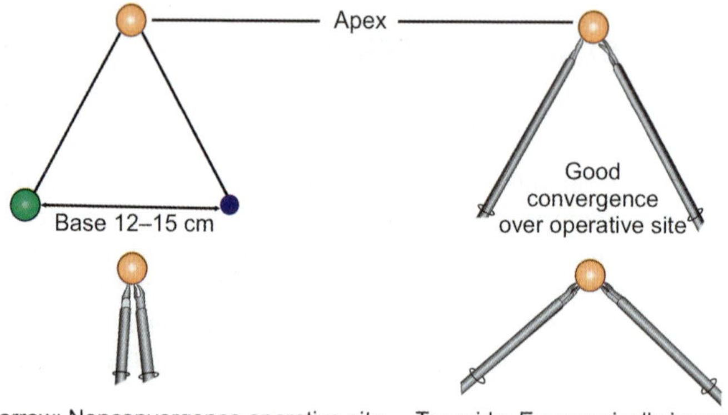

Fig. 15.4: Technique of intracorporeal suturing

Technique of Introduction of Needle and Suture Material into the Abdomen

After selecting the length of the suture material, the 5 mm lower ancillary cannula port is removed from its position. The needle driver is then introduced through this removed cannula. Then the suture material is grasped with the needle holder 2–3 cm away from the needle. Now the needle holder is reintroduced along with the suture material, needle and cannula through the same original ancillary port in the direction towards the hollow of pelvic cavity under the laparoscopic guidance. After the entry of the suture and the needle, the remaining suture material is pulled inside the abdomen under laparoscopic guidance (Figs 15.5A to C).

The needle is allowed to rest on the tissue and then it is grasped with the assisting needle grasper. The point to be grasped on the needle is the junction between the proximal and middle third of the needle. Needle can be

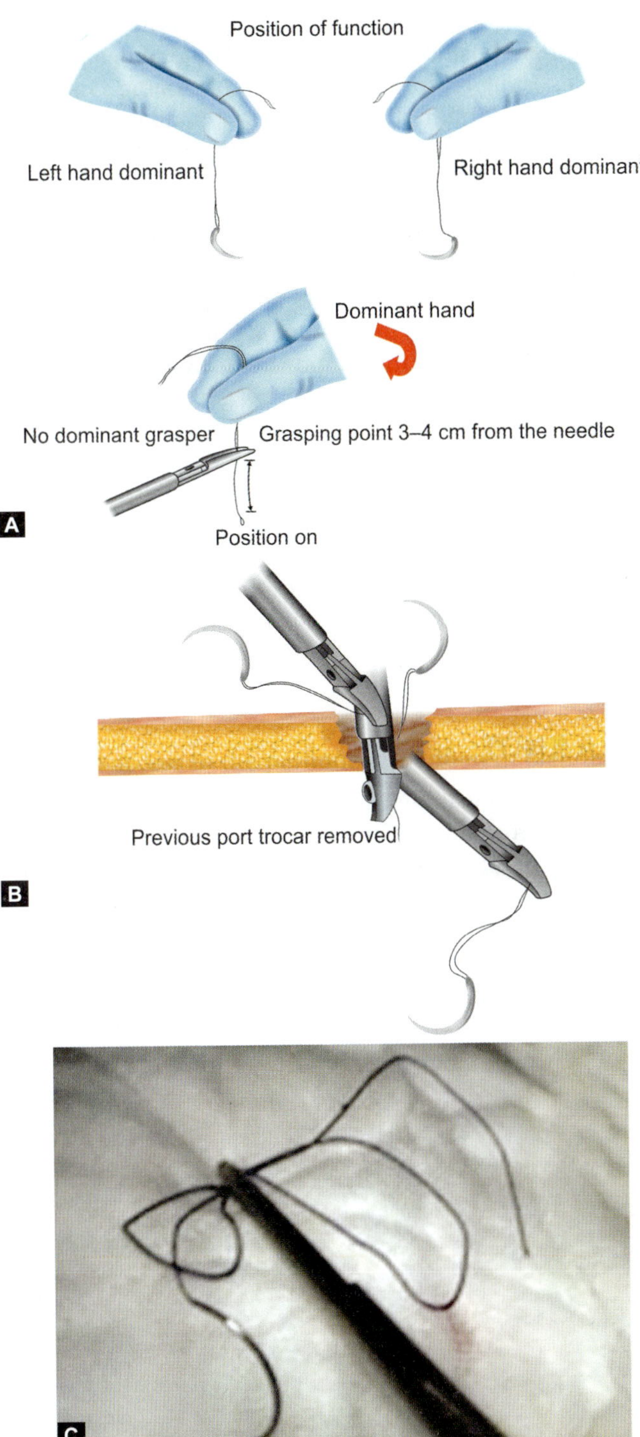

Figs 15.5A to C: Technique of inserting needle and suture

manipulated indirectly by manipulating the thread with the needle holder to achieve final upright position. Direct manipulation of needle by the needle driver and the assisting grasper may be time consuming. Once the needle is placed in upright position in the nondominant hand assisting grasper then it is handed over to the needle driver for its final position for suturing. This technique is similar to the technique of laparotomy suturing.

TAKING A BITE WITH NEEDLE

The elbow of the dominant hand should be abducted 60–90° away from the body followed by extension of the dominant hand laterally to penetrate the tissue; this is then followed by the rotation of the needle through the tissue. If you rotate the needle prematurely one will not get a good tissue bite reducing the suturing efficiency (Fig. 15.6).

At all times, the needle should be maintained in an upright position so its tip comes through the tissue freely. This allows grasping of the tip of the needle with the nondominant hand instrument without any interference. Once the needle has penetrated the tissue and the tip has reached the other side of the penetration, it is then grasped by the grasper and pulled out gently in the direction of the curvature of the needle. Keep pulling the suture till the tail is 2–3 cm only. Do not allow longer tail as it may interfere with the efficiency of the suturing.

PLACING A KNOT

While putting the surgical knot both the instruments should be moving simultaneously like the paddle of the bicycle near the tissue to be sutured. Do not go away from the tissue while placing the knot, which will again reduce the suturing process. Wrapping maneuver is accomplished using both hands (Figs 15.7A and B).

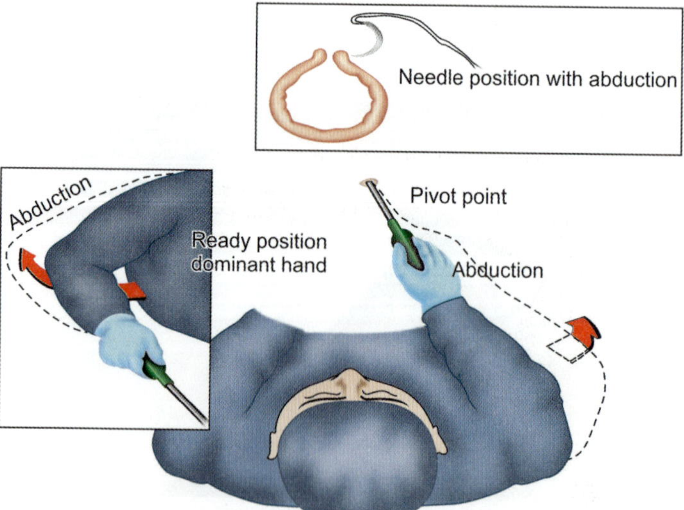

Fig. 15.6: Needle position in abduction

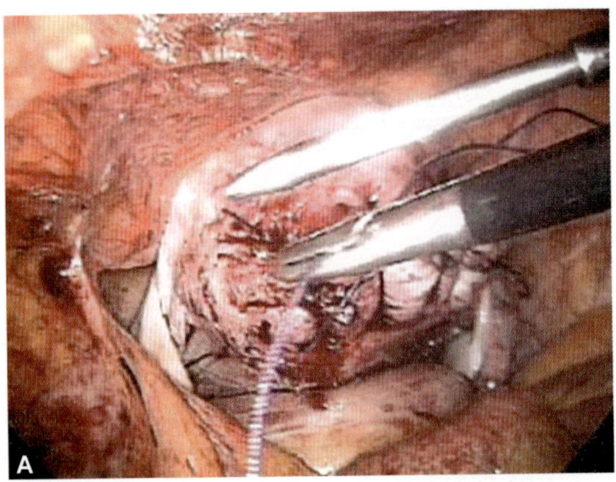

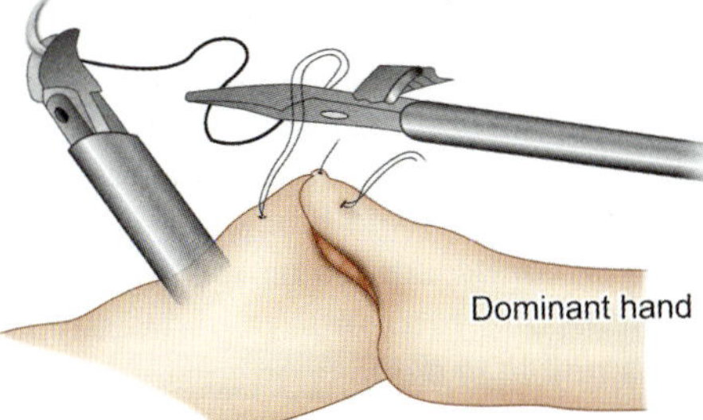

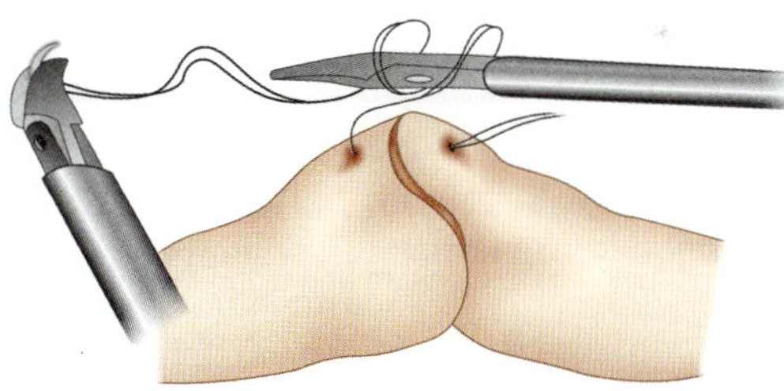

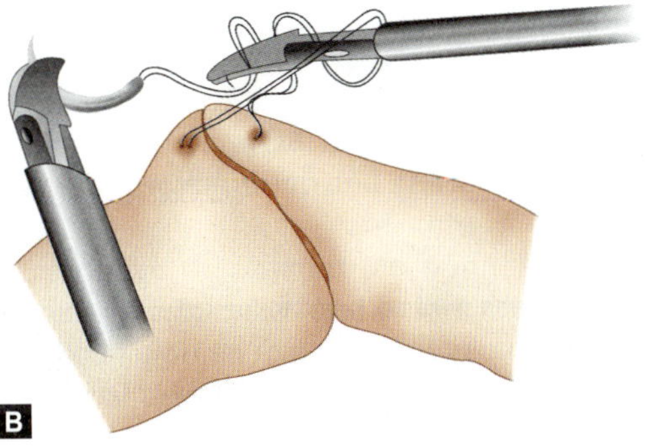

Figs 15.7A and B

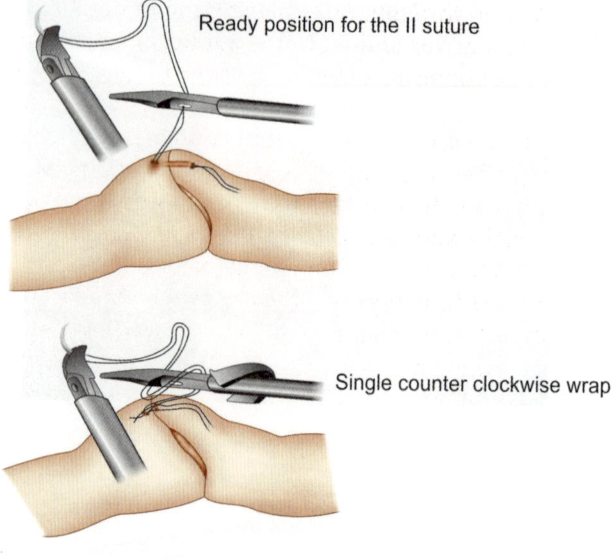

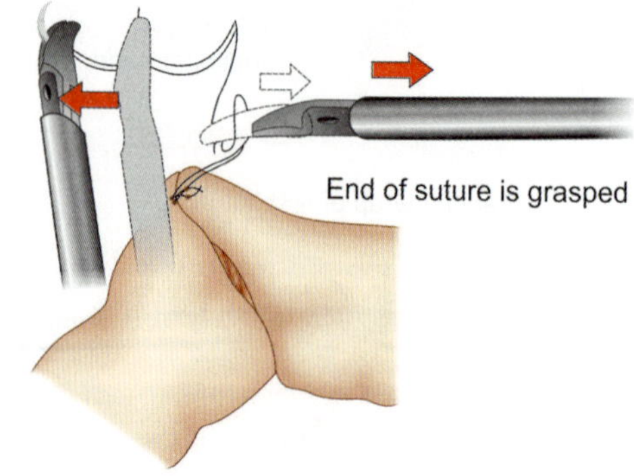

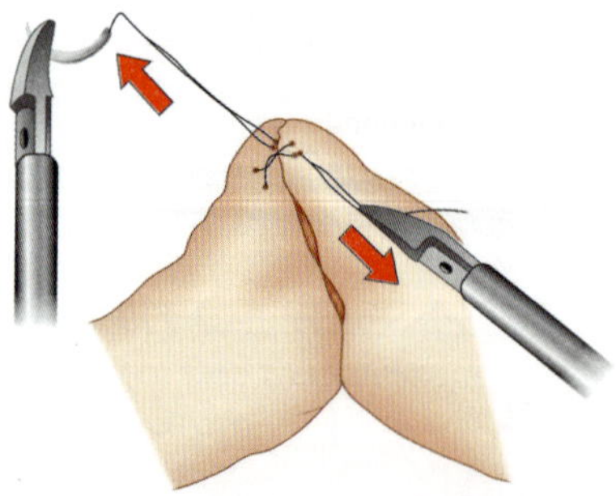

Fig. 15.7C

Figs 15.7A to C: Technique of putting knots

First place double through. After placing the double through hold the tail with the needle driver and place the surgical knot by pulling the two ends of the suture in opposite direction just like in the laparotomy suturing (Fig. 15.7C).

After the first clockwise wrap place single counter clockwise wrap and knot is tied by pulling the two instruments in opposite direction. This is followed by third wrap to complete the knotting process. Cut the suture and remove the needle by holding the suture 2–3 cm away from the needle. Always remove the needle immediately after the completion of the suturing process. Try and avoid parking the needle to the abdominal wall for later removal.

Laparoscopic suturing technique is the duplication of the laparotomy suturing technique. One needs to practice in order to master the technique as that of the laparotomy suturing.

16

3D Laparoscopy

Rakesh Sinha, Gayatri Rao, Shweta Raje

INTRODUCTION

Laparoscopy is now an essential part of gynecological surgery and is accepted as a safe, efficient and acceptable alternative to standard abdominal procedures.

Laparoscopy offers following benefits over conventional open surgery:

- Better magnified image by using telescope which increases the precision in surgery
- Minimal postoperative discomfort
- Shorter hospital stay
- Rapid convalescence
- Early return to the daily activities.

Laparoscopic surgeries are highly skill and technology dependent. Early pioneers in the field used instrumentation and optics that are primitive by today's standards, but technological advances have made the operations more efficacious and easier to perform. The advances in the field of electrosurgery, imaging techniques and robotic assistance have allowed surgeons to perform complex operations with improved confidence.

Despite the advances with technology, training remains a major issue in the field. Most gynecologists today completed their formal training before the wide dissemination of laparoscopic techniques, and even in today's academic climate there remain some teaching institutions that lack a dedicated laparoscopic or minimally invasive surgical program.

One of the largest challenges in laparoscopic surgical training is adaptation to a 2-dimensional (2D) flat view of the surgical field. In open surgery, surgeons rely on direct visual input to ascertain depth. In contrast, the monitors used in laparoscopy filter 3-dimensional (3D) cues from the operative field, resulting in a reduction of the depth.

The lack of depth perception is a significant sensory loss for the surgeon. The perception of depth during a laparoscopic surgery is critical to proper hemostasis and effective suturing. Although the challenges of lost depth perception can be overcome with a long experience of cases, most surgeons cannot depend on such a high volume over a short period.

Another limitation for laparoscopic surgeons due to the two-dimensional (2D) view provided by video monitors is video-eye-hand coordination which is further complicated by the diminished tactile feedback blunted by elongated instruments.

3D laparoscopy overcomes these problems by providing excellent depth perception, definition, and resolution. The relationships of structures are more easily defined, and instrument manipulation is easier, doing away with the need for touch and feel to determine instrument position.

Three-dimensional (3D) laparoscopic visual systems have been developed to augment laparoscopic skills. 3D displays are perceived to be more natural and possibly require less mental integration than 2D displays.

In recent years, robotic surgery has been introduced in urological surgery, general surgery, cardiac surgery and gynecological surgery. The Da Vinci surgical system (Intuitive surgical, Inc; sunnyvale, CA) provides robotic control of the laparoscope and all instrumentation. The Da Vinci surgical system has some advantages compared to conventional laparoscopic surgery, such as the 3-dimensional vision, better ergonomics, higher degree of freedom of the robotic instruments and reduction of tremor interference.

The system employs a 3D vision system and endowrist technology. Endowrist technology facilitates instrument rotation through tiny incisions. The robotic instruments replicate the surgeon's hand, wrist and finger movements. This allows for extended range of motion and improved manipulation while conducting laparoscopic procedures. Since most of the instruments of robotic surgery are disposable the recurring cost of every surgery is very high. On the other hand all the conventional straight instruments used in laparoscopy can be utilized when using a 3D laparoscope. There is no recurring cost and newer instruments can be used instantly.

It is acknowledged that the robot offers a potential advancement in minimally invasive procedures, particularly in complex or highly technical cases such as laparoscopic prostatectomy or certain cardiac cases. This value proposition tends to be offset when robotics is used in cases where traditional laparoscopic approaches can achieve the same clinical outcomes, but at far less cost to the hospital. Although subsequent generations of robots may represent the future, it is difficult economically to justify the use of robotic surgery for routine hysterectomies

The evolving literature on robot-assisted surgery in gynecology suggests that the surgical limitations of conventional laparoscopy can be overcome and that the skill level of the surgeon may be enhanced. At present, this seems to be the result of improved instrument, precision and dexterity and 3D imaging.

BRIEF HISTORY OF 3D VISION

The development of 3D cameras comes from the cinematographic industry. A 3D or S3D (stereoscopic 3D) film is a motion picture that enhances the illusion of depth perception and it derives from stereoscopic photography. Basically, a regular motion picture camera system is used to record the images as seen from two perspectives and the combination of these two views with projection hardware or eyewear provides the illusion of depth when viewing the film. Although 3D films have existed since many years ago, during the 1980s and 1990s they had a resurgence that culminated in the presentation of complete movies filmed in 3D after the 2000s.

The first surgical video-system employed 3D monitors with standard resolution and low visual ergonomics and single-channeled laparoscope. Surgeons found the quality of the images was poor because of the heavy active shutter glasses. They also experienced side effects: tiredness, headaches, ocular fatigue, and nausea. Moreover, earlier 3D system offered graded viewing conditions because of their lower resolution, brightness, and disparity plus the fact that the old software did not process 3D machine vision fast enough.

Recent technological advances have led to more flexible instruments, sophisticated high-resolution systems, and light polarizing glasses that are lighter and more comfortable.

The most recent instruments are quicker, more accurate, and precise for surgical tasks and help shorten the learning curve. Picture quality and resolution, as well as image separation are thus, improved not to mention the image refresh rate and brightness.

Cameras are also upgraded—lens system alignment, packing of photo-sensors, and digital image processing. Autostereoscopic glasses-free displays have also improved, as well as multi view autostereoscopic display which give a better depth perception thanks to multiple lenses.

The major manufactures in this field are Olympus® Tokyo, Japan; Storz® Tuttlingen, Germany; Vicking System® Westborough, Massachusetts and Aesculab®, Einstein Vision, Tuttlingen, Germany.

PHYSICS OF 3D

Principles of depth perception: Depth perception is the visual ability to judge the relative distance of objects and the spatial relationship of objects at different distances. As the 3-dimensional world projects onto a 2-dimensional retina, this projection on its own cannot provide depth information.

The brain has to combine various monocular and binocular cues given by the eyes to recover the depth, distance and 3-dimensional shape of objects.

Stereopsis is the most important cue for depth perception. It is the consequence of the inter papillary separation between the two eyes—6 cm, which causes each eye to have a slightly different view of the same scene. This is called 'retina disparity'. The brain is then able to combine the two views into a single 3D image—process is called stereopsis.

Stereoscopy (Greek: to look at a solid object) is the technique of creating or enhancing the illusion of depth in an image—by presenting two offset images separately to the left and right eye of the viewer. Both the 2D offset images are then combined in the brain to give the perception of depth.

STEREOSCOPIC VIEW

The way we perceive depth is complex, and based on two different group of mechanism. One is of depth clues that are monocular and very intuitive. Relative size, overlapping shade, color and movement analysis enable us to assess the distance of objects using 'flat' information, or only one eye. This is how we can watch movements and understand them. Today this is the information we use to operate. The other group is binocular information. Our brain receives two pictures from our eyes that are mot identical in angle, and minute differences are used to process a 3-dimensional picture in specialized areas in the visual cortex.

In order to mimic the process, several technologies to generate and display an artificial 3-dimensional image or rather a stereoscopic image, are used:

Image Generation

Dual Channel Video

In this technology, a dual channel optical scope is connected to two video cameras and delivers two pictures that are displayed to the viewer on a stereoscopic display.

An example to this is the system used in the intuitive robot da Vinci. The advantage of this technique is that it displays a very bright high-quality image generated from two-three chip camera. The disadvantages are common to many systems that implement similar techniques; the images generated by two scopes and two cameras are different not only in the picture angle but also in brightness color optical distortion and sharpness. Using current video and optic technology limit the size to a rather large cumbersome camera scope complex.

Also producing an angled scope becomes a major technical challenge especially if the scope is rotatable.

Dual Chip on the Tip

This closely related technology uses dual Channel video generated by two video chips that are mounted on the end of the scope. The two images created are digital and bypass the disadvantages of the optic distortions created by the optic scope. However, the problems with separated images still exist and the small distance between the chips enables to create a week 3D effect. In order to understand this drawback, the concept of disparity has to be explained.

The disparity of stereoscopic picture is a measure of how different from each other are the two images. This to a certain extent is what determines the accuracy and intensity of depth perception and is determined mostly by the distance between the two sources of the image which corresponds to the distance between our pupils.

When the technical barrier allows a small distance, the picture generated has weak 3D effect.

Shutter Mechanism

This technology used in the Storz 3D Scope relies on the fact that the camera is never absolutely still and that minor angle changes occur between frames.

The streaming video is thus divided by shutter mechanism into two, slightly different streaming videos and when displayed on a stereoscopic display device a stereoscopic image is created.

The advantages of this technology is that it can be generated using a single optic scope and there is no need to replace the whole system except for the camera and image processing unit. However, the small unpredictable changes that are generated by the cameras instability create an image with low disparity and the 3D perception is weak.

In addition the shutter mechanism creates of flicker that has user side-effects similar to those that accompany dual Channel video.

Insect Eye Technology

In this technology and microscope array of lenses is placed in front of a single video chip on the end of the scope, similar to the structure of an insect eye. The lens array creates many small slightly distorted images. When fed into a powerful image processing computer the images are divided into left and right images using a specialized algorithm add streaming stereoscopic video is generated. The disadvantages of this technology are that the image is generated from a single CCD, that is awaiting the difference between the 2 eyes and that it is the first system to truly generate an image that contains a volumetric information about the observed space. This ability harbors the potential of creating hybrid images using hybrid information like preoperative CT or MRI or online image and manipulating the image in many ways. The disadvantage is currently low picture intensity and system instability. A common problem with stereoscopic system is that they depend not only of the image generating technology, but on the display. Ideally the stereoscopic image should be displayed using a real 3D display or a multiplanar image such as a hologram.

Head-Mounted Display

Head-mounted display is based on small high-resolution liquid-crystal display (LCD) screens that display an image to each eye. The advantages are that the user is free to move and work in a relative ergonomic position and that each user can have his own display system.

There are several disadvantages to such systems: there is a need to wear a relatively heavy device and some users suffer from some degree of 'immersion' that is they are being cut off the real environment and lack the feel of what is happening around them. In addition, current LCD technology is limited in resolution and refresh rate, or the number of times the lines appear on the screen each second.

These limitations allow a medium resolution stereoscopic image and it may result in flicker and the resulting user side effects.

Polarizing Screens and Lenses

In this technology in the two images are projected simultaneously on the screen. The image to each eye is polarized to do a different angle by a polarizing screen placed in front of the projecting screen and when the viewer uses appropriate pair of passive polarizing lenses, each eye will see one corresponding image. The result is a stereoscopic image. The system is relatively cheap and allows adding multiple users at low cost. The main disadvantage is that at each polarization a substantial amount of light is filtered, and by the time the image reaches the eye, close to 75% of the light is filtered. The result is an image lower in intensity than usual, requiring a darker background environment (Fig. 16.1).

Active Shutter Glasses

This stereoscopic display technology uses a screen and synchronized glasses. Both screen and glasses have a polarizing screen that rapidly alternates between two polarized images, in a synchronized, rapid rhythm. The synchronization is usually achieved using infrared communication between the glasses and the screen. Each eye sees a dark screen or an image in a rapid sequence.

This allows the system to display alternatively a different image to each eye, resulting in a stereoscopic picture. Again, some loss of light exists. In addition, the glasses are somewhat cumbersome and suffer from some flickering.

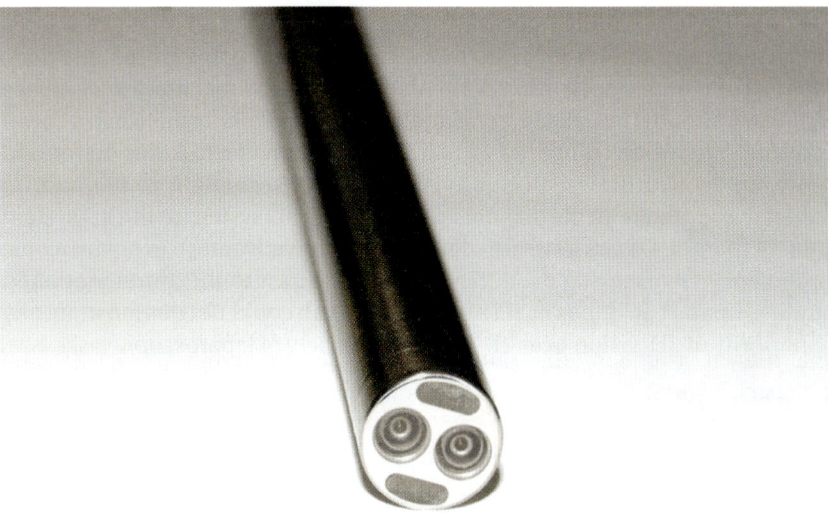

Fig. 16.1: Twin rod lens systems in the telescope

Autostereoscopic Displays

New developments in LCD technology allowed the creation of several systems that display stereoscopic images without using additional viewing devices.

The system is composed of two layers: the back layer is an illumination screen divided into numerous, very thin, bright lines that correspond to pixel columns in the LCD layer in the front.

Since our eyes view the screen from slightly different angels, the result is that each eye will view a different set of alternating lines. Thus, a stereoscopic image will be viewed from a certain distance and angel.

All laparoscopic surgeons using 2D images actually are operating with one eye closed. This is the reason that 2D laparoscopy is cerebrally intensive. The 3D-HD system has two cameras and two optical lens systems which transmit two offset images on the medical 3D monitor. When the surgeon wears circular polarized 3D glasses, the two images are merged by the brain into one and gives the perception of depth.

This gives the relationship of organs in the peritoneal cavity in real time suturing—especially intracorporeal stitching becomes very comfortable.

To date, the limited number of studies examining whether 3D systems have significant advantages over conventional 2D systems have failed to produce a consistent answer to this highly relevant question. Birkett et al. examined the efficacy of 3D laparoscopy in 9 participants who had to perform two exercises and concluded that the third visual dimension simplifies complicated procedures in laparoscopy. Wenzl et al. tested the application of 3D laparoscopy in 11 operations and suggested that 3D visualization improved orientation in the abdominal cavity, thereby reducing operative time. In a prospective randomized study, Peitgen et al. demonstrated that 3D imaging significantly improved speed ($P < 0.0001$) and other measures of performance in two separate tasks, regardless of participants' previous laparoscopic experience. Bhayani et al. demonstrated that among 24 novice laparoscopists, 3D visualization resulted in improved performance in a "bead transfer" task when compared with 2D visualization; the task was performed more rapidly with 3D visualization (108 versus 127 seconds, $P = 0.05$), and, on subjective evaluation, participants preferred the 3D system to the 2D system by a 2:1 margin. Others have also demonstrated an advantage in laparoscopic proficiency favoring 3D over 2D vision. In contrast to the aforementioned studies, Chan et al., Jones et al., and Mueller et al. could not demonstrate any superiority of 3D vision over 2D vision in a variety of laparoscopic tasks.

LEARNING CURVE

A learning curve is defined both by the time (quickness) as well as the number of cases (trials) necessary to attain proficiency.

The advent of new technology has brought new challenges and issues. The introduction of laparoscopy had posed the challenge of 2D images on a flat screen, i.e. as if viewing with one eye closed. Hence, laparoscopy was considered cerebrally intensive.

For the last one decade, robotic surgery with its 3D view revolutionized laparoscopic surgery. several publications discussed the benefits of 3D-HD view and improved surgeon performance.

Change and technology are the key words in surgery today; where is the future of surgery headed? Since the 'lap hysterectomy' revolution in 1989, no breakthrough has changed modern surgery more rapidly, definitively, or irrevocably than robotic and 3D laparoscopic surgery.

A preliminary testing has suggested that the new generation 3D system used will be helpful for developing skills in laparoscopy for the novice surgeon.

The learning curve for some gynecologists was approximately 50 cases to develop consistent operative times and predictable outcomes. These learning curves were dramatically less than those reported for general surgeons and urologists who report learning curves for robotic-assisted laparoscopic prostatectomy to be 150–200 cases.

We experienced much shorter learning curves with the new 3D-HD system. We took approximately 5 cases, i.e. 2 Or days to get used to the 3D vision on a 32" monitor using conventional instruments. This may also be due to the fact that our center is a dedicated gynecological endoscopy center with about 600 procedures being done every year. We have been operating for about 6 years now with 2D-HD system. But, our belief is that, the learning curve for 3D-HD system will be very short for all laparoscopic surgeons and this system will enhance the skills of good surgeons.

What we need to determine in the near future is how long will it take for a postgraduate to learn who is beginning laparoscopy. Will the 3D-HD system shorten his learning curve as compared to conventional laparoscopy; and to what degree?

Although some authors suggest that robotics can be useful method for shortening the learning curve in physicians performing minimally invasive gynecologic surgery.

Another study suggested that robotic surgery should not serve as a wholesale substitute for a skilled laparoscopic surgeon, especially in procedures where standard laparoscopy is routine (Figs 16.2 and 16.3).

COSTS

Another important consideration is that of higher hospital costs associated with robotic surgery is specific to perioperative and postoperative costs ($ 1446 more than conventional lap) and did not account for acquisition costs.

The robotic unit costs between $ 1 million and $ 2.3 million and is associated with annual higher maintenance costs of $ 180,000 a year (Intuitive surgical Investor presentation Q4-2009).

In comparison the total cost of the 3D-HD system, the acquiring costs is about $ 250,000 and lower annual maintenance costs while there is no recurring cost per patient.

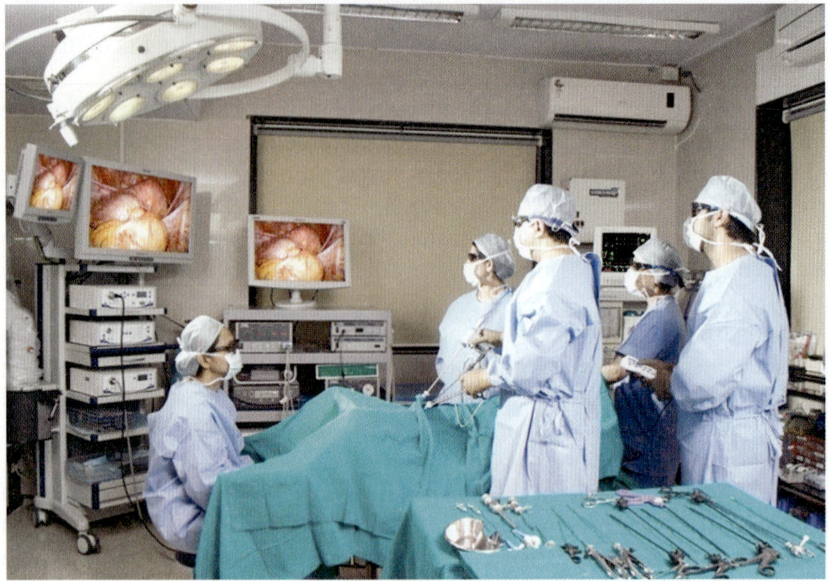

Fig. 16.2: Operation theater set-up

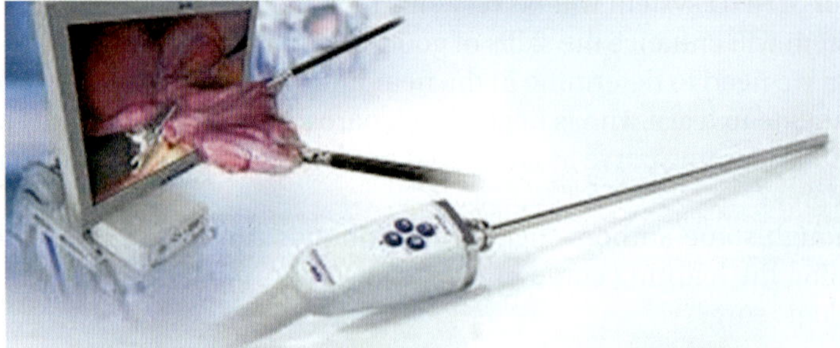

Fig. 16.3: Camera Head with light cable and telescope

CONCLUSION

Using 3D-HD for laparoscopic surgery has definitely improved the hand-eye coordination due to the remarkable depth perception while preserving the tactile feedback. It provides precise spatial orientation, eventually reducing the procedure time, blood loss and reduces surgeon fatigue. There is virtually no learning curve and any surgeon performing laparoscopic surgeries can adapt to this technique.

Benefits to the patients are in the form of improved safety, less complications, cost effectiveness, one day hospital stay and less time for surgery. Benefits to the surgeons are in the form of improved depth perception, precision, accuracy, high resolution 3D image reducing surgical and anesthesia time.

BENEFITS OF 3D LAPAROSCOPY

Restores Natural 3D Vision

- Provides depth perception while preserving tactile feedback
- Improves hand-eye coordination
- Provides precise spatial orientation.

Increases Theater Efficiency

- May help to reduce surgeon fatigue
- Helps to reduce procedure time
- 3D vision extends to entire surgical team
- Virtually no learning curve.

Helps Improve Clinical Outcomes

- Contributes to greater surgical precision
- Enhances dissection, grasping, suturing, and stapling skills.

Delivers Economic Value

- Multispecialty platform
- Helps to reduce procedure costs as compared to robotic surgery.

BIBLIOGRAPHY

1. Bhayani SB, Andriole GL. Three-dimensional (3D) vision: Does it improve laparoscopic skills? An assessment of a 3D head-mounted visualization system. Rev Urol. 2005;7:211-4.
2. Birkett DH, Josephs LG, Ese-McDonald J. A new 3-D laparoscope in gastrointestinal surgery. Surg Endosc. 1994;8:1448-51.
3. Chan AC, Chung SC, Yim AP, et al. Comparison of two dimensional vs three-dimensional camera systems in laparoscopic surgery. Surg Endosc. 1997;11:438-40.
4. Giulianotti PC, Coratti A, Angelini M, et al. Personal experience in a large community hospital. Arch Surg. 2003;138:777-84.
5. Izquierdo L, Peri L, Garcia-Cruz E, et al. 3D advances in laparoscopic vision. Eur Urol Rev. 2012;7(2):137-9.
6. Jones DB, Brewer JD, Soper NJ. The influence of three dimensional video systems on laparoscopic task performance. Surg Laparosc Endosc. 1996;6:191-7.
7. Mueller MD, Camartin C, Dreher E, et al. Gadget or progress? A randomized trial on the efficacy of three-dimensional laparoscopy. Surg Endosc. 1999;13:469-72.
8. Patel H, Ribal MJ, Arya M, Nauth-Misir R, Joseph JV. Is it worth revisiting laparoscopic three dimensional visualization? A validated assessment. Urology. 2007; 70(1)47-9.

9. Peitgen K, Walz MV, Holtmann G, et al. A prospective randomized experimental evaluation of three-dimensional imaging in laparoscopy. Gastrointest Endosc. 1996;44:262-7.
10. Reich H, Roberts L. Laparoscopic hysterectomy in current gynaecological practice. Rev Gynecol Pract. 2003;3:32-40
11. Resad P Pasic, John A Rizzo, Hai Fang, Susan Ross, Matt Moore, Candace Gunnarsson. Comparing robotic assisted with conventional laparoscopic hysterectomy: Impact on cost and clinical outcome. JMIG. 2010;17(6).
12. Talamini MA, Chapman S, Horgan S, Melvin W. A prospective analysis on 211 robotic assisted surgical procedure. Surgendosc. 2003;17:1521-24.
13. Wenzl R, Lehner R, Vry U, et al. Three-dimensional videoendoscopy: Clinical use in gynecological laparoscopy. Lancet. 1994;344:1621-2.
14. Wexner SD, Bergamschi R, Lacy A, et al. The current status of robotic pelvic surgery: results of a multidisciplinary consensus conference. Surgendosc. 2009;23:438-43.
15. Yamauchi Y, Shinohara K. Effect of binocular stereopsis on surgical manipulation performance and fatigue when using a stereoscopic endoscope. Stud Health Technol Inform. 2005;111:611-4.
16. Yu L Lee, Gokhan S Kilic, John Y Phelps. Medicolegal review of liability risks for gynecologists stemming from lack of training in robot assisted surgery. J Min Inv Gynec. 2011;18:512-5.

17

Laparoscopic Hysterectomy: Easy and Safe

Prakash Trivedi, Sandeep Patil, Animesh Gandhi, Soumil Trivedi

Abstract

A chronological evaluation has been undertaken in the method of Laparoscopic removal of uterus from 1993 to 2016. The transition has been from laparoscopic-assisted vaginal hysterectomy (LAVH) to laparoscopic hysterectomy (LH) to total laparoscopic hysterectomy (TLH), use of single chip, three chip, high definition and 3D camera, conventional laparoscopic surgery, single incision laparoscopic surgery and impact of robotic surgery. Further bipolar, endosuturing, harmonic and vessel-sealing devices, technique of ligating uterine artery at the origin for minimal blood loss are compared and evaluated. Though removal of uterus laparoscopically had started for simple to very complex cases, now with surgeon's expertise, a focus is kept on complications. A total of 2562 laparoscopic hysterectomy, 690 LAVH with bipolar with endosuturing, 430 LH with bipolar with endosuturing, 1242 TLH with vessel sealing and harmonic scalpel, 200 TLH with clipping of uterines direct at the origin done for various indications are evaluated. There were 7 bladder injuries, 5 ureteric injuries, 8 conversions to laparotomy and one unconnected mortality for medical reasons. 90% of the complications were managed laparoscopically. In the wake of recent controversies of morcellation in fibroid uterus, we also introduce the technique of In-bag morcellation for specimen of TLH to prevent inadvertent spread of unsuspected malignancy in the specimen.

INTRODUCTION

First laparoscopic hysterectomy was done by Harry Reich[1] in 1989, which hallmarked a big revolution and also generated controversies. Now TLH has established its place in modern gynecology. Also in early cervical and endometrial cancer, radical laparoscopic hysterectomy with pelvic lymph node removal has gained momentum especially with oncological endoscopists. Advent of new technology in terms of 3D camera, energy sources and even robotic surgery has simplified TLH, but has added cost to patient and also increased few ureteric injuries.

Newer techniques like tackling uterine artery at the origin for reducing blood loss during TLH, use of In-bag morcellation for prevention of the inadvertent spread of unsuspected malignancies are the latest advances in laparoscopic hysterectomy that will be elucidated in details in this chapter.

INDICATIONS OF LAPAROSCOPIC HYSTERECTOMY

- Fibroids and excessive bleeding
- Menometrorrhagia with enlarged uterus
- Excessive bleeding with adnexal pathology
- Adenomyosis and endometriosis
- Premalignant and early malignancy of endometrium

Our experience: Total number of hysterectomies—2562:

- Menorrhagia with bulky uterus with no laxity (DUB)—1285 Associated appendicitis -98 Associated SUI - 94 Associated enterocoele-5
- Fibroid uterus—1120
- Associated endometriosis—72
- Ovarian cysts/TO Mass/Tumours—80
- Pelvic lymphadenectomy for malignancy—5

Improvements in the Camera Systems

Olympus has a different tip with camera (Endoeye Flex) placed on the end, and it can be maneuvered to access difficult areas and view them from a completely different angle.

Robotics also uses 3D camera system and gives better visual comfort.

All these camera systems have definitely enhanced our anatomical visualization of structures, reduced strain on the surgeons during prolonged surgeries and also improved the accuracy of dissection and different surgical maneuvers.

BIPOLAR AND LAPAROSCOPIC SUTURING TECHNIQUE

For the cornual or infundibulopelvic ligament and other haemostasis a dedicated bipolar cautery at 30 watts is preferred. The uterine vessels are properly skeletonised and usually sutured with no. 1 Vicryl, intra- or extracorporeal. The specimen side is coagulated by bipolar cautery and uterine vessels are separated from the uterus to prevent avulsion bleeding. After cutting the uterosacral ligaments, the colpotomy is done by monopolar spatula and vagina is closed after removal of uterus vaginally or by morcellation, if bigger in size and if patient has previous cesarean sections (Fig. 17.1, Table 17.1).

LIGASURE AND HARMONIC SCALPEL

The initial vessel sealing devices were mainly of 10 mm size. Now all the vessel sealers come as 5 mm instruments. LigaSure technology delivers a

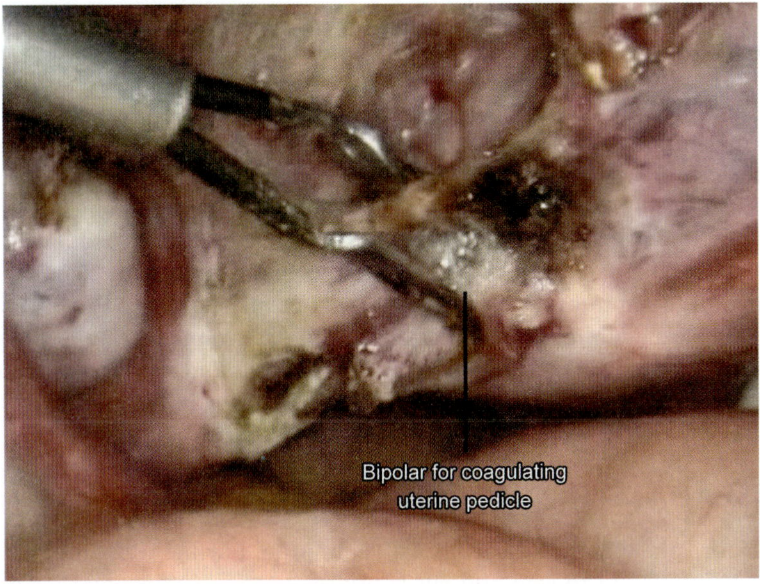

Fig. 17.1: Demonstrating use of bipolar

TABLE 17.1: Comparison of different hemostatic devices

Sr. No.	*Parameter*	*Bipolar with endo-suturing*	*LigaSure with harmonic scalpel*	*ENSEAL with harmonic scalpel*	*OLYMPUS THUNDERBEAT with harmonic scalpel*
1.	Average duration of surgery	115 min (80 to 240 min)	75 min (65–150 min)	70 min (60–127 mL)	64 mins (58–123 mL)
2.	Mean blood loss	160 mL (min 75–300 mL)	94 mL (min 20–320 mL)	80 mL (30–100 mL)	42 mL (24–88 mL)
3.	Complications	4 bladder injury all previous cesarean	Nil	Nil	Nil
4.	Conversion to laparotomy	5	Nil	Nil	Nil
5.	Average postoperative stay	38 hours (Range 36 to 72 hours)	32 hours (Range 30 to 51 hours)	30 hours (28–48 mL)	28 hours (26–42 hours)
6.	Postoperative analgesia requirement	For 3 days in 66%	For 2 days in 45% only	For 2 days in 40%	For 2 days in 18%

unique combination of pressure and energy to create a consistent seal for vessels up to 7 mm with each application. Feedback-controlled response system automatically discontinues energy delivery when the seal cycle is complete, eliminating the guesswork. Due to good and fast sealing, the cornual/infundibulopelvic ligaments and even the uterines were desiccated by the vessel-sealing device.

Harmonic scalpel is a unique device using a very different type of energy to work like a scalpel in laparoscopic surgeries. In it, electrical energy is converted to mechanical energy. The active blade vibrates at 55,000 times a second to simultaneously coagulate and cut tissue. This reduces tissue to a sticky coagulum, sealing vessel walls. The harmonic scalpel separated uterine vessels from uterus, incised the uterosacrals and also circumferential colpotomy is done on a silicon vaginal tube. Vagina is closed laparoscopically and suspended to the uterosacral ligaments (Fig. 17.2, Table 17.1).

ENSEAL AND HARMONIC SCALPEL

The port placement is like bipolar technique. Further Enseal is only 5 mm and efficient to seal and cut supports, uterine vessels and even the uterosacrals. The remaining part is finished with harmonic scalpel on a tube or a Koh's colpotomizer. The vagina is closed and supported by uterosacrals laparoscopically (Fig. 17.3, Table 17.1).

THUNDERBEAT AND HARMONIC SCALPEL

Here essentially everything is done by OLYMPUS-THUNDERBEAT instead of ENSEAL. THUNDERBEAT combines bipolar and ultrasonic energy which

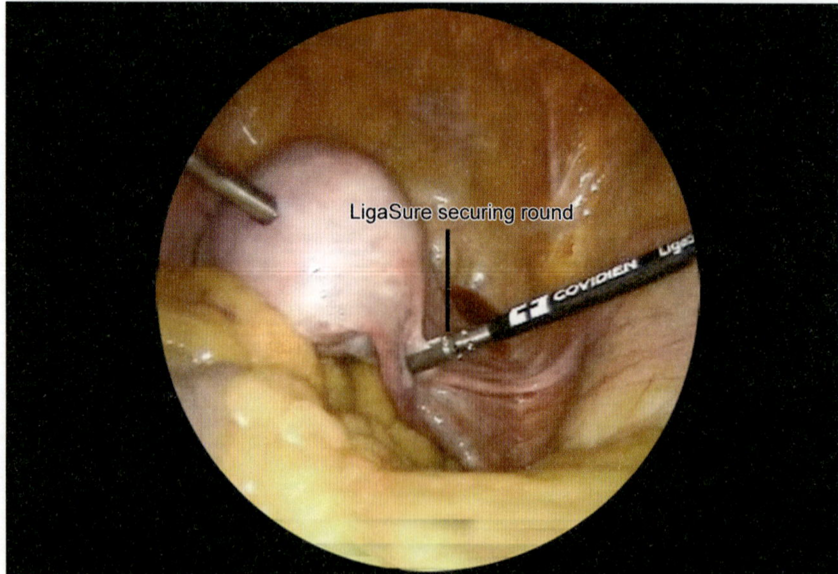

Fig. 17.2: Demonstrating use of LigaSure

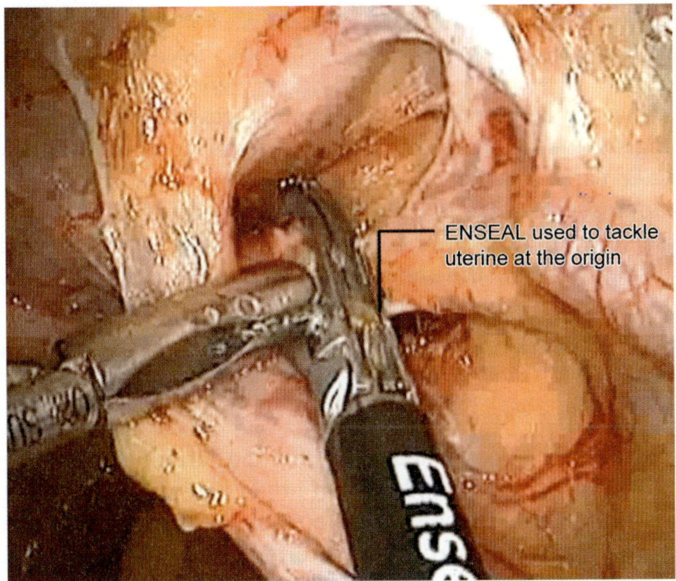

Fig. 17.3: Demonstrating use of ENSEAL

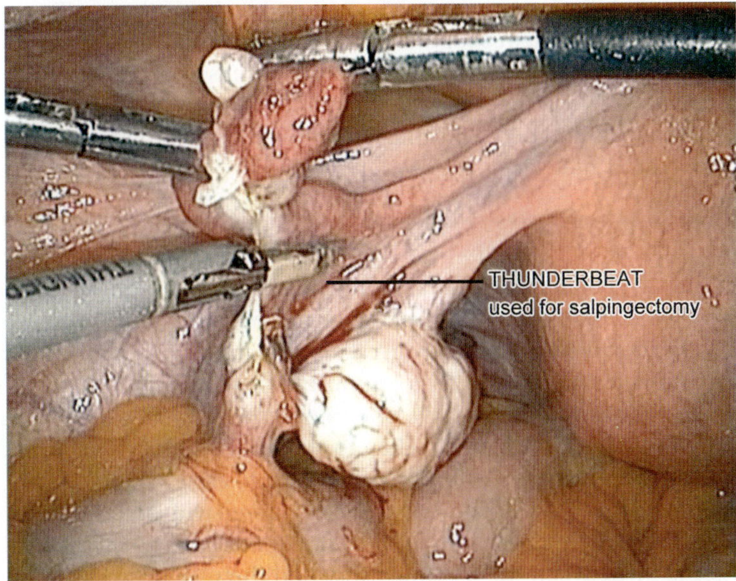

Fig. 17.4: Demonstrating use of THUNDERBEAT

is delivered simultanously from a single, multi-functional instruments. The combination delivers the widely recognized benefits of each types of energy. Rest of the steps is similar.

Earlier other energy devices like GYRUS PK, FORCE-TRIAD were used. But bladder and ureteric injuries were noted with GYRUS PK and hence it is not widely used now (Fig. 17.4, Table 17.1).

TACKLING THE UTERINE ARTERY AT THE ORIGIN

Lateral pelvic wall dissection is a gift from Onco-laparoscopists to routine gynecologists. With increased interaction and combined approach by both Gynec Laparoscopists and Oncosurgeons, more and more routine Gynec laparoscopists are mastering the dissection of lateral pelvic wall. The dissection mainly favors tackling uterine arteries at the origin and accurate visualization of the ureters in each case. This makes each dissection completely safe, if done properly and also reduces ureteric injuries to bare minimum (Figs 17.5A and B).

Anterior Approach

The round ligament is coagulated with either the harmonic scalpel or bipolar coagulation and cut. Both the leaves of broad ligament are separated and blunt dissection done directly below to reach the great pelvic vessels. The uterine artery originating from the anterior division of the internal iliac artery is identified separate from the other structures in the area by tracing it upwards to see the bifurcation of the common Iliac artery. Alternatively, the obliterated umbilical artery can be tugged and it shows the position of the uterine artery at the origin beautifully. The 5 mm vascular clips are applied to the uterine artery well away from the ureter which is easily identified due to the peristaltic movements seen at frequent intervals. Post-surgery also ureter can be visualized, and peristaltic movements can be recorded as a routine to document intact ureters.

Posterior Approach

The dissection begins from the area lateral to the sacral promontory after identifying the ureter crossing the pelvic brim. The peritoneum is held lateral to the ureter and divided vertically parallel to the ureter so that the ureter lies on the medial leaf of the cut peritoneum. The dissection is carried out with harmonic scalpel and the positive pneumoperitoneum aids the separation of the loose tissue. Care is to be taken to stay parallel to the ureter and the great vessels. The common iliac, its bifurcation into external and internal iliac arteries, the ureter crossing the iliac are all visualized with precision. The only structure crossing the field horizontally is the uterine artery. The ureter is seen going in-between the uterine artery and the uterine vein, and hence care has to be taken while applying the vascular clips.

Small vessel bleeding in the area can be managed with simple pressure by a gauze piece. Large vessel bleeds have to be meticulously avoided and may warrant management by the vascular surgeons. It may require conversion to open surgery.

With improved visualization of anatomy especially retroperitoneal and pelvic sidewall anatomy due to 3D camera systems, direct ligation/clipping of uterine artery at the origin is now done at our center on a regular basis.

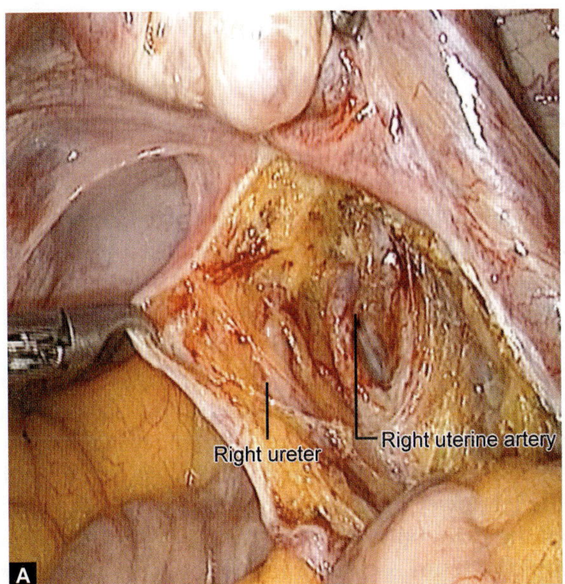

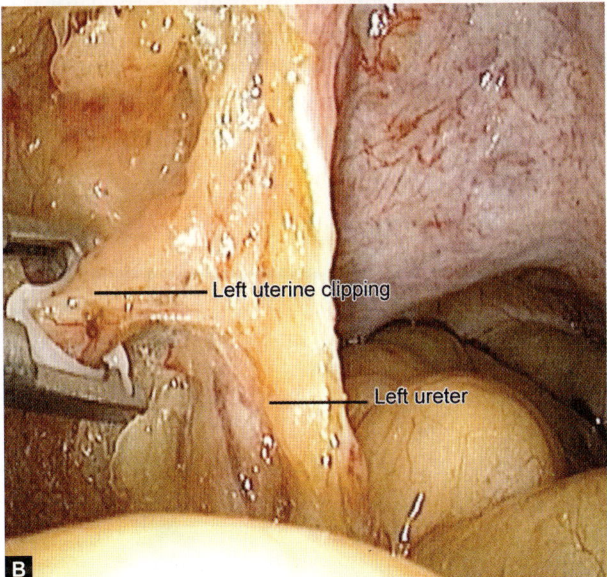

Figs 17.5A and B: Demonstrating direct uterine clipping at the origin from internal iliac artery

Distinct advantages over the earlier technique of tackling uterine at the isthmus:

- Bloodless surgery—especially for larger uteri
- Improved safety of the ureter as it is directly visualized and can be checked
- Lymph node dissection is facilitated

MORCELLATION CONTROVERSY AND THE SOLUTION

In 2014, a physician in the USA was diagnosed as uterine Leiomyoscarcoma (ULMS) after morcellation of the fibroid separated laparoscopically. This led to the controversy that culminated in the ban on use of power morcellators for the morcellation of fibroids by US-FDA. The American Congress of Obstetricians and Gynecologists (ACOG) issued a statement to counsel patients on the occurrence of the incidence of ULMS preoperatively and also cautioned against use of power morcellators.[4] The dilemma here is lack of proper diagnostic parameters pre-operatively for the ULMS. In the wake of this controversy, we introduced a unique technique of In- bag morcellation of specimen.[3] The TLH is done normally with use of the different energy sources available. For morcellation, we introduce a plastic (polyurethane) bag in the shape of a stomach. The specimen is put in it. The mouth of the bag is drawn out through the left lower port, and the other ear-shaped end of the bag is taken out from the main optic port and the laparoscope reintroduced from it. The pnumoperitoneum is created inside the bag and the morcellator is introduced from the left lower port. Morcellation is carried out as usual. Not a drop of blood or any specimen fragment spills over into the peritoneum. This reduces the chances of spread of ULMS. However, one should note that even after an open surgery for ULMS, the disease can recur as part of its natural course, thus showing that morcellation is not the only cause of the recurrence (Figs 17.6 and 17.7).

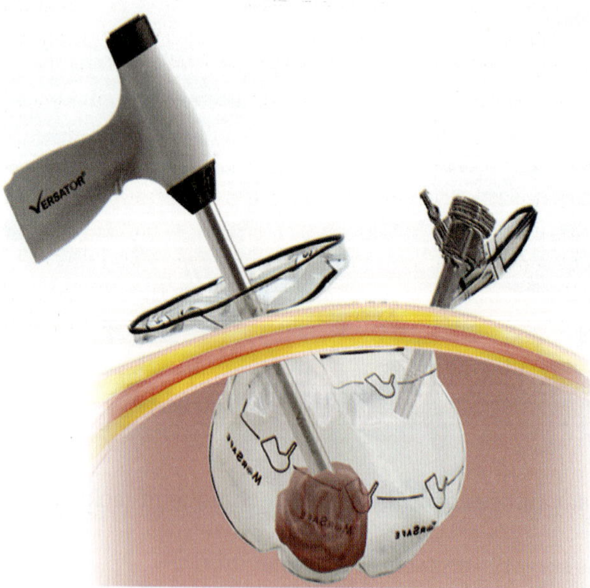

Fig. 17.6: Schematic representation of In-Bag Morcellation

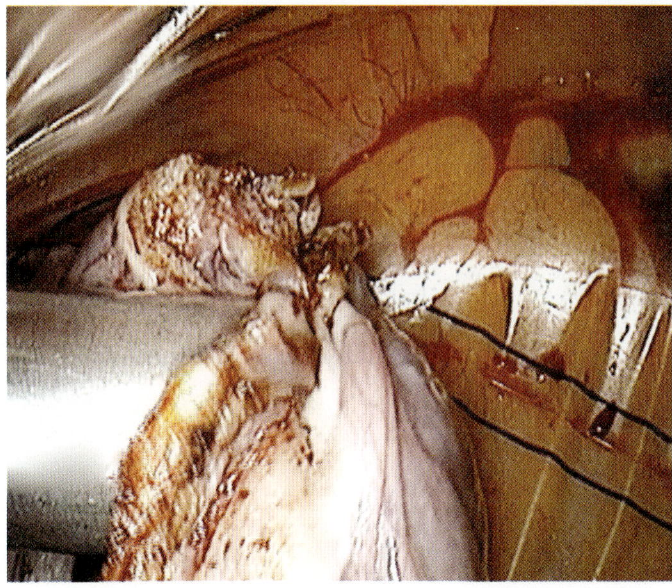

Fig. 17.7: Uterus being morcellated within insufflated bag

THE LATERAL WINDOW FOR DIFFICULT BLADDER DISSECTION

The much-acclaimed lateral window in cases of difficult bladder dissection like previous LSCS, laparotomies, dense anterior adhesions is a technique the world is cognizant with. Introduced by Dr Shirish Sheth popularly known as the Sheth's Space in vaginal surgery, the window is actually beautifully seen during laparoscopy rather than imaginarily felt during vaginal surgery. In such cases, after separating cornual structures and nowadays salpingectomy, the lateral window is identified just anterior and medial to the ascending uterine branch, just one layer above it. Dissection can be proceeded from lateral to medial, as most adhesions are in the midline and this is a free space. Surprisingly, the midline anterior adhesions may be left untouched, once dissection is carried out by this technique in the correct plane (Figs 17.8A and B).

SINGLE-PORT OR SINGLE-INCISION MULTIPLE-PORT TECHNIQUE

The single port or single incision multiple port TLH is a borrowed technique from surgeons who remove gallbladders, etc effectively. In gynecological situation, only simple or not a difficult hysterectomies are done by single port. An improper statement of "2.5 - 3 cm scar less single port/incision"

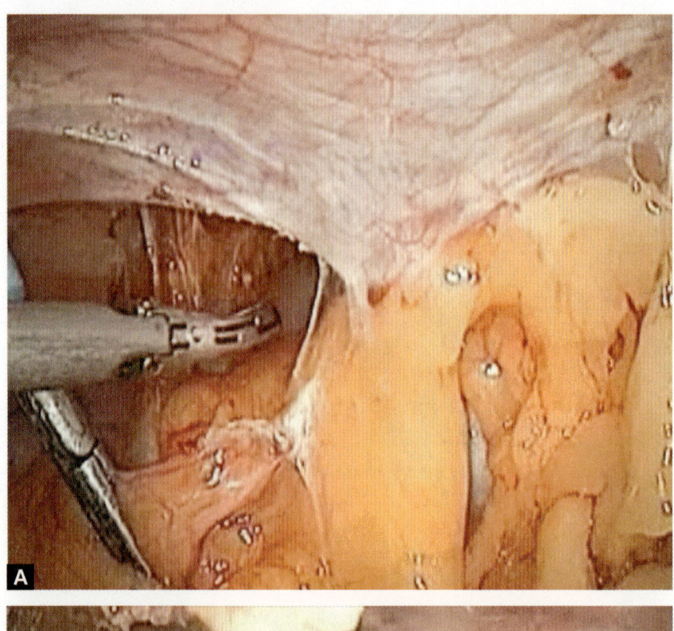

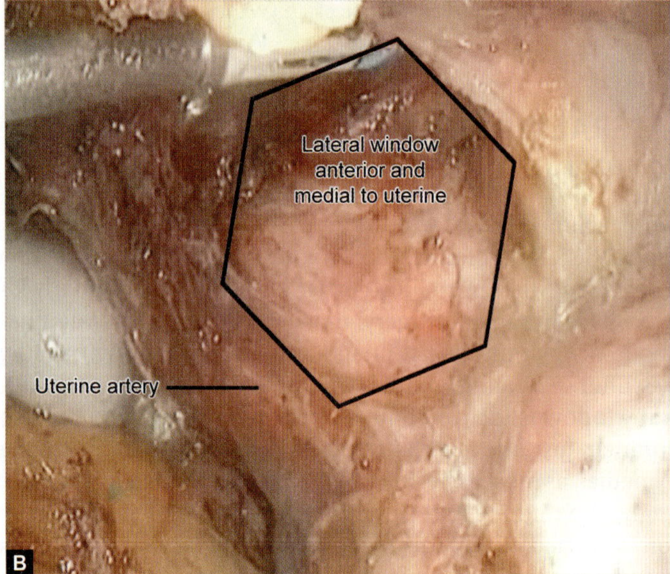

Figs 17.8A and B: Demonstrating dense adhesions being tackled by lateral window approach

is unscientific and complicating standard laparoscopic surgery for the only reason that a surgeon wants to do something different. At the cost of few more umbilical hernias, the cosmetic benefits only convinces the surgeon and nobody else.

ROBOTIC SURGERY FOR REMOVAL OF UTERUS[4,5]

First automated endoscopic system for optimal position (AESOP)[2]—was in 1994—voice activated robotic arm. The Da-Vinci system is currently cleared by FDA and a second generation Da-Vinci system S was released in 2006 which has narrower robotic arm, increased flexion-extension and lateral excursion with a sub-window of 3D screen for surgeon. This technique claims a lot of comfort and an advantage for the surgeon with movement at fingertip and wrist rather than strain on the shoulder. Robotic surgery comes at a much higher cost with occasional technical issues and at present taking longer time. Probably robotic surgery has advantage in radical hysterectomy with lymphadenectomy in hands of a trained surgeon. However, there are coned down indications like single port surgery to do as robotic surgery for removal of uterus. Most of the robotic hysterectomy data is a study of 50 cases maximum and retrospective (Advincula AP) with an additional cost of $ 1446 per patient.

COMPLICATIONS IN TLH

- Hemorrhage—minimized with newer methods like direct uterine, better vessel-sealing devices
- Urinary tract injuries—bladder injuries more in previous LSCS cases can be sutured laparoscopically. Ureter injuries—noted due to energy sources and the lateral spread associated with it.
- Bowel complications—seen in difficult cases like endometriosis, cancer.
- Trocar wounds getting infected–rare but serious with prolonged morbidity—Atypical mycobacteria.

SUMMARY AND CONCLUSION

Laparoscopic hysterectomy has undergone a sea change since 1989 when Harry Reich did the first one. There are changes in techniques every 2-3 years, few to simplify, few to make it safe and few to complicate the technique. Only those with a definite benefit for the patient will stand up especially, if cost effective. The current status of laparoscopic hysterectomy for benign pathology is as follows:

- In patients where vaginal hysterectomy is not possible or advised, laparoscopic hysterectomy replaced more than 90% of abdominal hysterectomies
- A simple bipolar cautery, scissors dissection and endosuturing are still a gold standard, minimizing complications in moderate case.
- Use of vessel-sealing devices and harmonic scalpel makes TLH fast and possible for difficult cases with a definite increase complications in early cases and late complications, especially injury to the right ureter for person standing on left side of the patient and vice-a-versa.
- The single port technique has limitations in simple suturing, instruments hitting each other and converts small multiple port laparoscopy into

single port larger incision technique. Quite often, it is the surgeon's desire to do something different and not a great advantage to patient. Also there is increased incidence of incisional hernia.

- The 3D camera vision definitely makes the surgery anatomical, fast and pleasure to watch with the same ancillary vessel-sealing devices, harmonic scalpel, etc. Few cost-effective uterine manipulators with colpotomizers have reached the state of maturity and safety, if properly used.
- Recording and relay has limits with 3D light camera as they have a single output. A 3D laparoscopy with heavy camera and a remote controlled arm is not robotic at all and too costly. However with two cameras for projection, relay is possible but effectivity and utility is debatable.
- The technique of tackling uterine artery at the origin is a giant leap in a laparoscopic gynecologists career that needs dedicated and deliberate learning effort under supervision and continued use of the technique. This step has the potential to reduce ureteric injuries to the bare minimum and the bloodless field that it offers is a reward in itself.
- In the wake of recent ban on power morcellators and raging controversy over ULMS and its diagnostic dilemmas, its prudent to use the technique of In-bag morcellation till some clear guidelines are made by competent bodies. The technique is simple and easy to incorporate in the daily routine TLH. Also its financially not taxing.
- The robotic laparoscopic hysterectomy is a logical progression which makes the surgeon perform TLH by sitting comfortably at a console. In routine or moderate cases, it is not cost effective. But in difficult cases and radical hysterectomy with lymphadenectomy, it may be a boon, obviously at much extra cost, with a smaller learning curve that unfortunately bypasses conventional laparoscopic training.
- In the era of gadgets, companies' promotion and technologies and also enthusiastic laparoscopists we should not forget the place of a safe vaginal hysterectomy in the hands of a skilled Indian surgeon and also to do an abdominal hysterectomy safely, is still acceptable over complex laparoscopic approach in the hands of unskilled or poorly trained laparoscopic surgeons.

REFERENCES

1. Reich H, DeCaprio J, McGlynnis F. Laparoscopic hysterectomy. Journal of Gynecological Surgery. 1989;5:213-6.
2. The American College of Obstetricians and Gynecologists (2014). Power morcellation and occult malignancy in gynecologic surgery. A Special Report
3. Trivedi PH, Patil SS, Parekh NA, Gandhi AC, Trivedi SP, Abreo MO. Laparoscopic Morcellation of Fibroid and Uterus In-Bag. JOGI. 2015;65(6):396-400.
4. Nathan CO, Chakradeo V, Malhotra K, D'Agostino H, Patwardhan R. The voice controlled robotic assist scope holder AESOP for the endoscopic approach to the sella. Skull Base. 2006;16(3):123-31.
5. Advincula AP, Song A. The role of robotic surgery in gynecology. Curr Opin Obstet Gynecol. 2007;19(4):331-6.

18

Office Hysteroscopy

Pratik Tambe, Pooja Bandekar

Abstract

Office hysteroscopy is a unique approach to identifying and treating intrauterine lesions. It is easy to learn and perform, is safe and accurate, provides immediate results under direct visualization and offers the additional benefit of histological confirmation while patient discomfort is minimal, tolerability and acceptance is high.

We examine the special features and details of the technique itself and its evolution over two decades. We describe the technique and instrumentation used, the indications of use, its incorporation in daily practice, its advantages over conventional surgery, and patient and clinician acceptability.

INTRODUCTION

Infertility and recurrent pregnancy loss are frequently associated with intrauterine pathologies such as endometrial polyps, fibroids and adhesions. The traditional method of tackling these has been the resectoscope; initially the monopolar and more recently, the bipolar resectoscope with their larger diameter requiring dilatation up to 9–10 Fr. This remains the gold standard even today but requires the use of anesthesia and an operating room.

Over the past two decades, advances in optics have led to production of smaller diameter telescopes with excellent vision via HD camera systems. The outer sheath required is of a smaller diameter i.e. 3–5 Fr including the operating channel, inflow and outflow systems. Owing to the refinements in the use of bipolar underwater energy systems, saline can now be used as a non-ionic distension medium, reducing the incidence of operative complications owing to fluid over load and energy spread through tissues.

Consequently, both diagnostic and operative procedures can now be performed in the office setting with minimal analgesia without cervical dilatation, which truly represents a technological advancement in technique and a minimally invasive approach to treating intrauterine pathology.

OPERATIVE PROCEDURE

Among the pioneers of the technique of office hysteroscopy, Stefano Bettocchi stands head and shoulders above the rest.

Over a 7-year period from 1995–2002, he performed 7256 office hysteroscopy procedures at Bari, Italy.[1] All procedures were performed during the proliferative phase of the cycle using a transvaginal approach sans the use of a speculum or tenaculum using normal saline as a distension medium and a 2.9 mm rod lens Karl Storz telescope with a 30° view, the outer sheath being just 5 mm. The continuous flow sheath incorporates a 5 Fr working channel for grasping forceps and scissors.

Electrosurgical systems including the Versapoint from Gynecare Ethicon with a dedicated bipolar generator and dedicated electrodes are available for precise and controlled vaporization of targeted tissues. The Twizzle electrode with a setting of 50 watts and vapor cutting mode VC3 is recommended.

TECHNOLOGICAL IMPROVEMENTS

De Angelis et al. at the Sapienza University of Rome in 2003.[2] Performed a randomized controlled trial comparing traditional hysteroscopy utilizing a 5 mm telescope (Group A, 100 patients) versus mini-hysteroscopy (Group B, 100 patients) using a 3.3 mm telescope.

A marked reduction in the mean pelvic pain score during office hysteroscopy was seen in group B (2.3 +/- 2.1) as compared with group A (4.6 +/- 2.2) ($P<0.0001$). This result was also confirmed when using an alternative approach and a visual analog score (VAS). A significant reduction was observed in the incidence of moderate and severe pelvic pain in group B at the end of the examination ($P = 0.001$) and 5–10 min later ($P<0.05$).

They concluded that the use of mini-hysteroscopes (3.3 mm with diagnostic sheath) lowers considerably the level of pelvic pain the patients feel: it is halved in comparison with traditional caliber hysteroscopes. Furthermore, the outpatient hysteroscopy failure rate is less than half (2%) with the minihysteroscope compared with the traditional 5 mm hysteroscope (5%). As for side-effects and hemodynamic parameters, no differences were observed except for an increase ($P<0.05$) in bradycardia in group B.

The advantage of this technique is self-evident, if the patients' compliance is taken into account: in many cases the introduction or withdrawal of the vaginal speculum was reported as the greatest discomfort.

RELIABILITY AND FEASIBILITY

Cicinelli E et al. in 2003.[3] Published data on 6017 outpatient diagnostic hysteroscopies with a minihysteroscope (2.7-mm outer diameter (OD) telescope with 3.5-mm OD single-flow diagnostic sheath) and 4,204 with traditional hysteroscope (4-mm OD telescope with 5-mm OD single-flow diagnostic sheath). All hysteroscopies were performed using a vaginoscopic approach and saline to distend the uterus.

In the minihysteroscopy, group rates of successful introduction and satisfactory examinations were significantly higher than in the traditional hysteroscope group (99.52% vs.72.53% and 98.53% vs. 92.33%, respectively), while pain and vagal reactions were significantly lower (0.10 +/- 0.34 vs.1.09 +/- 0.53 and 2.25% vs.17.12%, respectively). They concluded that hysteroscopy with lens-based minihysteroscopes was easier, less painful, more reliable, and safer than with 5-mm hysteroscopes. Minihysteroscopy with a vaginoscopic approach is a very well-tolerated, effective, and safe outpatient procedure.

OPERATIVE OFFICE HYSTEROSCOPY

In a landmark paper in 2002, Bettocchi presented a series of 501 cases wherein benign intrauterine pathologies were treated using an office hysteroscopic procedure without anesthesia or analgesia (Fig. 18.1).[1] A Versapoint 5 Fr electrical generator was used to treat endometrial polyps up to 4.5 cm as well as submucous and partly intramural myomas up to 2 cm.

445 endometrial polyps were removed, either intact or using a slicing technique. The average operating time was 17 min. 49 submucous myomas were removed, requiring on average 22 min. No failures or major complications took place during the procedures.

On evaluating treatment efficacy and patient compliance, the uterine cavity was found to be normal in all patients at follow-up without recurrence or persistence of pathology. 47–80% of the patients underwent the procedure without discomfort (Fig. 18.2).

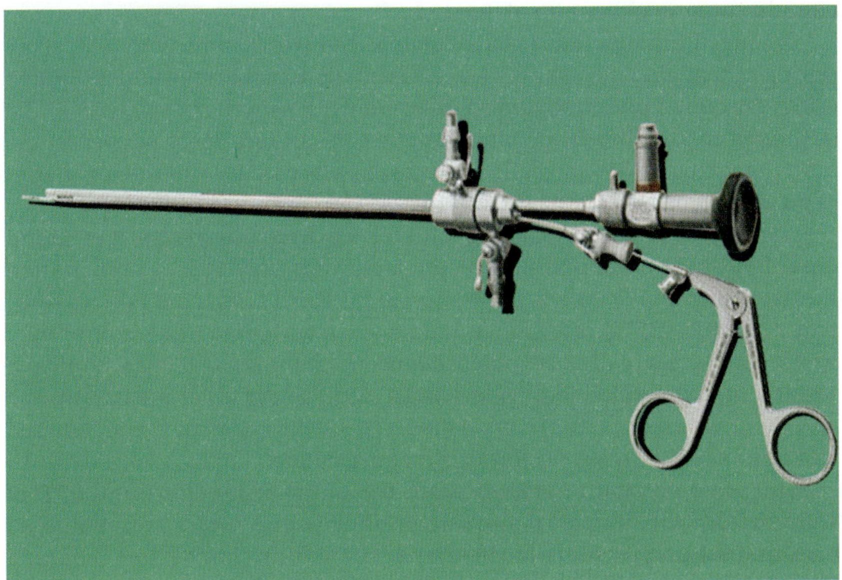

Fig. 18.1 Office hysteroscopy Stefano

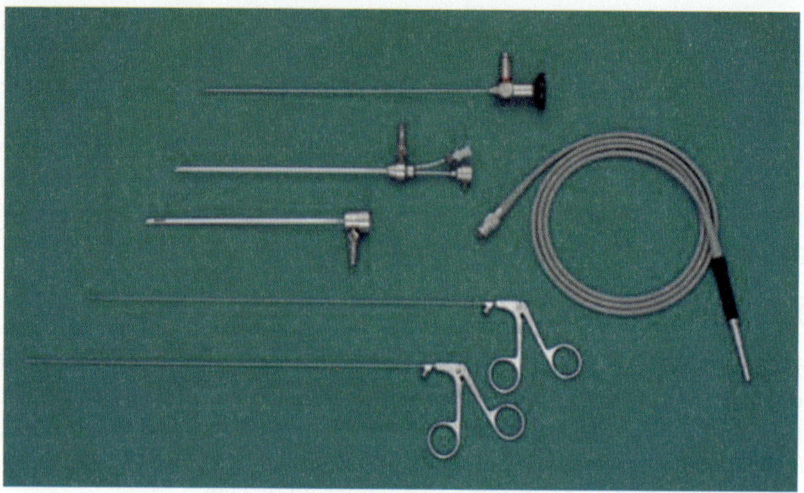

Fig. 18.2 Instrument set

COMPARISON WITH DAYCARE HYSTEROSCOPY

Marsh FA et al, from Leeds, UK reported in 2006.[4] A randomized controlled trial comparing outpatient versus daycare endometrial polypectomy.

The majority of women from both cohorts were premenopausal (62.5%), parous (85%) and in paid employment (62.5%). One woman allocated to outpatient polypectomy had cervical stenosis and dilatation was unsuccessful in the outpatient setting. There were no other intra- or postoperative complications in either arm of the study.

The mean intraoperative visual analog style (0–100 mm) VAS pain score during outpatient polypectomy was 23.7 mm (1–62). A proportion of women (20%) described no intraoperative discomfort; however, the majority (75%) described mild or moderate intraoperative discomfort. More women in the outpatient cohort (58%) described themselves as pain free for the remainder of the day than in the daycase cohort (28%) (P= 0.09).

The day after the procedure, all women from the outpatient group described slight or no discomfort compared with only 41% of women from the daycase group (P= 0.02). All women undergoing outpatient polypectomy had a significantly shorter mean time away from home (3.24 hours) than women undergoing daycase polypectomy (7.42 hours), $P<0.0005$. Similarly, women from the outpatient cohort had a significantly faster mean return to preoperative fitness (1 [0–4] day versus 3.2 [1–13] days; P= 0.001) and required less postoperative analgesia than the daycase cohort.

Ninty-five percent of women from the outpatient cohort and 82% of women from the daycase cohort stated they would prefer to undergo an endometrial polypectomy in the outpatient setting should they require a further polyp removal. They concluded that endometrial polypectomy can be successfully performed in the outpatient setting with minimal intraoperative

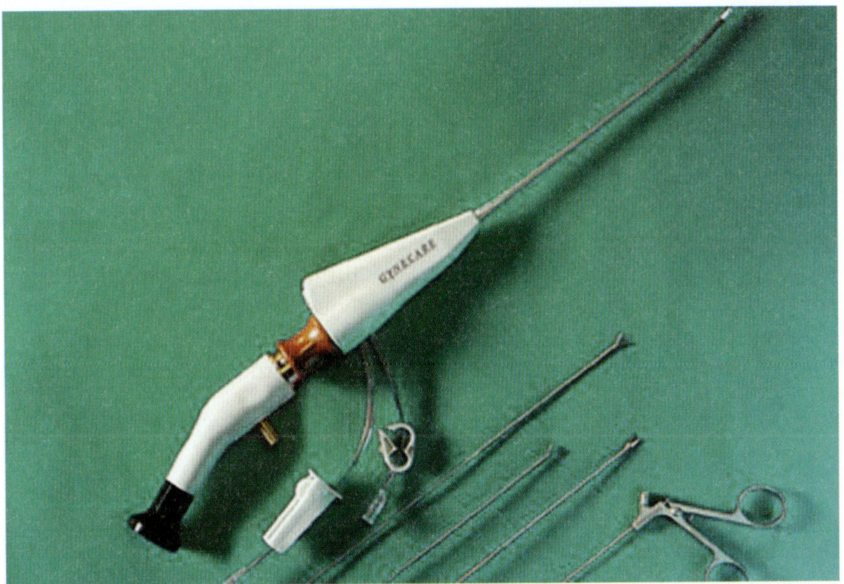

Fig. 18.3 The GyneCare versascope

discomfort, a significantly shorter time away from home and faster recovery and is preferred by women when compared with daycase polypectomy (Fig. 18.3).

OPERATIVE OFFICE HYSTEROSCOPY WITHOUT ANESTHESIA

Bettocchi et al. in 2004 published their analysis of 4863 cases of operative hysteroscopy without anesthesia using mechanical instrumentation.[5]

They used 5F mechanical instruments (scissors, grasping forceps) to treat cervical and endometrial polyps ranging between 0.2 and 3.7 cm, as well as intrauterine adhesions and anatomic impediments. From 71.9% to 93.5% of women underwent the procedure without discomfort for all pathologies treated except endometrial polyps larger than the internal cervical os, for which 63.6% experienced low or moderate pain.

They concluded that simple instruments enable us to perform many operative procedures in an office setting with excellent patient satisfaction, provided that the indications are correct.

PAIN RELIEF DURING OUTPATIENT HYSTEROSCOPY

Cicinelli E performed a review on the need for anesthesia or analgesia during hysteroscopy in 2010[6] and says this is still a matter of debate. Many factors explain the lack of agreement about anesthesia in hysteroscopy depending on the instrumentation, technique employed, need of performing surgical procedure, operator skill and patients' characteristics.

Diagnostic minihysteroscopy (3.5 mm or less in size) is less painful and easier to perform than hysteroscopy performed with instruments sized around 5 mm. Thanks to miniaturized instruments, office hysteroscopy allows a growing number of women to be treated in an office setting avoiding the operating room.

Intrauterine surgical procedures involving only the endometrial mucosa (biopsies, adhesiolysis, cervical and endometrial polyectomies) are not painful. For endometrial polypectomy size of polyps (<2.2 m) and duration of the procedure (more than 15 min) are limiting factors. Most literature suggests that office hysteroscopy in experienced hands is a well-tolerated technique and requires the use of analgesics only in selected patients like women with previous cesarean section, history of chronic pelvic pain, anxiety and in menopause.

COCHRANE META-ANALYSIS

Ahmad G, et al. in a Cochrane Database Systematic review 2010[7] addressed the question of pain relief during outpatient hysteroscopy.

24 RCTs were identified involving a total of 3155 participants, with 15 studies included in the review. Meta-analysis (9 RCTs, 1296 participants) revealed a significant reduction in the mean pain score for the use of local anesthetics during the procedure compared with placebo (SMD -0.45, 95% CI -0.73 to -0.17, I(2) = 82%). Meta-analysis (4 RCTs, 454 participants) demonstrated a significant reduction in the mean pain score for the use of local anesthetics within 30 minutes after the procedure compared with placebo (SMD -0.51, 95% CI -0.81 to -0.21, I(2) = 54%).

There was no significant reduction in the mean pain score with the use of NSAIDs or opioid analgesics compared with placebo during or within 30 minutes after the procedure. There was no significant reduction in the mean pain score with the use of local anesthetics, NSAIDs or opioid analgesics compared with placebo more than 30 minutes after the procedure.

There was no significant difference between the number of incidents of failure to complete the procedure due to cervical stenosis between the intervention and control groups (OR 1.31, 95% CI 0.66 to 2.59; 6 RCTs, 805 participants). There were significantly fewer incidents of failure to complete the procedure due to pain in the intervention group than in the control group (OR 0.29, 95% CI 0.12 to 0.69; 2 studies, 330 participants). Meta-analysis demonstrated no significant difference between the intervention and placebo groups with regards to adverse effects.

They concluded that there was a significant reduction in the mean pain score with the use of analgesia during and within 30 minutes after outpatient hysteroscopy.

POSTMENOPAUSAL BLEEDING

Cordeiro A, et al. from Lisbon, Portugal reported a series of 245 women with postmenopausal bleeding and thickened endometrium on ultrasound.[8]

The women were evaluated for age, hormonal therapy, hysteroscopic findings, procedure duration, complications and associated pain, and histological diagnosis. Symptomatic patients were older and had longer procedure duration. The most frequent hysteroscopic finding was endometrial polyp in both groups. Pain was subjectively assessed in a numeric scale from 0 to 10 and median value was 4. There were no complications reported.

The global neoplasia rate was 2.9% for asymptomatic patients and 16.4% for symptomatic ones ($p < 0.05$). Thickened endometrium with postmenopausal metrorrhagia gave patients a significantly higher risk for neoplasia and hyperplasia.

PRE-IVF OFFICE HYSTEROSCOPY

Hinckley MD, et al. from Stanford, USA in 2004.[9] Published data on 1000 patients subjected to an office hysteroscopy prior to undergoing an IVF cycle. 62% of patients had a normal uterine cavity, while 32% had endometrial polyps. Other pathology included submucous fibroids (3%), intrauterine adhesions (3%), polypoid endometrium (0.9%), septum (0.5%) retained products of conception (0.3%), and bicornuate uterus (0.3%). The pathology was treated in all patients without complication.

They concluded that when hysteroscopy is routinely performed prior to *in vitro* fertilization, a significant percentage of patients have uterine pathology that may impair the success of fertility treatment. Patient tolerance, safety, and the feasibility of simultaneous operative correction make office hysteroscopy an ideal procedure.

RECURRENT IMPLANTATION FAILURE

Hosseini MA, et al. 2014 reported the use of hysteroscopy in the cycle preceding treatment in women with recurrent implantation failure.[10] As an aid to improving treatment outcomes.

Of 353 women in the trial, the results of hysteroscopy were normal in 103 women (72.5%), and they revealed inflammation in 22 (15.5%), polyp in 16 (11.3%) and Asherman syndrome in one patient (0.7%).

Chemical pregnancy occurred in 58.5% of women in the hysteroscopy group versus 34.1% of control women (OR: 2.7; 95% CI: 1.7–4.2; P < 0.001). Clinical pregnancy occurred in 50.7% and 30.3% of women in the hysteroscopy and control groups, respectively (OR: 2.4; 95% CI: 1.5–3.7; P < 0.001). Delivery rate was 35.5% in hysteroscopy group and 21.1% in the controls (OR: 1.9; 95% CI: 1.2–3.1; P = 0.008).

The authors concluded that hysteroscopy in the menstrual cycle before ovarian stimulation in fresh cycles and before endometrial preparation in frozen thawed cycles in women experiencing recurrent implantation failure with apparently normal uterine cavity significantly increases the pregnancy rates in fresh and frozen cycles, respectively.

CONCLUSION

With advancements in technology and continuous refinement of telescope and camera systems coupled with operator expertise, office hysteroscopy has largely begun to replace standard daycare hysteroscopy in the majority of the developed world.

In appropriately selected cases, it is safe, effective and a reasonably pain-free procedure in the vast majority of patients with excellent pain scores and postprocedure feedback.

Consequently, both diagnostic and operative procedures can now be performed in the office setting with minimal analgesia without cervical dilatation and represents a truly minimally invasive approach to treating intrauterine pathology.

It has found application in a variety of clinical scenarios including evaluation of abnormal uterine bleeding, prior to ART procedures and as a unique means of improving treatment outcomes in recurrent implantation failure.

REFERENCES

1. Bettocchi S, Ceci O, Di Venere R, Pansini MV, et al. Advanced operative office hysteroscopy without anaesthesia: analysis of 501 cases treated with a 5 Fr bipolar electrode. Human Reproduction. 2002;17,2435-38.
2. De Angelis C, Santoro G, Re ME, Nofroni I. Office hysteroscopy and compliance: mini-hysteroscopy versus traditional hysteroscopy in a randomised trial. Human Reproduction. 2003;18(11):2441.
3. Cicinelli E, Parisi C, Galantino P, Pinto V, Barba B, Schonauer S. Reliability, feasibility, and safety of minihysteroscopy with a vaginoscopic approach: experience with 6,000 cases. Fertil Steril. 2003;80(1):199.
4. Marsh FA, Rogerson LJ, Duffy SR. A randomised controlled trial comparing outpatient versus daycase endometrial polypectomy. BJOG. 2006;113(8):896.
5. Bettocchi S, Ceci O, Nappi L, Di Venere R, et al. Operative office hysteroscopy without anesthesia: analysis of 4863 cases performed with mechanical instruments. J Am Assoc Gynecol Laparosc. 2004;11(1):59-61.
6. Cicinelli E. Hysteroscopy without anesthesia: review of recent literature. J Minim Invasive Gynecol. 2010;17(6):703-8.
7. Ahmad G, O'Flynn H, Attarbashi S, Duffy JM, et al. Pain relief for outpatient hysteroscopy. Cochrane Database Syst Rev. 2010;(11):CD007710. doi: 10.1002/14651858.CD007710.pub2.
8. Cordeiro A, Condeco R, Leitao C, Sousa F. Office hysteroscopy after ultrasonographic diagnosis of thickened endometrium in postmenopausal patients. Gynecol Surg. 2009;6:317-22.
9. Hinckley MD, Milki AA. 1000 office based hysteroscopies prior to in vitro fertilisation: feasibility and findings. JSLS. 2004;8(2):103.
10. Hosseini MA, Ebrahimi N, Mahdavi A, Aleyasin A, et al. Hysteroscopy in patients with repeated implantation failure improves the outcome of assisted reproductive technology in fresh and frozen cycles. J Obstet Gynecol Res 2014;40(5):1324-30.

19

Hysteroscopy in Asherman's Syndrome

Neeta Warty, Rajkishor Sawant

INTRODUCTION

Asherman's syndrome (AS), also called "uterine synechiae" or intrauterine adhesions (IUA), is a condition characterized by the presence of adhesions and/or fibrosis within the uterine cavity due to scars. Other terms have been used to describe the condition and related conditions include: traumatic intrauterine adhesions, uterine/cervical atresia, traumatic uterine atrophy, sclerotic endometrium and endometrial sclerosis.

It was first described in 1894 by Heinrich Fritsch (Fritsch, 1894)[1] and further characterized by the gynecologist Joseph Asherman in 1948.[2] Hence, it is also known as Fritsch syndrome, or Fritsch-Asherman syndrome (Figs 19.1 and 19.2).

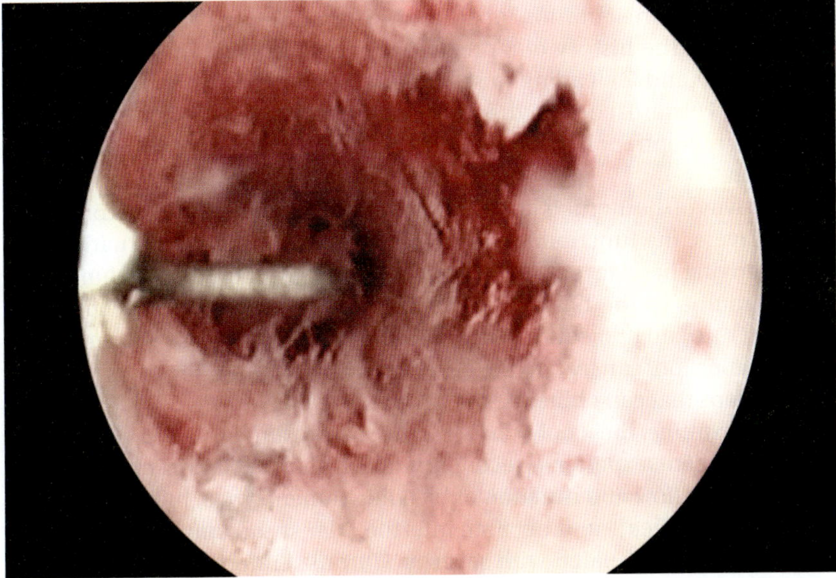

Fig. 19.1: Dense intrauterine adhesions

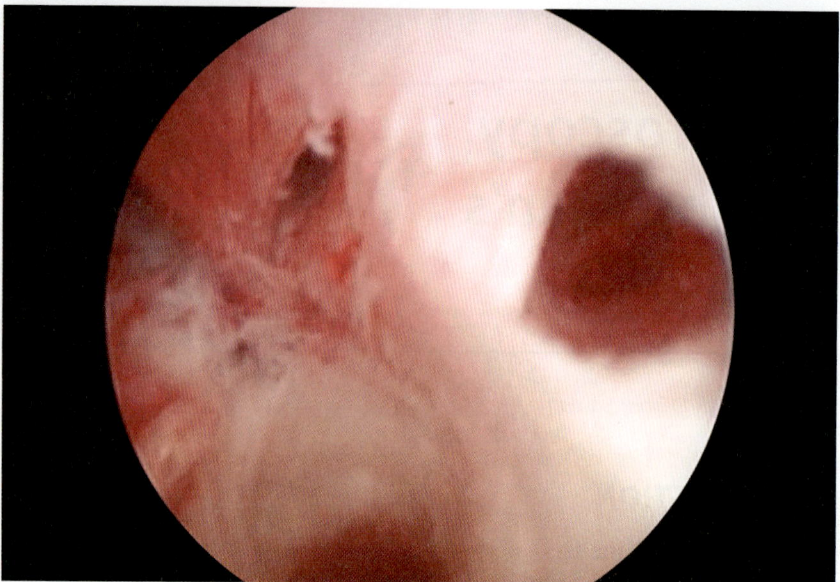

Fig. 19.2: Another case of severe Asherman syndrome

INCIDENCE

The condition was found in 1.5% of women undergoing HSG[3] and between 5% and 39% of women with recurrent miscarriage.[4-6]

ETIOPATHOLOGY

The common presentation of intrauterine adhesions is infertility and amenorrhea. The history of a pregnancy event followed by a dilation and curettage (D and C) leading to secondary amenorrhea or hypomenorrhea is typical. Hysteroscopy is the gold standard for diagnosis.[7] Imaging by sonohysterography or hysterosalpingography will reveal the extent of the scar formation.

The cavity of the uterus is lined by the endometrium. This lining is composed of two layers, the functional layer which is shed during menstruation and an underlying basal layer, which is necessary for regenerating the functional layer. Trauma to the basal layer, typically after a dilation and curettage (D and C), a blind procedure performed after a miscarriage, or delivery, or for elective abortion, can lead to the development of intrauterine scars resulting in adhesions that can obliterate the cavity to varying degrees.

In the extreme, the whole cavity can be scarred and occluded.

Often, patients experience secondary menstrual irregularities characterized by changes in flow and duration of bleeding (amenorrhea, hypomenorrhea, or oligomenorrhea)[8] and become infertile. Menstrual anomalies are often but not always correlated with severity. Chronic endometritis from genital tuberculosis is an important cause of severe intrauterine adhesions in the

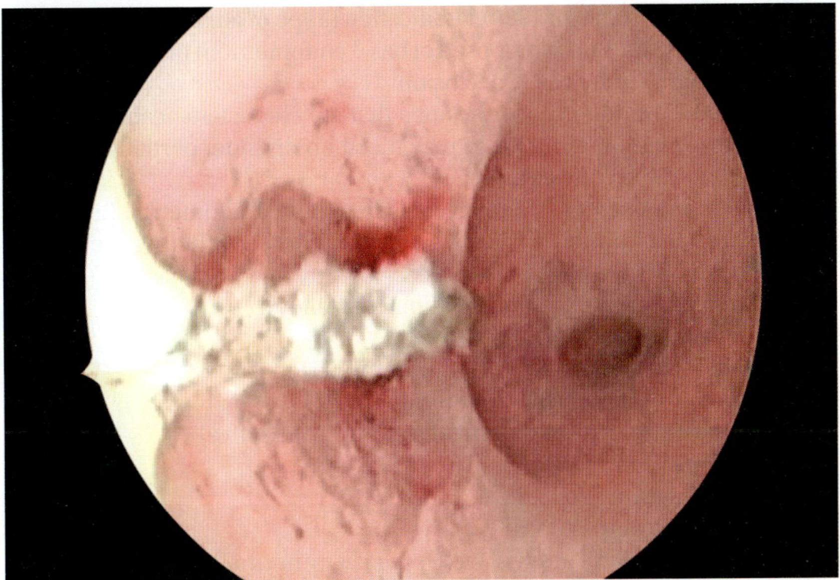

Fig. 19.3: Areas of endometrial lining

developing world.[9] Adhesions restricted to only the cervix or lower uterus may result in cryptomenorrhoea. Asherman's syndrome can also result from other pelvic surgeries including Cesarean sections.[10,11] Removal of fibroid tumors (myomectomy) and from other causes such as IUDs, pelvic irradiation, schistosomiasis[12] and genital tuberculosis (Fig. 19.3).[13]

CLASSIFICATION

Grades of Asherman's Syndrome Severity

From European Society for Hysteroscopy and settled in 1989 (Site of adhesions):

- Thin or filmy adhesions easily ruptured by hysteroscope sheath alone, cornual areas normal
- Singular firm adhesions connecting separate parts of the uterine cavity, visualization of both tubal ostia possible, cannot be ruptured by hysteroscope sheath alone
- Occluding adhesions only in the region of the internal cervical os. Upper uterine cavity normal
- Multiple firm adhesions connecting separate parts of the uterine cavity, unilateral obliteration of ostial areas of the tubes
- Extensive scarring of the uterine cavity wall with amenorrhea or hypomenorrhea
- Combination of III and IIIa
- Extensive firm adhesions with agglutination of the uterine walls. Both tubal ostial areas occluded.

Valle and Sciarra's table of 1988 classification (Type of adhesions):

- *Mild*: Filmy adhesions composed of basal endometrium producing partial or complete uterine cavity occlusion
- *Moderate*: Fibromuscular adhesions that are characteristically thick, still covered by endometrium that may bleed on division, partially or totally occluding the uterine cavity
- *Severe*: Composed of connective tissue with no endometrial lining and likely to bleed upon division, partially or totally occluding the uterine cavity.

Donnez and Nisolle (1994) classification is as follows:

- Central adhesions
  - Thin filmy adhesions (Endometrial adhesions)
  - Myofibrous (Connective adhesions)
- Marginal adhesions (Always myofibrous or connective)
  - Wedge-like projection
  - Obliteration of one horn
- Uterine cavity absent on HSG
  - Occlusion of the internal os (Upper cavity normal)
  - Extensive agglutination of uterine walls (Absence of uterine cavity—true Asherman's syndrome).

RELEVANT ANATOMY

For any hysteroscopic procedure, the surgeon must understand the thickness of the uterine wall allowing the surgeon to manipulate the surgery on the basis of the area of surgery. Table 19.1 lists the wall thickness for each area of the uterus.

ROLE OF HYSTEROSCOPY

Modalities

Diagnostic Hysteroscopy

Plain distention of the uterine cavity with a hysteroscope can itself lyse flimsy adhesions. Blunt dissection with a flexible hysteroscope is effective for maintenance of cavity patency after primary treatment of intrauterine adhesions.

TABLE 19.1 Thickness of the uterine wall

Location	*Mean (mm)*	*Range (mm)*
Anterior wall	22.5	17–25
Posterior wall	21	15–25
Fundus	19.5	15–22
Isthmus	10	8–12
Corpus	5.5	4–7

Monopolar Current

The resectoscope is a specialized instrument used with a monopolar electrode and a trigger device for use in hypotonic, nonconductive media such as glycine. The current cuts and coagulates tissue by contact coagulation. The current settings usually involve the use of pure cutting current of 90–100 watts (Fig. 19.4).

Bipolar

This system again uses the bipolar circuitry for electrosurgery in isotonic media. The versapoint system is a similar system which includes a spring tip for hemostatic vaporization, and a twizzle tip for hemostatic resection (Figs 19.5 and 19.6).

Laser

Nd-YAG: Laser energy is delivered to the tissues via a fiber inserted through operating hysteroscope. The laser energy provides a tissue penetration of 5–6 mm. Two techniques are commonly described. The dragging technique requires the laser fiber to be in constant contact with the endometrium which ultimately results in vaporization of the tissue and the blanching technique in which the fiber does not come in contact with the endometrium. Both the techniques require constant motion to minimize risk of perforation. Choice of distention media includes normal saline or Dextran 70 (Fig. 19.7).

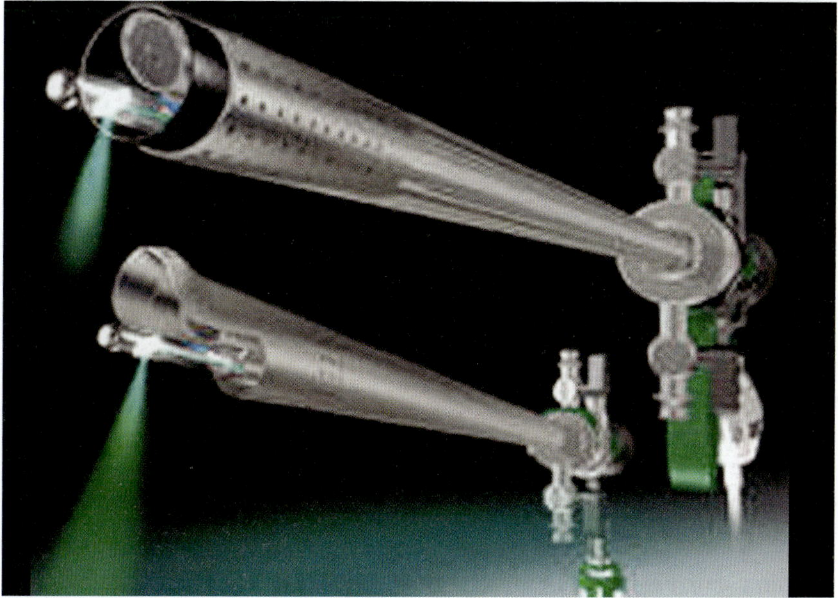

Fig. 19.4: The resectoscope

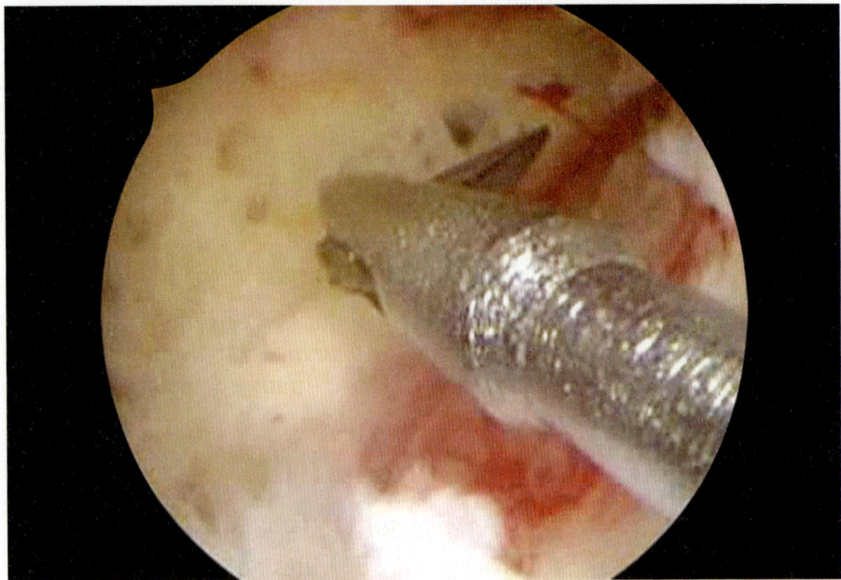

Fig. 19.5: Hysteroscopic scissors for adhesiolysis

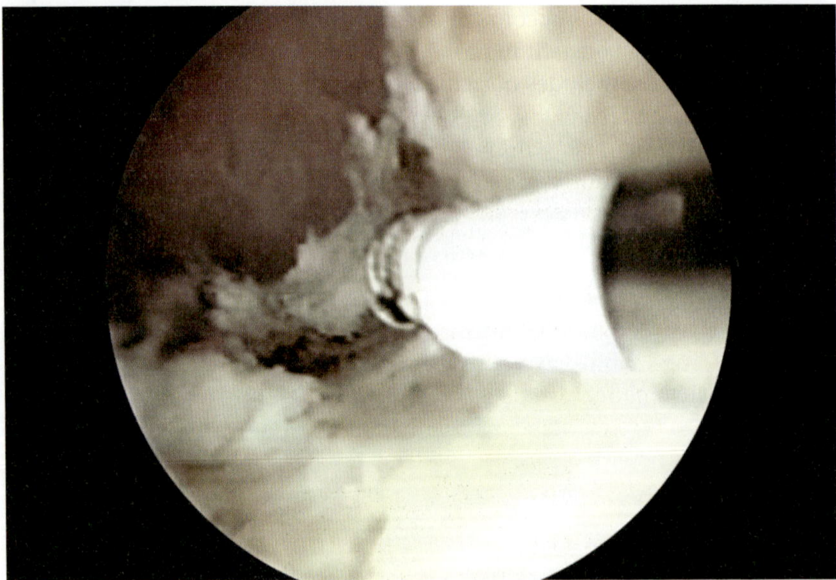

Fig. 19.6: Bipolar twizzle electrode for adhesiolysis

Scissors

Scissors can be used for mechanical cutting of the visible adhesions (Fig. 19.5).

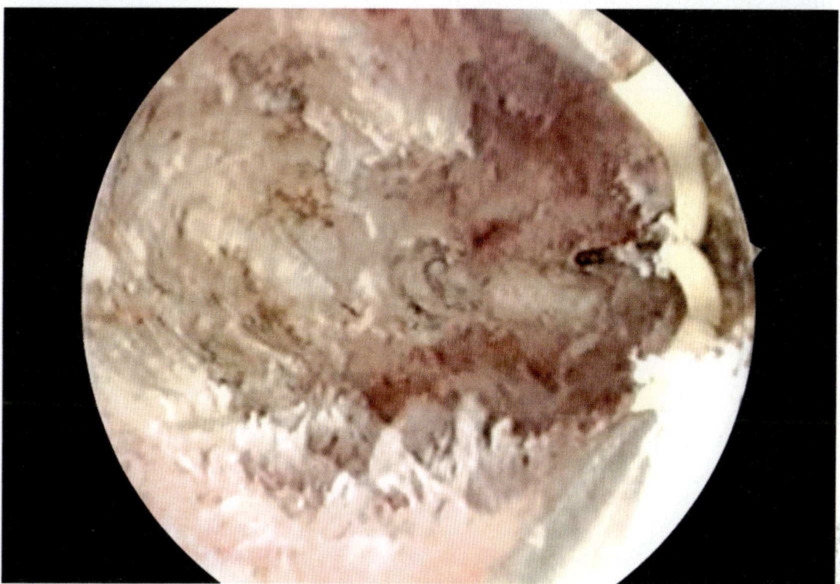

Fig. 19.7: Endometrial cavity after adhesiolysis

Preparation of Nulliparous Cervix

In patients with known cervical stenosis or tortuous cervical canals preoperative vaginal or oral misoprostol (200 µg) 2–4 hours prior to the procedure is known to increase ease of dilatation, reduce the need for mechanical cervical dilatation and lower the rate of cervical laceration and false passage formation, especially, in cases of severe intrauterine adhesions.

Role of Estrogens

Preoperative administration of estrogens is beneficial in cases of severe Asherman's syndrome so as to allow proliferation of the endometrial lining and allow better visualization of the cavity lining especially so when associated with cervical stenosis and ultrasound-guided resection.

Postoperative Estrogen Therapy

Conjugated estrogens 5 mg for 25 days with medroxyprogesterone for the last 5 days. The purpose of the estrogen is to limit the amount of postoperative bleeding due to vasoconstriction of the small blood vessels and to rapidly rejuvenate the endometrial lining (Fig. 19.8).

OPTIMIZING RESULTS AND PREVENTING RECURRENCE

Postprocedure adhesion dissection can be technically difficult and must be performed with care in order to not create new scars and further exacerbate

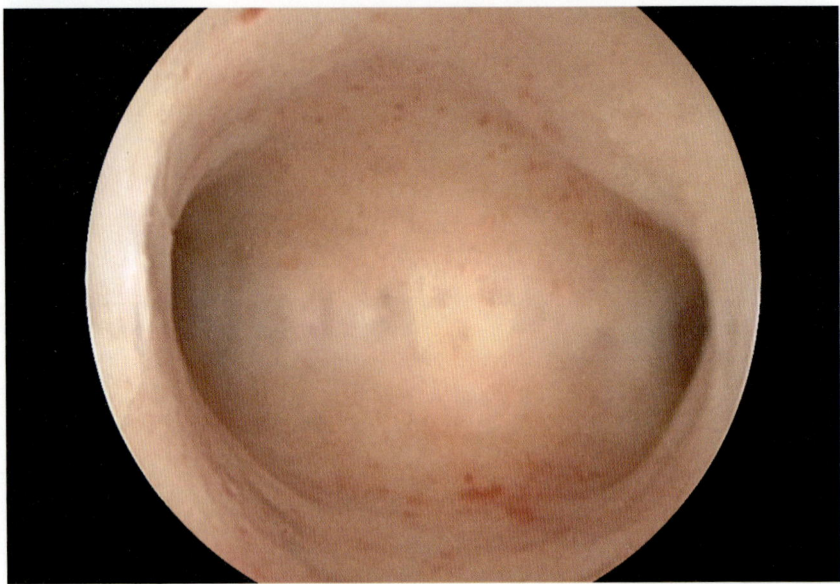

Fig. 19.8: Normalized cavity after adhesiolysis and estrogen therapy

the condition. In more severe cases, adjunctive measures such as laparoscopy are used in conjunction with hysteroscopy as a protective measure against uterine perforation. Microscissors are usually used to cut adhesions. Electrocauterization is not recommended.[14]

As intrauterine adhesions (IUA) frequently reform after surgery, techniques have been developed to prevent recurrence of adhesions. Methods to prevent adhesion reformation include the use of mechanical barriers (Foley's catheter, saline-filled Cook medical balloon uterine stent, IUCD) and gel barriers (Seprafilm, Spraygel, Autocrosslinked hyaluronic acid gel hyalobarrier) to maintain opposing walls apart during healing (Tsapanos, 2002); (Guida, 2004); (Abbott, 2004), thereby preventing the reformation of adhesions. Antibiotic prophylaxis is necessary in the presence of mechanical barriers to reduce the risk of possible infections. A common pharmacological method for preventing reformation of adhesions is sequential hormonal therapy with estrogens followed by a progestin to stimulate endometrial growth and prevent opposing walls from fusing together (Roge, 1996).

Additionally, an early second look hysteroscopy (2–4 weeks) postoperatively may facilitate treatment of new adhesions at an earlier, more amenable stage.

Amnion graft over an inflated Foley's balloon for 2 weeks also seems to be a promising procedure for decreasing recurrence of adhesions and encouraging endometrial regeneration.

To prevent recurrence of intrauterine adhesions after effective lysis, an 8 Fr pediatric Foley's catheter with a 3 mL balloon can be inserted into the uterus and left in place for 7–10 days after surgery.[15-18] Insertion of an intrauterine device (IUD) immediately after adhesiolysis has been used successfully to prevent recurrence of adhesions[15] but it may not be as effective as placement of a pediatric Foley[18] and has fallen from favor.

OUR EXPERIENCE

There are certain protocols that we maintain for all the cases of Asherman's syndrome treated at our center:

- Routine preoperative investigations along with an ultrasonography to determine endometrial integrity
- Patients are started on tab estradiol valerate 8–16 mg/day at least 2 weeks prior to surgery
- Patients are administered misoprostol tablets (200 μg) 4 hours prior to the procedure either orally or vaginally. The vaginal route is preferred due to avoidance of systemic symptoms of chills, abdominal cramps, bleeding
- Monopolar current with resectoscope with settings of 110 watts pure cutting current and 80 watts coagulation current with 1.5 percent glycine as distending medium is used
- The type of anesthesia preferred is general anesthesia either with a laryngeal mask or endotracheal intubation
- The patient is in lithotomy position with return electrode in close proximity to the operative site
- The tubings and the wires are so arranged so as to allow free movement of the apparatus throughout the procedure
- A special absorbent mat with fluid reservoir attached so as to get an exact estimation of the spilled fluid
- The cervix is held with 2 tenaculum type towel clips so as to minimize space occupied and also to secure a firm grip over the cervix
- The cervix is dilated a size more than that required for the regular resectoscope of 26 Fr (Hegar's dilator no. 10.5) to allow free movement of the resectoscope throughout the procedure
- The procedure is performed as per requirement with periodic reorientation so as to avoid any errors in reshaping the cavity
- The procedure is stopped just short of reaching the myometrial layer as evidenced by the appearance of pink myometrium or vascular channels
- The outflow tubing is placed in a labelled container. This gives us an estimate of the fluid flowing out allowing us to monitor inflow/outflow difference continuously during the procedure. The deficit has a bearing on the safety of the procedure
- A constant watch is kept all throughout the procedure on the inflow and the outflow by one personnel dedicated to the job who periodically informs the anesthetist and the surgeon the fluid deficit status
- Early administration of furosemide as soon as a large fluid deficit is anticipated
- Close postoperative monitoring of vital parameters
- Serum electrolytes and serum ammonia whenever increased fluid deficit especially over 1000 mL and the necessary correction postoperatively
- Patients are usually discharged on the same day if procedure uneventful.

POSTPROCEDURE

Patients are administered estradiol valerate 8–16 mg per day for 25 days along with medroxyprogesterone (10 mg) for the last 5 days from day 21 to day 25 for 2 or 3 cycles as per the individual findings. In cases of severe adhesions, estrogens are administered continuously without a break for a period of 2–3 months. Followed by a second look hysteroscopy with further adhesiolysis, if required. Of all the adhesion prevention modalities like insertion of a Foley's catheter post-procedure, placement of an inert IUCD and postoperative estrogens, we have found that the best results are obtained with priming of the endometrium with estrogens and continuous or sequential estrogen support from 1 month to 3 months postprocedure.

We perform cervical os tightening only in indicated cases as per the clinical and ultrasonological findings and not as a routine.

Our results correlate well with the world statistics in terms of live pregnancy rates, return of menstruation, rate of abortion, etc.

IRRIGATION MODALITIES

The potential cavity inside the uterus requires the application of pressure to separate the uterine walls. The minimum required pressure to produce satisfactory degree of distention is 40–50 mm Hg. This can be achieved by:

Hydrostatic Pressure

A bag of infusion fluid suspended 150 cm above the uterus allowing the fluid to enter the cavity with a pressure of 45 mm Hg. Varying the height of the bag above the patient will clearly alter this infusion system for controlling the inflow pressure.

Pressure Cuff

Pressure cuff can be placed around the soft-walled infusion bag and the cuff inflated to a suitable level. Infusion rates can be varied by altering the pressure around the cuff.

Pressure Controlled Pump

Hamou has developed a pressure-limited rotatory pump (Hysteromat). The rate of infusion can be altered by varying the pressure the pump can produce (Garry,1995).

Special Fluid Pump

A fluid pump is used to distend the uterus which includes a blood pressure monitor which preselects the maximum pressure for the pump at or slightly below the mean arterial pressure for the patient (awaiting patent).

COMPLICATIONS

The most alarming complications after hysteroscopy are due to fluid overload, bleeding and uterine trauma. An accepted range of complications during surgical hysteroscopy is 3.8%.

Mechanical Complications

Mechanical complications include perforation and cervical trauma. Risk factors include cervical stenosis, severe uterine anteflexion or retroflexion, infection, myomas of the lower uterine segments and synechiae.

A proper clinical examination and determination of the cervical angle and position of the uterus may limit the complications associated with cervical dialatation. Alternately a vaginoscopic-guided or an ultrasonic-guided entry may limit the said complication.

Uterine perforations can occur during operative maneuvers especially the region of the cornua. In general, a small midline or fundal injury with a blunt instrument with minimal bleeding may be of no grave significance but lateral rents or injuries of the lateral walls, or injuries with electrosurgical instruments may need diagnostic laparoscopy or interventional radiology or angiography to evaluate injury to the uterus as well as to the surrounding viscera.

Whenever electrical or laser injury to the viscera is suspected, laparoscopy or laparotomy is required for complete evaluation. For procedures in which electrical or laser energy is used, the surgical tip should be always kept in direct view to avoid inadvertent thermal injury.

In cases of electrosurgical energy being used, especially monopolar energy, proper grounding of the current is a must to prevent distal site injuries to the patient though the newer generation of electrosurgical units are programmed to stop function in the event of faulty grounding of current.

Media-Related Complications

Fluid Overload

Risk factors for clinically significant intravasation of fluid include prolonged operative procedures, use of large volumes of low-viscosity media, resection of large fibroids or adhesiolysis for advanced Asherman's syndrome involving the opening up of uterine venous channels or unidentified perforations.

Intravasation can occur when the intrauterine pressure is greater than the patient's mean arterial pressure.

Nonelectrolyte hypotonic media which are nonconductive are most often used for the prolonged complicated electrosurgical procedures. These media have serious adverse effects especially when large volumes of these solutions are absorbed, hyponatremia, hypervolemia, hypotension, pulmonary edema, cerebral edema and cardiovascular collapse can occur. Accurate monitoring of the input and output of the media is the key to prevent overload as also early detection of the signs of overload (parotid sign).

For every liter of hypotonic media absorbed the patient's serum sodium decreases by 10 mEq/L. If the patient's sodium level is less than 120 mEq/L changes due to hyponatremia such as cerebral edema, seizures, even death can occur. In general, if the fluid deficit is greater than 1500 mL or if the sodium level is less than 125 mEq/L the procedure should be terminated. Forced diuresis with furosemide, fluid restriction and administration of 3% sodium chloride at a rate to correct hyponatremia by 1.5–2 mOsm/L/h may be instituted.

In cases with evidence of pulmonary edema, corrective medical measures along with a delayed extubation may be indicated. Serum ammonia levels may also be needed to be monitored as ammonia is a byproduct of glycine in the body. Temporary visual disturbances have also been reported in cases of glycine overload.

Gas Embolism

Gas embolism is one of the major complications reported; though using carbon dioxide gas in hysteroscopy as distention medium is not so popular as the other distention media available; when used, the intrauterine pressure should be maintained below 100 mm Hg with maximal flow rates less than 100 mL/min.[19] Air embolism can occur even with the use of other media especially when the circuits show presence of air which is inadvertently pushed under pressure.

When gas embolism occurs circulatory collapse can occur. If an embolus is suspected because of a change in patient's vital signs (hypotension, tachycardia, desaturation, decreased end tidal CO_2), the hysteroscope should be removed, patient's positioned on the left side and an intravenous bolus of sodium chloride solution should be delivered as a first line treatment. Further evaluation with echocardiography and cardiopulmonary resuscitation are attempted. Percutaneous aspiration of the embolus has been reported.

Uterine Trauma, Perforation and Bleeding

Bleeding during or after surgery is the second most common complication of hysteroscopy (0.25%). Distention media themselves may yield enough pressure to cause hemostasis during a procedure. In addition, the coagulating effects of surgical instruments can aid in controlling the bleeding.

If the bleeding persists after surgery, Foley's catheter filled with 15–30 mL of fluid can be inserted into the cavity and removed 24 hours later. Vasopressin and misoprostol are alternate medications that can help with vasoconstriction and uterine contractions. As the last resort embolization of the uterine artery or hysterectomy is an option for definitive management.

SEQUELAE

Reformation of Adhesions

Follow-up tests (USG monitoring of endometrial lining, hysteroscopy) are necessary to ensure that adhesions have not been reformed. Further, surgery may be necessary to restore a normal uterine cavity. According to a recent study among 61 patients, the overall rate of adhesion recurrence was 27.9% and in severe cases, this was 41.9%.[21] Another study found that postoperative adhesions reoccur in close to 50% of severe AS and in 21.6% of moderate cases.[7] Mild intrauterine adhesions, unlike moderate-to-severe synechiae, do not appear to reform.

Abnormal Placentation

Patients who carry a pregnancy even after the treatment of intrauterine adhesions, may have an increased risk of having abnormal placentation including placenta accreta,[20,22] where the placenta invades the uterus more deeply, leading to complications in placental separation after delivery. Abnormal adherent placenta (placenta accreta, increta) may require a cesarean hysterectomy. Premature delivery,[21] second-trimester pregnancy loss[22] and uterine rupture[23,24] are other reported complications. They may also develop incompetent cervix.

Weakening of the Uterine Wall

There are certain studies which mention that the scarred uterus following treatment for Asherman's syndrome is more prone to uterine rupture during delivery but more definitive studies are required to support this. As most of the pregnancies following Asherman's syndrome correction are cases of infertility; they are most often delivered by elective cesarean section.

Role of Lateral Metroplasty

Palmer and Meylan (1964) described three types of uterine hypoplasia:

1. *Simple hypoplasia*: The form of the uterus is normal, but it is small-scaled.
2. *Elongated hypoplasia*: The uterus has a normal or elongated length, but it has a narrow fundus.
3. *Malformative hypoplasia*: Arcuate fundus, T-shaped (seen in 31% of cases), or a Y-shaped uterus (has the worst prognosis). Moreover, restrictions in the form of a constriction ring may be seen in the mid-uterus in addition to the coexistence of irregular uterine contours, dilatations, adhesions, rudimentary horns, and diverticulae. The enlarging hysteroscopic metroplasty is performed early in the follicular phase. The principle is based upon incising with a hook the lateral spurs (including the myometrium) and the arcuate fundus to a depth of 7 mm in order to obtain an increase in the size of the uterus and ameliorate its shape while avoiding as much as possible the perforation of the uterus or the fundus.

Garbin et al. (1998) published the reproductive outcome results before and after the enlarging hysteroscopic metroplasty performed on 24 cases. We can see a decrease in the rates of abortion from 88% to 12.5%. And the rates of term deliveries were increased from 3% to 87.5%.

Similarly, Barranger et al. (2002) evaluated the reproductive outcome on 29 cases; 21 women (72.4%) had 30 pregnancies (follow-up for 13–67 months). Thirteen of them gave birth to 16 live infants. In this study, the rates of delivery increased from 3.8% to 63.2%.

After 18 years of publishing his results in 1998, Garbin O et al. (2006) believe that the enlarging hysteroscopic metroplasty should not be proposed as a first-line treatment in patients having a dysmorphic uterus except in specific cases such as before enrollment in an Assisted Reproductive Technique Program, in order to decrease the possibility of implantation failure, or in the case of a nulligravida of advanced age.

Sequelae

In fact, the enlarging hysteroscopic metroplasty is not innocuous. Since it may create cervical fragilization (Garbin, 1998) apart from the cervical incompetence, thus, necessitating the insertion of a cervical cerclage in order to prevent 2nd trimester pregnancy loss. Moreover, the incision on the myometrium weakens the uterus and makes it more prone to uterine rupture. So, pregnancy in such a uterus must be considered a high-risk pregnancy.

Of course, complications are not limited to the enlarging hysteroscopic metroplasty alone, since the hysteroscopic septoplasty may be complicated by uterine perforation which occurs either during dilatation of cervix, or during the resection of septum. There is also a risk of visceral burns if perforation is not detected. For this reason, some authors recommend a concomitant intraoperative sonography or laparoscopy.

Sentilhes L et al. (2006) observed that the time interval between hysteroscopic septoplasty and a subsequent pregnancy varied from one month to 5 years with an average delay of 16 months. Uterine rupture occurred in pregnancies between 19 weeks and 41 weeks of gestation, even in the absence of labor (in 12 out of the 18 cases reported) thus, exposing the maternal and fetal prognosis to high-risks. In his study, he denoted that the two most important factors that may increase the likelihood of uterine rupture are—the use of monopolar electrosurgery and perforating the uterus while resecting the septum. So, instead of using monopolar electrosurgery, he encourages the use of a coaxial bipolar electrode for a safer resection.

In addition to the mechanical complications already mentioned, post-hysteroscopic endometritis occurs in 1–5% of cases, thus justifying the systematic use of intraoperative prophylactic antibiotics. In order to avoid during hysteroscopy, the intravascular passage of a significant quantity of irrigation fluid which can lead to hemodilution, adherence to the procedural protocol is essential with a meticulous monitoring of the inflow and outflow of fluids.

DISCUSSION

Hysteroscopic adhesiolysis is a safe and effective procedure for restoring the normal menstrual pattern and fertility.[25,26]

The initial severity of the adhesions appears to correlate best with the reproductive outcome. Adhesions after suturing the uterine cavity after open myomectomy or open surgery seem to cause maximum damage and yield poor results in both hysteroscopic correction and reproductive performance.

The outcome of hysteroscopic adhesiolysis for Asherman's syndrome is significantly affected by recurrence of intrauterine adhesions. Further research in Asherman's syndrome should be directed toward reduction of adhesion reformation with a view to improving outcome. The extent of adhesion formation is critical. Mild-to-moderate adhesions can usually be treated with success.

Extensive obliteration of the uterine cavity or fallopian tube openings (ostia) and deep endometrial or myometrial trauma may require several surgical interventions and/or hormone therapy or even be uncorrectable. Pregnancy and live birth rate has been reported to be related to the initial severity of the adhesions with 93, 78, and 57% pregnancies achieved after the treatment of mild, moderate and severe adhesions, respectively and resulting in 81, 66, and 32% live birth rates, respectively.[7] The overall pregnancy rate after adhesiolysis was 60% and the live birth rate was 38.9% according to one study.[27]

Age is another factor contributing to fertility outcomes after treatment of Asherman's syndrome. For women under 35 years of age treated for severe adhesions, pregnancy rates were 66.6% compared to 23.5% in women older than 35.[21]

After successful lysis of intrauterine adhesions, normal menstruation resumes in 78–92% of women; another 8–9% may have menses relatively light or short in duration (hypomenorrhea).[27] The incidence of spontaneous abortion after lysis of intrauterine adhesions (15–43%) is generally lower than that reported before the treatment (24–87%).[28,29] The incidence of preterm delivery (2%), placenta previa (1%), stillbirth (1%), postpartum hemorrhage or retained placenta (4%) is generally low.

HYSTEROSCOPY UNDER GUIDANCE

Laparoscopy

Laparoscopy is a commonly used method for monitoring hysteroscopic adhesiolysis. When the uterine wall becomes unduly thin, it will permit transmission of light across the uterine wall, and there will be a bulge over the remaining serosal layer, which signifies that further hysteroscopic surgery must immediately stop. It has the advantage of detecting the perforation immediately, preventing any further trauma to pelvic organs. Laparoscopy may also provide an opportunity to inspect the pelvis, to diagnose and treat any concurrent pathology such as endometriosis or adhesions.

Fluoroscopic Control

Broome and Vancaillie[30] described a fluoroscopically guided hysteroscopic division of adhesions for an obliterated uterine cavity where several isolated pockets were located near the fundus. This technique provides an intraoperative fluoroscopic view of pockets of endometrium behind an otherwise blind-ending endocervical canal in women with severe Asherman syndrome.

Gynecoradiologic Uterine Resection (GUR)

One group[31,32] reported the use of a special catheter inserted into the cavity through the cervix with a balloon attached to its tip. Radioopaque dye was injected through a side channel of the catheter to delineate the uterine cavity with its adhesions and hysteroscopic scissors were introduced through a central channel of the catheter to divide the adhesions. This was described as an ambulatory technique resulting in minimal discomfort; however, the effectiveness of this procedure needs to be further evaluated The disadvantage of this method relates to radiation exposure.

Transabdominal Ultrasound Guidance

When there are severe adhesions in the uterine cavity, it may be very difficult to identify the cavity without ultrasound. Transabdominal ultrasonography provides efficient monitoring of the Hysteroscopic procedure and guiding the scope toward the uterine cavity even when the adhesions may have completely or almost completely obliterated the uterine cavity.

OTHER TECHNIQUES

Pressure Lavage Under Guidance (PLUG)

Coccia et al.[33] developed a technique based on sonohysterography, in which a continuous intrauterine injection of saline solution led to mechanical disruption of intrauterine adhesions. This technique may be more suitable for patients with mild adhesions.

Conversion of a "Blind" Hysteroscopic Procedure to a "Septum" Division

McComb and Wagner [34] used a variant hysteroscopic technique in patients with severe intrauterine adhesions. The indication in all the cases was lack of communication between the cornua and the cervical canal as shown by HSG. This method was performed hysteroscopically with concomitant laparoscopic guidance. A 5 mm hysteroscope was introduced with fluid used as the distending medium. A Pratt cervical dilator (gauge 13F) was passed through the cervix with the curved tip pointing laterally toward the uterine cornu. The dilator was aligned with the plane of the uterine corpus. The limit of passage was determined by the bulging of the cornua as seen by laparoscopy. This maneuver was performed bilaterally for a completely obliterated cavity. Thus, bilateral passage of the cervical dilator converted the obliterated uterine cavity into the configuration of a uterine "septum."

The scar was cut with hysteroscopic scissors in side-to-side swaths, from one lateral passage to the other, until the fundus was reached and the uterine cavity had been liberated.

Myometrial Scoring Technique

Protopapas et al.[35] and Capella-Allouc et al.[36] reported a myometrial scoring technique for the treatment of severe Asherman syndrome associated with the presence of dense intrauterine adhesions and marked reduction in the size of the uterine cavity. This technique aims to restore the normal size and shape of the uterine cavity and uncover functional endometrium by making six to eight 4 mm deep longitudinal incisions into the myometrium with two or three lateral incisions from the fundus to the isthmus on both the sides and two or three transverse incisions at the fundus. The procedure stops at that point even if the ostia are not visible. The surgery is monitored by either concomitant laparoscopy or abdominal ultrasound scan. At the end of the surgery, the cervix is dilated up to Hegar 12–18 to reduce the likelihood for postoperative cervical stenosis.

Balloon fluoroscopy as treatment for intrauterine adhesions: a novel approach.[37]

Hysteroplasty, using standard interventional radiographic techniques, may provide an alternative treatment modality for patients with intrauterine adhesions and lower uterine defects from prior cesarean deliveries in select cases.

REFERENCES

1. Fritsch H, Ein Fall von volligem. Schwaund der Gebormutterhohle nach Auskratzung. Who Named It? Zentralbl Gynaekol. 1894;18:1337-42.
2. Asherman JG. Traumatic intra-uterine adhesions. J Obstet Gynaecol Br Em. 1948;55(2):2-30.
3. Dmowski WP, Greenblatt RB. Asherman's syndrome and risk of placenta accreta. Obstet Gynecol. 1969;34(2):288-99.
4. Rabau E, David A. Intrauterine adhesions: etiology, prevention, and treatment. Obstet Gynecol. 1963;22:626-9.
5. Toaff R. Some remarks on post-traumatic uterine adhesions in French. Rev Fr Gynecol Obstet. 1966;61(7):550-52.
6. Ventolini G, Zhang M, Gruber J. Hysteroscopy in the evaluation of patients with recurrent pregnancy loss: a cohort study in a primary care population. Surg Endosc. 2004;18(12):1782-4.
7. Valle RF, Sciarra JJ. Intrauterine adhesions: hysteroscopic diagnosis, classification, treatment and reproductive outcome. Am J Obstet. 1988;158(6Pt1):1459-70.
8. Klein SM, Garcia C-R. Asherman's syndrome: a critique and current review. Fertility and Sterility. 1973;24(9):722-35.
9. Bukulmez O, Yarali H, Gurgan T. Total corporal synechiae due to tuberculosis carry a very poor prognosis following hysteroscopic synechialysis. Hum Reprod. 1999;14(8):1960-1.

10. Schenker JG, Margalioth EJ. Intrauterine adhesions: an updated appraisal. Fertility and Sterility. 1982;37(5):593-610.
11. Rochet Y, Dargent D, Bremond A, Priou G, Rudigoz RC. The obstetrical outcome of women with surgically treated uterine synechiae (in French). J Gynecol Obstet Biol Reprod. 1979;8(8):723-6.
12. Krolikowski A, Janowski K, Larsen JV. Asherman syndrome caused by schistosomiasis. Obstet Gynecol. 1995;85(5Pt2):898-9.
13. Netter AP, Musset R, Lambert A, Salomon Y. Traumatic uterine synechiae: a common cause of menstrual insufficiency, sterility, and abortion. Am J Obstet Gynecol. 1956;71(2):368-75.
14. Kodaman PH, Arici AA. Intrauterine adhesions and fertility outcome: how to optimize success? Curr Opin Obstet Gynecol. 2007;19(3):207-14.
15. Schenker JG. Etiology of and therapeutic approach to synechia uteri. Eur J Obstet Gynecol Reprod Biol. 1996;65:109-13.
16. Knopman J, Copperman AB. Value of 3D ultrasound in the management of suspected Asherman‘s syndrome. J Reprod Med. 2007;52:1016-22.
17. Doyle MB, Lavy G. Intrauterine synechiae and pregnancy loss. Infertil Reprod Med Clin North Am. 1991;2:91-103.
18. Orhue AAE, Aziken ME, Igbefoh JO. A comparison of two adjunctive treatments for intrauterine adhesions following lysis. Int J Gynecol Obstet. 2003;82:49-56.
19. Morrison DM. Management of hysteroscopic surgery complications. AORN J. 1999;69(1):194-7,199-209;quiz 210,213-5,21.
20. Yu D, Li T, Xia E, Huang X, Peng X. Factors affecting reproductive outcome of hysteroscopic adhesiolysis for Asherman's syndrome. Fertility and Sterility. 2008;89(3):715-22.
21. Fernandez H, Al Najjar F, Chauvenaud-Lambling, et al. Fertility after treatment of Asherman‘s syndrome stage 3 and 4. J Minim Invasive Gynecol. 2006;13(5):398-402.
22. Roge P, D‘ercole C, Cravello L, Boubli L, Blanc B. Hysteroscopic management of uterine synechiae: a series of 102 observations. Eur J Obstet Gynecol Reprod Biol. 1996;65(2):189-93.
23. Capella-Allouc S, Morsad F, Rongieres-Bertrand C, et al. Hysteroscopic treatment of severe Asherman‘s syndrome and subsequent fertility. Hum Reprod. 1999;14(5):1230-3.
24. Deaton JL, Maier D, Andreoli J. Spontaneous uterine rupture during pregnancy after treatment of Asherman‘s syndrome. Am J Obstet Gynecol. 1989;160 (5Pt1):1053-4.
25. Pabuçcu R, Atay V, Orhon E, Urman B, Ergün A Hysteroscopic treatment of intrauterine adhesions is safe and effective in the restoration of normal menstruation and fertility. Fertil Steril. 1997;68(6):1141-3.
26. Siegler AM, Valle RF. Therapeutic hysteroscopic procedures. Fertil Steril. 1988;50(5):685-701.
27. Goldenberg M, Sivan E, Sharabi Z, et al. Reproductive outcome following hysteroscopic management of intrauterine septum and adhesions. Hum Reprod. 1995;10:2663-5.

28. Cooper JM, Brady RM. Late complications of operative hysteroscopy. Obstet Gynecol Clin North Am. 2000;27:367-74.
29. Sandridge DA, Councell RB, Thorp JM. Endometrial carcinoma arising within extensive intrauterine synechiae. Eur J Obstet Gynecol Reprod Biol. 1994;56:147-9.
30. Broome JD, Vancaillie TG. Fluoroscopically guided hysteroscopic division of adhesions in severe Asherman syndrome. Obstet Gynecol. 1999;93:1041-3.
31. Gleicher N, Pratt D, Levrant S, Rao R, Balin M, Karande V. Gynaecoradiological uterine resection. Hum Reprod. 1995;10:1801-3.
32. Karande V, Levrant S, Hoxsey R, Rinehart J, Gleicher N. Lysis of intrauterine adhesions using gynecoradiologic techniques. Fertil Steril. 1997;68:658-62.
33. Coccia ME, Becattini C, Bracco GL, Pampaloni F, Bargelli G, Scarselli G. Pressure lavage under ultrasound guidance: a new approach for outpatient treatment of intrauterine adhesions. Fertil Steril. 2001;75:601-6.
34. McComb PF, Wagner BL. Simplified therapy for Asherman's syndrome. Fertil Steril. 1997;68:1047-50.
35. Protopapas A, Shushan A, Magos A. Myometrial scoring: a new technique for the management of severe Asherman's syndrome. Fertil Steril. 1998;69:860-4.
36. Capella-Allouc S, Morsad F, Rongieres-Bertrand C, Taylor S, Fernandez H. Hysteroscopic treatment of severe Asherman's syndrome and subsequent fertility. Hum Reprod. 1999;14:1230-3.
37. Rebecca J. Chason, Eric D. Levens, Belinda J, Yauger, Mark D Payson, Kenneth Cho, Frederick W. Larsen Balloon fluoroscopy as treatment for intrauterine adhesions: a novel approach. Fertility and Sterility - November 1, 2008.

20

The Incompetent Cervix

Ameya Purandare

A stitch in time saves nine

—An English proverb

Obstetricians often think that the problem of the incompetent cervix is solved. The diagnosis is made without proper examination and at times with history alone. An indiscriminate cerclage of cervix is carried out with a high rate of failure. The psychological impact of repeated fetal wastage is felt by both, the physician and the couple involved. Nicholas Eastman, when he was the editor of Obstetrics and Gynecological Survey commented, "Because cerclage is a simple matter, let not our enthusiasm cloud our diagnostic judgement, otherwise many a cervix will be sutured unnecessarily and to no avail."

HISTORY

The "Torn Cervix" was recognized as the cause of repeated abortions as early as in the 17th century. The term "Cervical Incompetence" was first coined by Gream in 1865, in Lancet, In 1902, Herman[1] reported successful pregnancies in 2 or 3 women treated with Emmet trachelorrhaphy operation. It was in 1948, that Palmer[2] in Europe and in 1950, Lash and Lash[3] in America defined the "Incompetent Cervix". The most important break through occurred in 1955, when Shirodkar[4] reported his first series of cerclage operations during pregnancy using homologous fascia lata. Prior to this, the treatment of incompetent cervix was undertaken only in the nonpregnant state. Within 3 years, in 1957, McDonald[5] simplified the cerclage operation by using nonabsorbable suture at a lower level. In 1965, Benson[6] advocated abdominal approach for cases not suitable for vaginal route because of the loss of cervical lips. Numerous modifications have been devised but in principle the operation can be classified as high or low cerclage, and that performed with tape or string.

DEFINITION

The cervix is labeled "Incompetent" when it is unable to retain an intrauterine gestation until term because of deficiency in structure or function. The physiology of cervical competence is not well understood till the date. The mechanism involves a complex physiological process of uterine muscle rearrangement as well as biochemical changes in the cervix. Equally baffling is the response to trauma. With similar type of trauma the cervix may not produce any physiological alteration in subsequent pregnancy in some cases while in same, it may lead to classical incompetence and yet in others the end result may be stenosis and cervical dystocia.

ETIOLOGY

Cervical incompetence can occur in primigravidae or multigravidae but is more common in the latter. The reported incidence is 1 in 500 to 1 in 2,000 pregnancies although at referral centers it can be as high as 1 in 125 pregnancies. Trauma to the cervix, as judged by retrospective history, forms the main etiologic factor. In the present times, instead of the traumatic labor, the trauma caused by induced abortion or gynecological surgery as a cause, is rising. Congenital malformations of the uterus may be associated with cervical incompetence even when the malformation does not involve the cervical canal. Low placental attachment tends to open up the cervix early. Congenital cervical adenosis and diethylstilbestrol (DES) exposure in intrauterine life have recently been observed as the coexistent factors in a few cases. However, there will remain about 30% cases in which no obvious cause can be pinpointed (Table 20.1).

The modern understanding of cervical incompetence is as follows:

The cervical competence is *an active*, not passive, phenomenon. It is a specific entity involving not just an abnormality or defect of cervical collagen, but is also due to either:

- Absence of the usual cervical musculature in cases of congenital cervical incompetence

TABLE 20.1: Etiological factors for cervical incompetence
Idiopathic (most cases).
Congenital disorders (müllerian duct abnormalities viz. Septate uterus, Bicornuate uterus)
DES exposure in utero.
Connective tissue disorder (Ehlers- Danlos syndrome)
Surgical trauma:
Conization and amputation (resulting in substantial loss of connective tissue, cone biopsy and Fohergill's repair)
Traumatic damage to the structural integrity of the cervix: (repeated forced cervical dilatation associated with D & C)

OR

- Injury or damage to the cervical musculature caused by previous trauma.

PATHOGENESIS

The function of the cervix during pregnancy depends on the regulations of connective tissue metabolism. Collagen is the principal component in the cervical matrix

Others are: Proteoaminoglycans, elastin, fibronectin, etc.

The biochemical events implicated in the cervical ripening are:

- Decrease in total collagen content
- Increase in collagen solubility
- Increase in collagenolytic activity.

DIAGNOSIS

The classical history of a case of cervical incompetence is painless cervical dilatation in the midtrimester with bulging membranes. The membranes later rupture without painful uterine contractions, with the fetus expelled out almost painlessly, being usually alive at birth. In some cases the signs and symptoms may be clear but not so in every instance. Hence, the differential diagnosis from causes of midtrimester fetal loss is extremely important. It is essential to remember that cervical dilatation is the terminal phase of all pregnancy losses and mere presence does not necessarily mean cervical incompetence (Table 20.2).

Preconception diagnosis and correct obstetric history is very important. The accepted sign is an internal os dilated to 8 mm and allowing No. 8, Hegar dilator through without resistance or pain. The other signs like measurement of internal os diameter by hysterography or with rubber balloon test have also been used. However, it is important to remember that none of these signs can be an indicator of incompetent cervix during subsequent pregnancy.

TABLE 20.2: Diagnostic criteria for cervical incompetence
Factors on History
• Painless cervical dilatation with preterm delivery
• Forceful cervical dilatation and evacuation
• *Obstetric trauma:* Cervical lacerations, prolonged second stage followed by CS
• Prior cervical surgery: Cone, loop, amputation
• DES exposure in utero
Cervical sonography
• Short cervical length
• Cervical funneling

The diagnosis is at present largely *subjective* and *retrospective*. If possible, an *objective* (i.e. measurable) diagnosis, made before pregnancy or in the early stages (1st or early 2nd trimester) would provide:

- An accurate incidence of cervical incompetence
- Allow treatment to be targeted appropriately
- Provide the basis for definitive trials of treatment.

Transvaginal ultrasonography is extremely useful in the diagnosis. TVS has provided a reproducible method of evaluating the cervix. In pregnancy it is important to establish a high-risk group with the suspected diagnosis of "Incompetent Cervix". Serial clinical and ultrasonographic examinations are to be carried out after 10 weeks gestation every fortnightly until the 28th week. By transvaginal ultrasonography, the cervix is usually studied in the sagittal longitudinal plane, wherein the endocervical canal will become the most prominent structure. This will outline the anterior-posterior and lateral diameters of the internal os and the length of the closed cervical canal.

For vaginal ultrasonography, the bladder should completely be empty, while for transabdominal ultrasonographic evaluation of internal os diameters the bladder should not be overdistended. At 8th to 10th week, a mean diameter of internal os more than 15 mm or a closed cervical canal less than 20 mm length would be a warning sign. Repeat ultrasonography at the 14th week indicating the internal os diameter more than 20 mm or closed cervical canal length less than 30 mm is a definite parameter for the correct diagnosis and would indicate the need for cerclage operation. At 14th week of gestation, transabdominal ultrasonography and as early as 10th week of gestation, transvaginal ultrasonography will also facilitate the visualization of any congenital fetal anomaly and localization of placenta. If the patient is first seen at 20th week of gestation or latter, an internal os diameter of more than 25 mm and cervical canal length of less than 20 mm will indicate a cervical incompetence. After 28th week of gestation the open cervix is not a criterion of incompetent cervix unless the cervical canal is less than 20 mm in length and the membranes are bulging.

Advantage of Diagnostic Ultrasound

With the aid of ultrasound, accurate measurement of the internal os diameter in its natural condition is possible by taking the mean of anterior-posterior and lateral diameters at the level of internal os. Measurement of the length of closed cervical canal and the lips of the cervix can give a far better prediction of cervical effacement. The digital palpation by an enthusiastic obstetrician may overstretch the soft cervical canal during pregnancy thus giving a false impression of incompetence. Internal os may dilate earlier than the external os in the congenital type. It is difficult to judge the cervical effacement without sonography especially with the cervix torn into small tags. Postoperative digital palpation is painful and inconclusive and herein lies the importance of the ultrasonography for follow-up. Finally, consistent standard norms can

TABLE 20.3: USG criteria for cervical incompetence
• Funneling of the cervix with the changes in forms T, Y, V, U (correlation between the length of the cervix and the changes in the cervical internal os) (Fig. 20.1)
• Cervix length < 25 mm
• Protrusion of the membranes
• Presence of fetal parts in the cervix or vagina

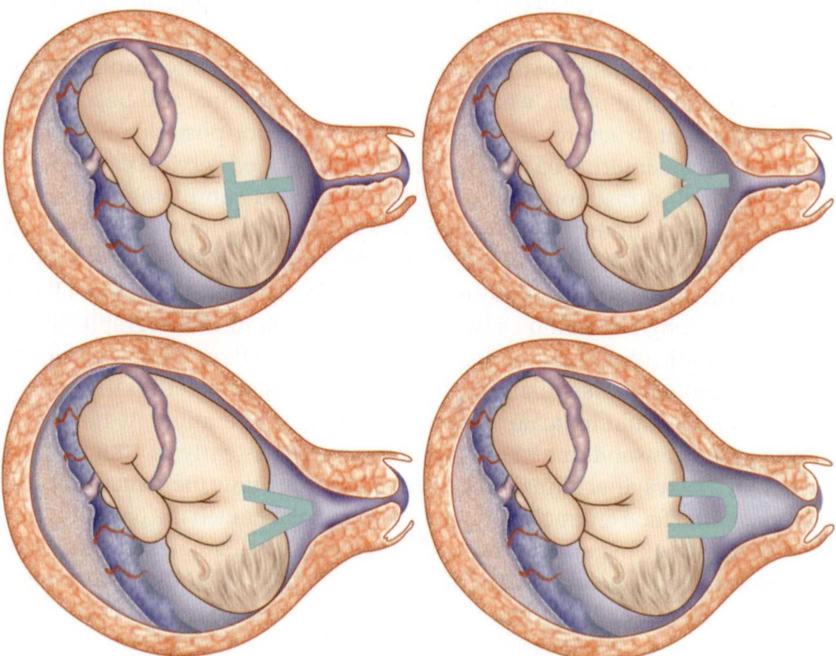

Fig. 20.1: Funneling of the cervix with the changes in forms

be maintained for repeated evaluation with photographic records, while undertaking serial ultrasonographies. Sonography also has the advantage of being a noninvasive procedure.

Iam's et al.[7] suggested that cervical competence is a continuous variable and is indicated indirectly by measurement of the length of the cervix (Table 20.3).

Funneling' or 'Breaking' of the internal cervical os (at rest or particularly in response to trans-abdominal pressure on the uterine fundus) is characteristic of cervical incompetence. USG serial evaluation (every 2 wks) of the cervix for funneling and shortening in response to transfundal pressure has been found to be useful in the evaluation of incompetent cervix.[8]

METHODS OF TREATMENT

Surgical approach to cervical incompetence still remains the mainstay of treatment.

A planned cerclage after definite diagnosis should be the aim of treatment rather than the emergency procedure, as the latter is associated with high failure rate (Table 20.4).

Cerclage should never be performed when the membranes have ruptured; painful uterine contractions have set in, presence of bleeding, evidence of fetal anomaly, and also when the cervix is dilated up to 5 cm or more (Table 20.5).

Amongst these the most commonly performed are the McDonald and Shirodkar cerclages (Table 20.6).

An ideal cerclage suture should have good tensile strength, should be nonirritant, and must not cut through the soft pregnant cervix. It must not slip down allowing effacement of the cervix should easily be identifiable for easy removal and must have elastic memory, to maintain the occlusion. The mersilene (polyester) tape is the best available suture till date, but needs improvement, as it has no elastic memory. Mixing polyester fibers with nylon in desired proportion can produce the adequate elastic memory. The tape

TABLE 20.4: Indications of cerclage
• History compatible with incompetent cervix and
• USG changes or
• Clinical evidence of extensive trauma to cervix

TABLE 20.5: Contraindications of cerclage
• Uterine contractions.
• Uterine bleeding
• Chorioamnionitis
• Premature rupture of membranes (PROM)
• Severe maternal disease
• Fetal anomaly incompatible with life

TABLE 20.6: Types of cerclage procedures		
• McDonald procedure 1957	1957	(Low)
• Shirodkar operation	1955	(High)
• Wurm procedure (Hefner cerclage)	1961	
• Transabdominal cerclage	1965	(High)
• Lash procedure	1950	

TABLE 20.7: Modern classification of cerclage

Terms	*Newer nomenclature*
• Prophylactic, elective	• History-indicated
• Therapeutic, salvage	• USG-indicated
• Rescue, emergency, urgent	• Physical exam indicated

cerclage is superior to the string cerclage as the string invariably cuts through the soft cervical tissue and the high cerclage at the level of internal os gives better result.

TECHNICAL DETAILS (TABLE 20.7)

High Cerclage (Figs 20.2 and 20.3)

The operation is carried out under general anesthesia or low spinal anesthesia. Injection of vasopressin in normal saline keeps the field dry. A transverse incision is made at the cervicovaginal junction in the anterior fornix. The vesicocervical fascia is incised completely and the bladder pushed away from the front of the cervix and retracted up. The ectocervix is exposed up to the level of internal os in the midline as well as laterally. A similar incision is made posteriorly and the rectum pushed down without opening the cul-de-sac peritoneum. A needle carrying the tape is passed by the side of the cervix from anterior to posterior side as high up near the internal os level as possible. The other end of the strip is passed in similar manner on the other side of the cervix taking care that the levels of the needle entry on each side of the cervix is the same in relation to the axis of the cervical canal. Only by this way will the tape be at a right angle to the axis of the cervix. It will have sufficient amount of the parametrium below it to prevent it from slipping down and the thickness of the tape prevents it from cutting through the cervix. The tape ends are tied posteriorly with a surgical knot and the ends kept long for later identification. The vaginal incisions are then closed with absorbable suture material.

Low Cerclage (Fig. 20.4)

The operation is simpler and may even be carried out under local analgesia in cooperative patients. The mersilene string suture no. 4 mounted on a cutting needle is passed submucosally around the cervix at the level of the cervicovaginal junction. The suture is started anteriorly and with five or six bites and returned to its anterior position for tying. The suture ends are kept long for easy removal. Controversy exists about the efficiency of one procedure over the other, which has never been evaluated in prospective controlled trials. In the author's practice, high cerclage has consistently given better results than the low cerclage.

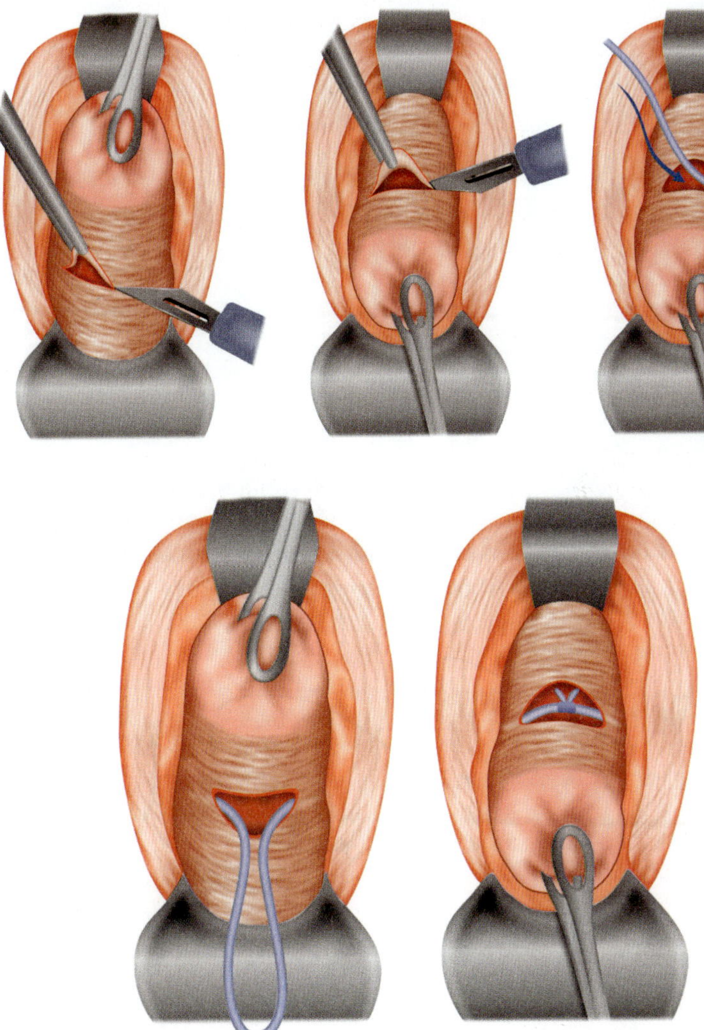

Fig. 20.2: High cerclage Shirodkar's method

Abdominal Cerclage (Figs 20.5 and 20.6)

In cases with absent or badly torn cervical lips the vaginal route is not feasible. Abdominal cerclage as described by Benson could be used whenever indicated by 14th week of gestation. Since the procedure requires gentle levering out the gravid uterus an adequate vertical abdominal incision is preferred. The uterovesical fold of peritoneum is picked up, divided and the bladder retracted down. On the lateral aspect of internal os, one would notice many dilated veins which tend to drain off with the elevation of fundus.

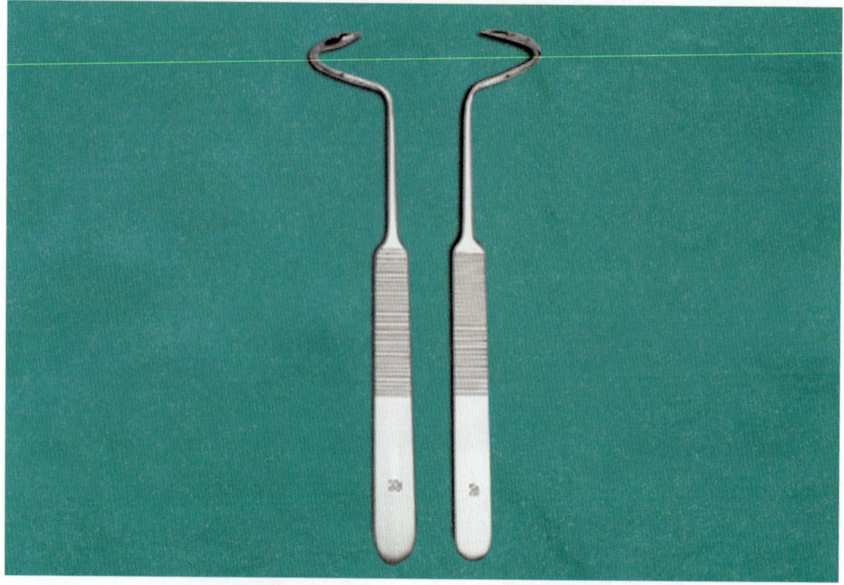

Fig. 20.3: Shirodkar's cerclage needles

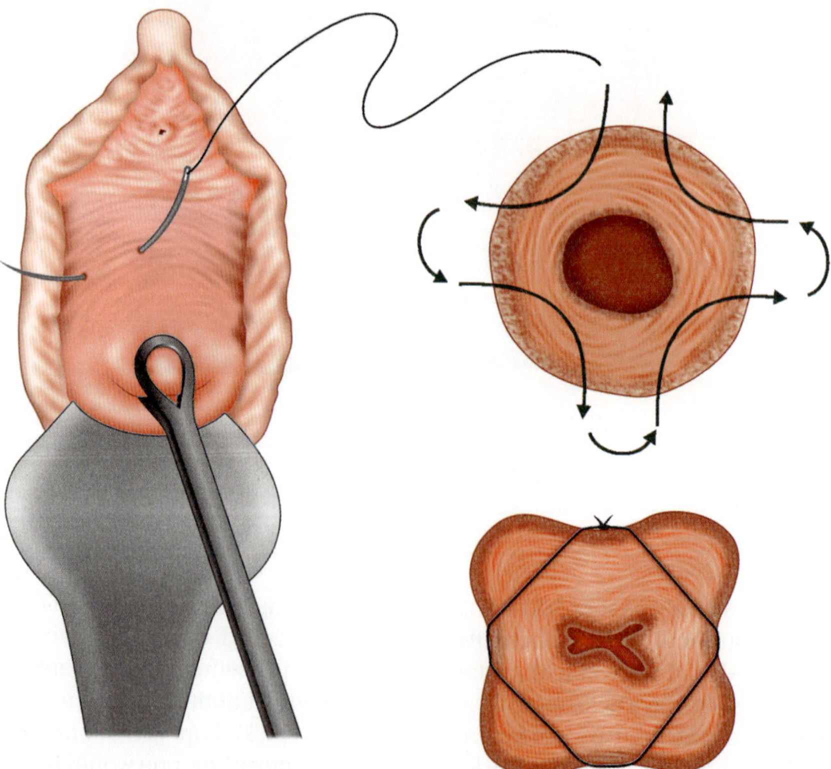

Fig. 20.4: Low cerclage McDonald's method

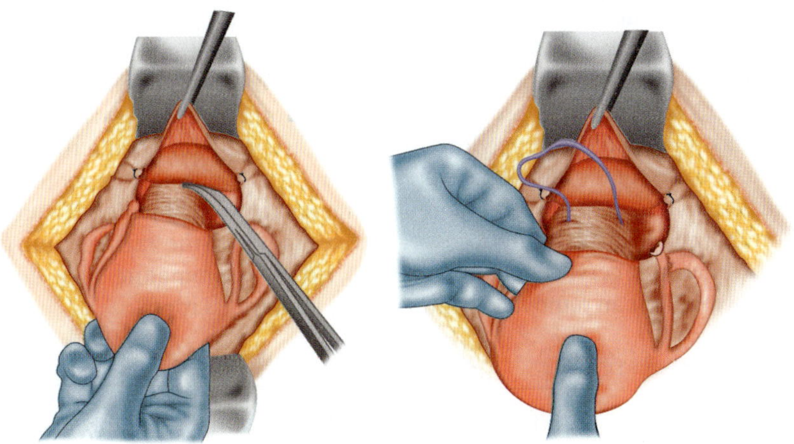

Fig. 20.5: Abdominal cerclage

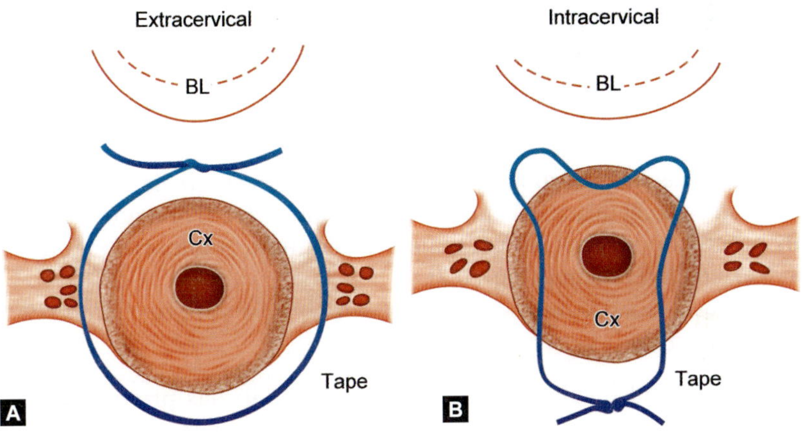

Figs 20.6A and B: Abdominal cerclage includes diagram from present

Careful dissection is performed between the blood vessels and lateral wall of the uterus at the level of the internal os. By placing two fingers of the operator behind the posterior leaf of broad ligament and retraction of the vessels by a retractor a safe puncture of the posterior leaf by curved hemostat is possible. The tape should be tied medial to the blood vessels to prevent their postoperative occlusion and congestion. It is important to note that the tape should be at the same level on each side of the cervix or truly at right angle to the uterine axis. The fundus is then reposited in the abdominal cavity and the tape ends pulled upwards, so that the membranes recede upwards, which is also aided by the assistant's two fingers, milking up the lower portion of the uterus. After knotting the tape with a surgical knot, the ends are anchored to sides and the peritoneum closed. One should never try to push the hemostat bluntly through the leaves of broad ligament, at it would lead to damage to the thin-walled veins on the side of cervix producing torrential uncontrollable hemorrhage, often precipitating uterine contractions. Benson in his original report of 13 cases encountered two cases of serious hemorrhage; recently, Arias[9] has modified the procedure by passing the tape on needle through the musculature of the lateral part of the cervix. This avoids any injury to the blood vessels lateral to the cervix and the surgery is usually bloodless. Usually abdominal cerclage has high success rate as compared to the vaginal route in the worst cases of cervical incompetence. If, however, premature labor does set in, it would mean removal of suture by the abdominal route.

Complications of Cerclage Operation

Cervical cerclage operation can by itself lead to infection, more so, if performed as an emergency. Complications include rupture of membranes, premature onset of labor, placental separation and even rupture of the uterus. Cervical tear or detachment of cervical lip can occur when string suture is used. Strangely enough, in some cases, cervical dystocia is noted after removal of the ligature, needing a Cesarean operation. This shows the unpredictable nature of the cervix.

Emergency Cerclage (Wurm Procedure)

The Hefner cerclage, also known as the Wurm procedure, is used for well advanced cervical dilatation and is usually done with a U or mattress suture. This procedure is especially of benefit when there is minimal amount of cervical length remaining (Fig. 20.7).

Prophylactic Cerclage

Of late the good results of the cerclage operation has prompted many obstetricians to utilize it as prophylaxis for twin pregnancies,[10] for low placental attachment, in cases with past history of premature labors but without cervical signs of incompetence and in cases with open cervix at 28 weeks without evidence of effacement. Prophylactic cerclage is not indicated and its usefulness has not been proved in properly controlled trials. Indeed in one trial[11] it was shown that the untreated cases went further to maturity and the treated cases terminated earlier (20%); 2% aborting immediately due to the operation itself. Prophylactic cerclage gives a false sense of security as the unidentified main etiologic factor will produce abortion in spite of the cerclage. The success rate of cerclage will actually fall by its indiscriminate use. It would be wise to remember that if the only tool you have is a hammer, you tend to see every problem as a nail.

LASH Procedure (Fig. 20.8)

This procedure is to be performed in the non-pregnant state. It is done when cervical trauma has caused an anterior anatomical defect.

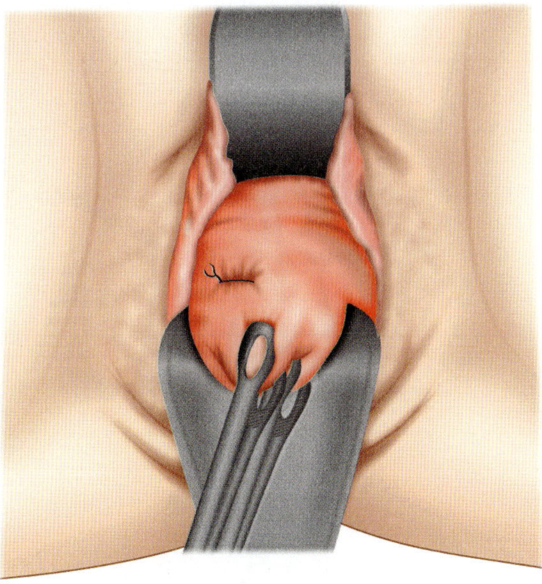

Fig. 20.7: Hefner cerclage

Other alternatives to cerclage that have been considered have included:

- Bedrest, for which little evidence of effectiveness exists
- The use of vaginal pessaries to elevate and close the cervix.

Occlusion Suture (Double Cerclage) (Figs 20.9 and 20.10)

Cervical malfunction may occur in varying degrees, with mechanical, physiological, and immunological factors playing their own parts in maintaining cervical barrier integrity. It is possible that a suture at the level of the internal os may not be sufficient to create an adequate barrier against the ascent of opportunistic organisms, particularly in the presence of a dilated cervical canal. The cervical mucus plug acts as an immunological gatekeeper, protecting the fetoplacental unit against infection from the vagina and plays an important role in preventing the ascent of vaginal organisms that would otherwise predispose to preterm birth. The cervical mucus plug is often lost under these circumstances, prior to the onset of labor. Therefore, insertion of an additional suture at the level of the external os may be of benefit in such cases.

Total cervical occlusion (TCO) was first documented by Saling et al.[12] In 1984 as an effective intervention for women at risk of preterm birth. Subsequently, Shirodkar cerclage and lower cervical occlusion was performed by Professor P Steer[13] and McDonald and lower cervical occlusion was used by McCormack and NJ Secher.[15] Their results demonstrated a 80% chance of live birth in those who underwent cervical occlusion.[12-15]

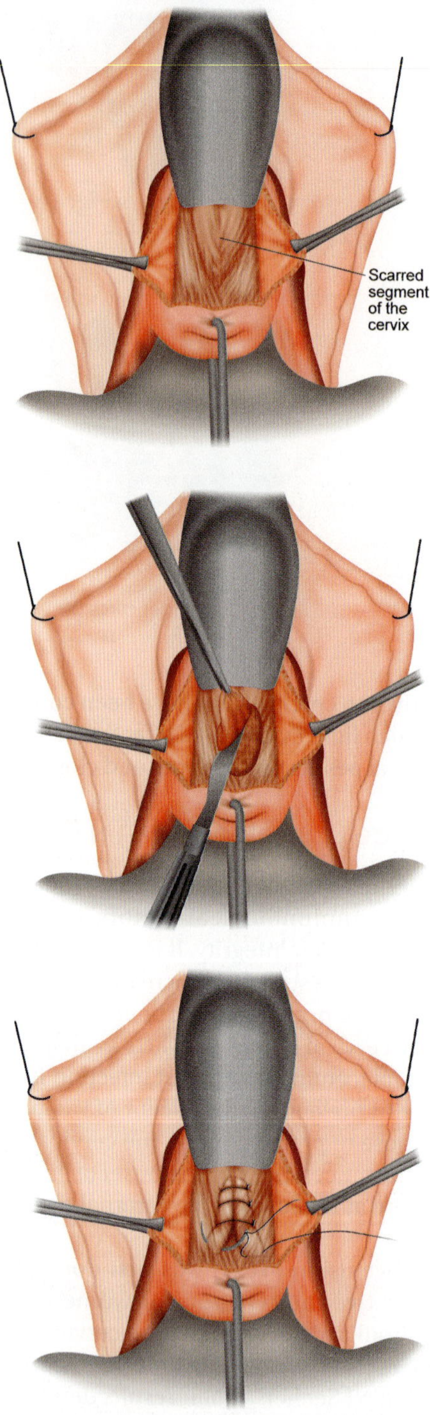

Fig. 20.8: LASH procedure

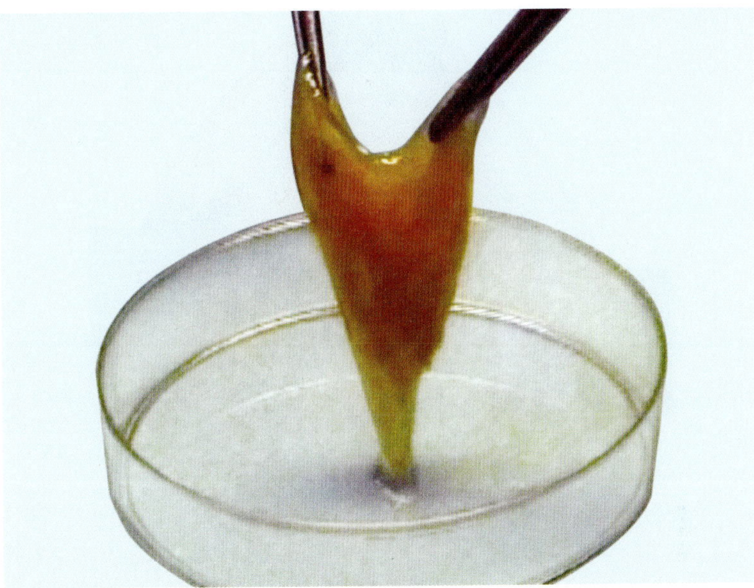

Fig. 20.9: Cervical plug—the gatekeeper for ascending infection

However, confirmation of the value of the procedure can only be achieved with an appropriately designed prospective randomized trial. Such a multicenter trial is now underway in Copenhagen.

EVIDENCE-BASED MEDICINE—RCOG TRIAL

Final report of the multicenter randomized trial of cervical cerclage carried out by Medical Research Council/Royal College of Obstetricians and Gynaecologists (MRC/RCOG Working Party on Cervical Cerclage.) was published in 1993.[14]

The objective of this study was to assess whether cervical cerclage in women deemed to be at increased risk of cervical incompetence prolongs pregnancy and thereby improves fetal and neonatal outcome. Hospitals in the United Kingdom, France, Hungary, Norway, Italy, Belgium, Zimbabwe, South Africa, Iceland, Ireland, the Netherlands and Canada participated in this trial. 1292 pregnant women whose obstetricians were uncertain whether to recommend cervical cerclage, most of whom had a history of early delivery or cervical surgery. Cervical cerclage was compared with a policy of withholding the operation unless it was considered to be clearly indicated.

The results were as follows:

- The overall preterm delivery rate was 28%.
- There were fewer deliveries before 33 weeks in the cerclage group (13% vs 17%), and this difference reflected deliveries characterized by features of cervical incompetence (painless cervical dilatation and prelabor rupture

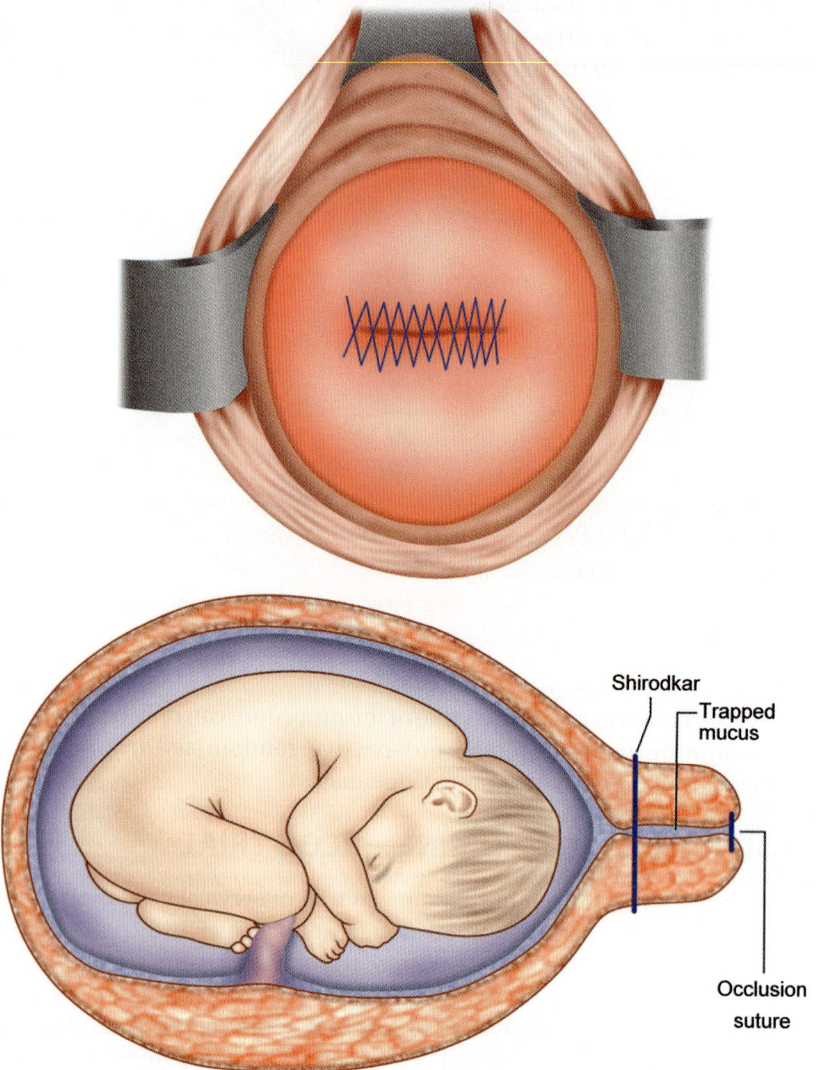

Fig. 20.10: Occlusion procedure

of the membranes). There was a corresponding difference in very low birth weight deliveries (10% vs 13%).

- The difference in the overall rate of miscarriage, stillbirth or neonatal death (9% vs 11%) was less marked and was not statistically significant.
- The use of cervical cerclage was associated with increased medical intervention and a doubling of the risk of puerperal pyrexia.

These results suggest that the operation had an important beneficial effect in 1 in 25 cases in the trial (95% confidence interval (CI) 1 in 12 to 1 in

300 sutures). Its use is associated with increased medical intervention and puerperal pyrexia. Nevertheless, this trial suggests that, on balance, cervical cerclage should be offered to women at high-risk, such as those with a history of three or more pregnancies ending before 37 weeks gestation.

POSSIBLE DEVELOPMENTS

Further research in the physiology of the cervix during pregnancy and labor is badly needed.

The wider use of ultrasonography, preferably with a vaginal probe, to greatly help the diagnostic accuracy.

An ideal suture for cerclage needs to be perfected.

A nonsurgical cervix occluder during pregnancy for cervical incompetence needs to be designed.

To summarize, serial ultrasonography today plays an important role in the early diagnosis and follow-up of treatment. A planned high cerclage rather than an emergency procedure with polyester tape (intermingled with nylon fibers) and use of abdominal route whenever indicated should give a success rate much higher than ever achieved.

REFERENCES

1. Herman CF. Notes on Emmet's operation as a prevention of abortion. Jrnl Obs gynecol Br Commonwealth. 1902;2:256.
2. Palmer R. Lacomme M. Ls beance de L'orifice intene cause d'avortement a repitition? Gynec Obstetrics (Paris). 1948;47:905.
3. Lash AF, Lash SR. Habitual abortion. The incompetent internal os of the cervix. Am J Obstet Gynecol. 59;68-78.
4. Shirodkar VN. A new method of operative treatment for habitual abortions in the second trimester of pregnancy. Antiseptic. 1955;52:299.
5. McDonald IA. Suture of the cervix for inevitable miscarriage. Jrnl Obstet Gynecol Br Emp. 1957;64:346.
6. Benson RC, Durfee RB. Trans-abdominal cervico-uterine cerclage during pregnacy for the treatment of cervical incompetency. Obslet Gynecol. 1965;25:145-55.
7. Iams JD, et al. Cervical competence as a continuum: a study of ultrasonographic cervical length and obstetric performance. Am J Obstet Gynecol. 1995;172(4 Pt 1):1097-103; discussion 1104-6.
8. Guzman ER, et al. A comparison of ultrasonographically detected cervical changes in response to transfundal pressure, coughing, and standing in predicting cervical incompetence. Am J Obstet Gynecol. 1997;177(3):660-5.
9. Arias F. High Risk Pregnacy and Delivery. The Mosby Co. St. Louis, 1984.
10. Dor I, Shaley J, Mashich S, et al. Elective cervical suture of twin pregnancies diagnosed ultrasonographically in the first trimester following induced ovulation. Gynecol Obset Invest. 1982;23:55.
11. Lazar P, Gueguen S. Multi centered controlled trial of cervical cerclage in women at moderate risk of prelerm delivery. Br J Obstet Gynecol. 1984;191:731.

12. Saling E. Prevention of prematurity. A review of our activities during the last 25 years. J Perinat Med. 1997;25:406–17.
13. Noori M, Helmig R, Hein M, Steer P. Could a cervical occlusion suture be effective at improving perinatal outcome? BJOG. 2007;114:532-6.
14. Final report of the Medical Research Council/Royal College of Obstetricians and Gynaecologists multicentre randomised trial of cervical cerclage. MRC/RCOG Working Party on Cervical Cerclage. Br J Obstet Gynaecol. 1993;100(6):516-23.
15. Secher NJ, Weber T, McCormack CD, Hein M, Helmig RB. Cervical occlusion in women with cervical insufficiency: protocol for a randomized controlled trial with cerclage, with and without cervical occlusion. BJOG. 2007;114:649.

21

Operative Vaginal Delivery

Nozer K Sheriar, Ameya Purandare

INTRODUCTION

The second stage of labor is a dynamic event that may require assistance when maternal efforts fail to effect delivery or when there are non-reassuring fetal heart rate patterns. Therefore, the ability to perform an operative vaginal delivery with forceps or vacuum remains a vital skill for those who provide maternity care. The World Health Organization considers operative vaginal delivery to be a critical part of basic emergency obstetric care.[1]

Operative vaginal delivery refers to a delivery in which the operator uses forceps or a vacuum device to assist the mother in transitioning the fetus to extrauterine life. The instrument is applied to the fetal head and then the operator uses traction to extract the fetus, typically during a contraction while the mother is pushing.

Contemporary trends in operative vaginal delivery show increasing numbers of vacuum deliveries and decreasing numbers of forceps deliveries worldwide. Primary drivers of such trends include concerns over neonatal and maternal safety as well as lesser number of modern day obstetricians skilled in forceps use.

Both the American College and the Royal College of Obstetricians and Gynecologists continue to support the use of both vacuum and forceps and strongly encourage residency programs to incorporate the teaching of these skills into their curricula.

PREVALENCE OF USE

Operative vaginal delivery rates have stabilized at between 10% and 13% in the UK, yielding safe and satisfactory outcomes for the majority of mothers and babies.[2,3] Although the overall rates of operative vaginal delivery are dropping, vacuum has emerged as the most popular delivery instrument in the United States. The rate of operative vaginal delivery fell 45%, from 9.4% of live births in 1994 to 5.2% in 2004. Vacuum deliveries comprised 4.1% of all live births in 2004, whereas forceps deliveries dropped dramatically, from 5.5% of births in 1989 to 1.1% in 2004.[4]

Training in forceps use also has decreased, with one study showing that only one half of graduating obstetrics and gynecology residents surveyed felt comfortable performing forceps deliveries in their practice.[5]

However, there has been an increasing awareness of the potential for morbidity for both the mother and the baby. The increased risk of neonatal morbidity in relation to operative vaginal delivery is long established although with careful practice overall rates of morbidity are low. In 1998, the US Food and Drug Administration issued a warning about the potential dangers of delivery with vacuum extractor.[6]

Cesarean section in the second stage of labor is an alternative approach but also carries significant morbidity and implications for future births.

The goal should be to minimize the risk of morbidity and, where morbidity occurs, to minimize the likelihood of serious harm while maximizing maternal choice.

CLASSIFICATION

A standard classification of operative vaginal delivery should be used (Table 21.1). This will enable bench marking, audit and comparison between studies. The American College of Obstetricians and Gynecologists classifications are generally used and define the delivery by station and position.[7]

INDICATIONS AND CONTRAINDICATIONS

The indications and contraindications of operative vaginal delivery are given in Tables 21.2 to 21.4.

PREREQUISITES (TABLE 21.5)

For deliveries in the delivery room, verbal consent should be obtained before an operative vaginal delivery and the discussion documented in the notes. If circumstances allow, written consent may also be obtained. Written consent should be obtained for trial of operative vaginal delivery in theater.

Women should be informed in the antenatal period about operative vaginal delivery, as part of routine antenatal education, particularly women having their first baby when the risk of requiring a forceps or ventouse delivery is higher. This information should include the strategies known to be effective in reducing the need for operative vaginal birth. The birth plan of the mother, including any preferences for or objections to a particular instrument, should be taken into account and discussed.[14]

The goal of operative vaginal delivery is to mimic spontaneous vaginal birth, thereby expediting delivery with a minimum of maternal or neonatal morbidity.

TABLE 21.1: Classification for operative vaginal delivery
Outlet
• Fetal scalp visible without separating the labia
• Fetal skull has reached the pelvic floor
• Sagittal suture is in the anteroposterior diameter or right or left occiput anterior or posterior position (rotation does not exceed 450)
• Fetal head is at or on the perineum
Low
• Leading point of the skull (not caput) is at station plus 2 cm or more and not on the pelvic floor
Two subdivisions
• Rotation of 450 or less from the occipito-anterior position
• Rotation of more than 450 including the occipito-posterior position
Mid
• Fetal head is no more than 1/5th palpable per abdomen
• Leading point of the skull is above station plus 2 cm but not above the ischial spines
Two subdivisions
• Rotation of 450 or less from the occipitoanterior position
• Rotation of more than 450 including the occipito-posterior position
High
Not included in the classification as operative vaginal delivery is not recommended in this situation where the head is 2/5th or more palpable abdominally and the presenting part is above the level of the ischial spines

Adapted from the American College of Obstetrics and Gynecology, 2000.[7]

TABLE 21.2: Indications for operative vaginal delivery[8]
Fetal
• Fetal distress
Maternal
• Maternal fatigue/exhaustion
• To shorten and reduce the adverse effects of the second stage of labor on medical conditions (e.g. cardiac disease NYHA Class III or IV, hypertensive crises, myasthenia gravis, spinal cord injury patients at risk of autonomic dysreflexia, proliferative retinopathy)
• Inadequate progress
– Nulliparous women – lack of continuing progress for 3 hours (total of active and passive second-stage labor) with regional anesthesia, or 2 hours without regional anesthesia
– Multiparous women – lack of continuing progress for 2 hours (total of active and passive second-stage labor) with regional anesthesia, or 1 hour without regional anesthesia
Operators should note that no indication is absolute and should be able to distinguish 'standard' from 'special' indications

TABLE 21.3: Contraindications to operative vaginal delivery[9]
Relative
• Unfavorable attitude of fetal head
• Rotation >45° from occiput anterior or occiput posterior (vacuum)
• Mid-pelvic station
• Fetal prematurity
Absolute
• Non-vertex or brow
• Unengaged head
• Incomplete cervix dilation
• Clinical evidence of cephalopelvic disproportion
• Fetal coagulopathy

TABLE 21.4: Contraindications to use of vacuum for operative vaginal delivery[10]
• Cephalopelvic disproportion
• Fetal head not engaged
• Gestational age less than 34 weeks
• Known fetal conditions that affect bone mineralization or bleeding disorder
• Noncephalic or face presentation
Blood-borne viral infections of the mother are not a contraindication to operative vaginal delivery. However, difficult operative delivery should be avoided where there is an increased chance of fetal abrasion or scalp trauma. It has been suggested that vacuum extractors should not be used at gestations of less than 34 weeks because of the risk of subgaleal and intracranial hemorrhage[11]

Obstetric trainees should receive appropriate training in operative vaginal delivery. Competency should be achieved before conducting unsupervised deliveries and should be monitored regularly thereafter.

An experienced operator, competent at mid-cavity deliveries, should be present from the outset for all attempts at rotational or mid-cavity operative vaginal delivery.

Operative vaginal births that have a higher risk of failure should be considered a trial and conducted in a place where immediate recourse to cesarean section can be undertaken.

Higher rates of failure are associated with [15]:

- Maternal body mass index over 30
- Estimated fetal weight over 4,000 g or clinically big baby
- Occipitoposterior position
- Mid-cavity delivery or when 1/5th of the head palpable per abdomen.

TABLE 21.5: Prerequisites for operative vaginal delivery

- Full abdominal and vaginal examination
  - Head is ≤1/5th palpable per abdomen, vertex presentation
  - Cervix is fully dilated and the membranes ruptured
  - Exact position of the head can be determined so proper placement of the instrument can be achieved
  - Assessment of caput and moulding
  - Pelvis is deemed adequate
  - Irreducible moulding may indicate cephalopelvic disproportion
- Preparation of mother
  - Clear explanation should be given and informed consent obtained
  - Appropriate analgesia is in place for mid-cavity rotational deliveries. This will usually be a regional block. A pudendal block may be appropriate, particularly in the context of urgent delivery
  - Maternal bladder has been emptied recently. In-dwelling catheter should be removed or balloon deflated
  - Aseptic technique
- Preparation of staff
  - Operator must have the knowledge, experience and skill necessary
  - Adequate facilities are available (appropriate equipment, bed, lighting)
  - Back-up plan in place in case of failure to deliver. When conducting mid-cavity deliveries, theater staff should be immediately available to allow a cesarean section to be performed without delay (less than 30 minutes). A senior obstetrician competent in performing mid-cavity deliveries should be present if a junior trainee is performing the delivery
  - Anticipation of complications that may arise (e.g. shoulder dystocia, postpartum hemorrhage)
  - Personnel present that are trained in neonatal resuscitation

* Adapted from the Society of Obstetricians and Gynaecologists of Canada 2004[12] and the Royal Australian and New Zealand College of Obstetricians and Gynaecologists 2009[13,14]
Safe operative vaginal delivery requires a careful assessment of the clinical situation, clear communication with the mother and healthcare personnel and expertise in the chosen procedure.

CHOICE OF INSTRUMENT: FORCEPS VS VACUUM

There are over 700 different models of forceps. There have been no randomized controlled trials comparing different forceps types and it is recognized that the choice is often subjective. The operator should choose the instrument most appropriate to the clinical circumstances and their level of skill.

Rotational delivery with the Kielland forceps carries additional risks and requires specific expertise and training. Alternatives to Kielland forceps include manual rotation followed by direct traction forceps or rotational vacuum extractor.[16] There have been no randomized controlled trials comparing these approaches and the operator should choose an appropriate approach within their expertise. Maintenance of skills in this area may reduce the need for second-stage cesarean section and training should be encouraged.

The relative merits of vacuum extraction and forceps have been evaluated in a Cochrane systematic review of ten randomised controlled trials, involving 2923 primiparous and multiparous women.[17]

Vacuum extraction compared with forceps is:

- More likely to fail delivery with the selected instrument (or 1.7; 95% Ci 1.3–2.2)
- More likely to be associated with cephalhematoma (OR 2.4; 95% CI 1.7–3.4)
- More likely to be associated with retinal hemorrhage (or 2.0; 95% Ci 1.3–3.0)
- More likely to be associated with maternal worries about baby (or 2.2; 95% Ci 1.2–3.9)
- Less likely to be associated with significant maternal perineal and vaginal trauma (or 0.4; 95% Ci 0.3–0.5)
- No more likely to be associated with delivery by cesarean section (or 0.6; 95% Ci 0.3–1.0)
- No more likely to be associated with low 5-minute apgar scores (or 1.7; 95% Ci 1.0–2.8)
- No more likely to be associated with the need for phototherapy (OR 1.1; 95% CI 0.7–1.8).

FORCEPS

Structure (Fig. 21.1)

Forceps have 4 major parts:

1. Blades
2. Shanks
3. Lock
4. Handles

- Blades
  - The blades grasp the fetus.
  - Each blade has a curve to fit around the fetal head (Cephalic curve).
  - The blades are oval or elliptical and can be fenestrated (with a hole in the middle) or solid.
  - Many blades are also curved in a plane 90° from the cephalic curve to fit the maternal pelvis (Pelvic curve).
- Shanks (Fig. 21.2)
  - The shanks connect the blades to the handles and provide the length of the device.
  - They are either parallel or crossing.

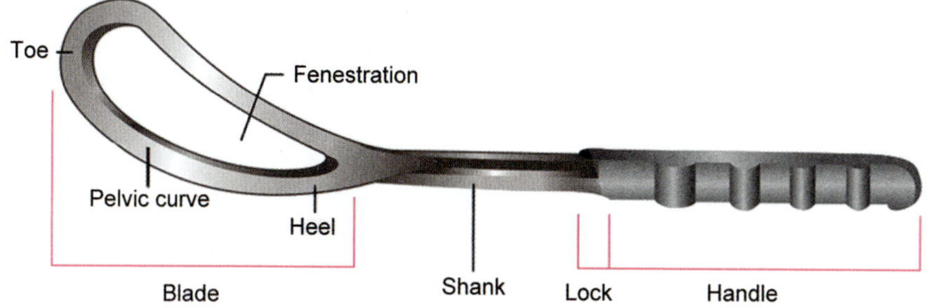

Fig. 21.1: Structure of forceps

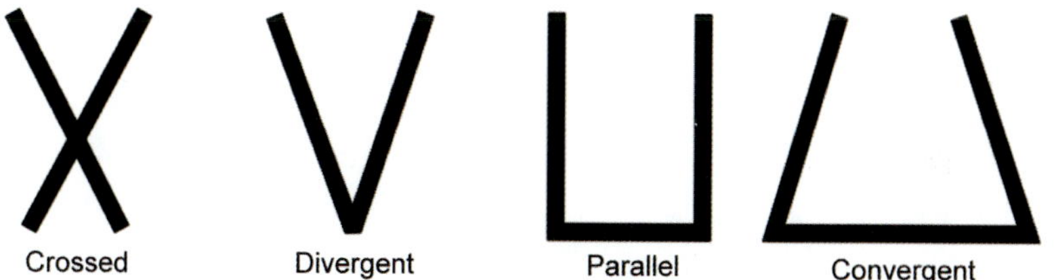

Fig. 21.2: Types of shanks

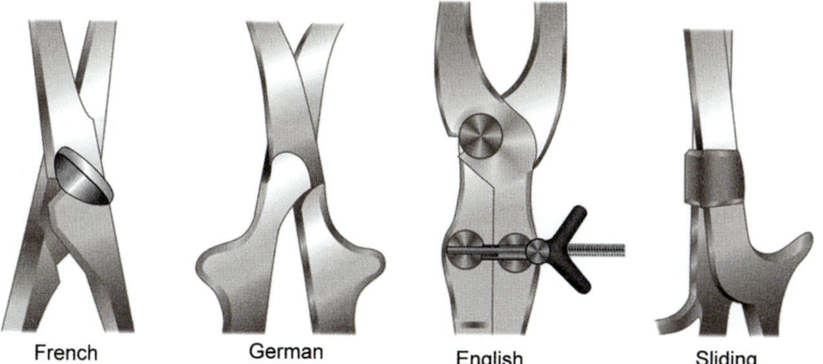

Fig. 21.3: Types of locks

- Lock (Fig. 21.3)
  - The lock is the articulation between the shanks.
  - Many different types have been designed.
- Handles (Fig. 21.4)
  - The handles are where the operator holds the device and applies traction to the fetal head.

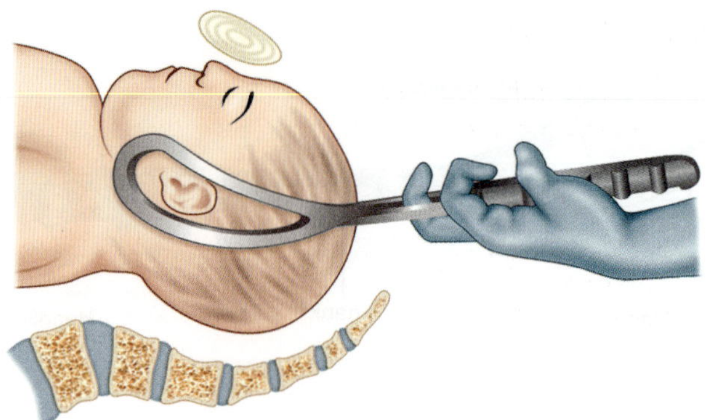

Fig. 21.4: Handle of forceps

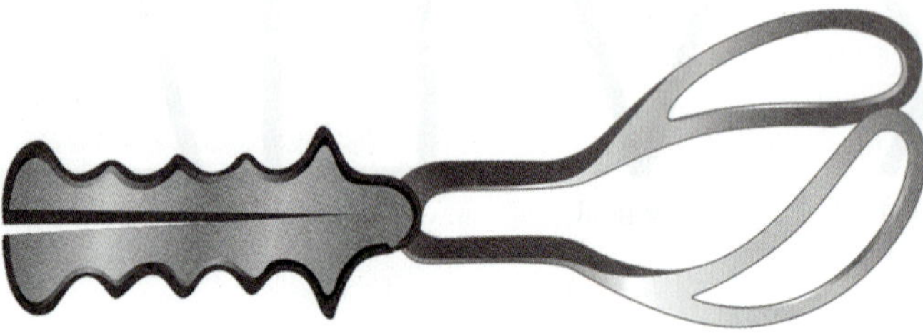

Fig. 21.5: Simpson forceps

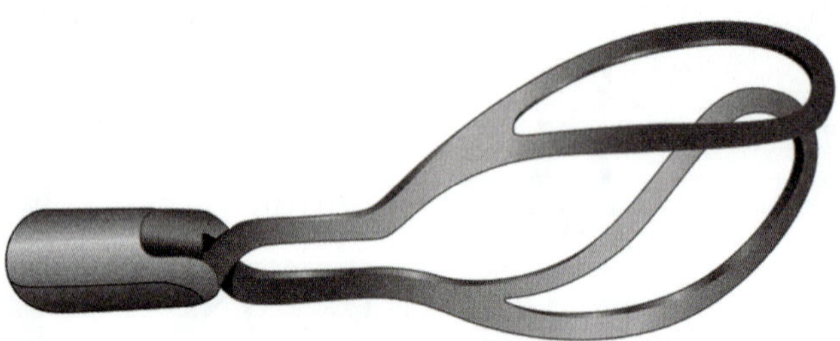

Fig. 21.6: Wrigley forceps

Types of Forceps

More than 700 types of obstetric forceps have been described.

Each of the three main types (outlet, midcavity,or rotational forceps) is appropriate to specific situations and requires differing levels of expertise.

Classical Instruments

- Originally designed by James Young Simpson, Wrigley and George L. Elliot Jr in mid 19th century (Figs 21.5 and 21.6)
- They are commonly used for outlet and low pelvic rotational delivery.

Specialized Instruments

Designed for specific indications like:

- Keilland's forceps for mid-pelvic rotation and correction of asynclitism (Fig. 21.7).
- Piper's forceps for delivery of aftercoming head in breech (Fig. 21.8).
- Laufe's forceps with divergent or parallel blades so designed to limit fetal cranial compression (Fig. 21.9).
- Barnes-Neville and Haig-Ferguson's forceps for axis traction (Figs 21.10 and 21.11).

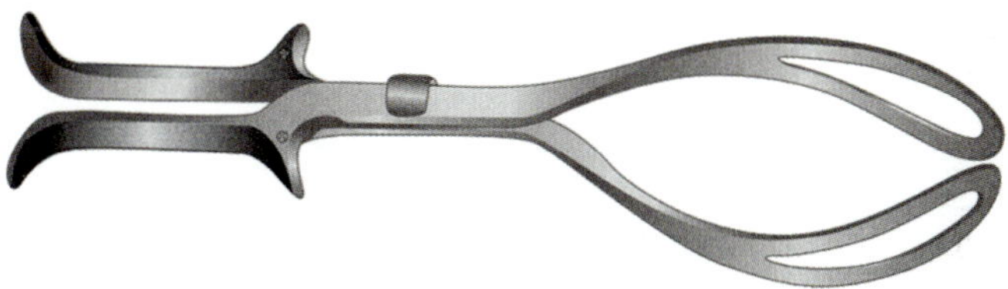

Fig. 21.7: Kielland's forceps

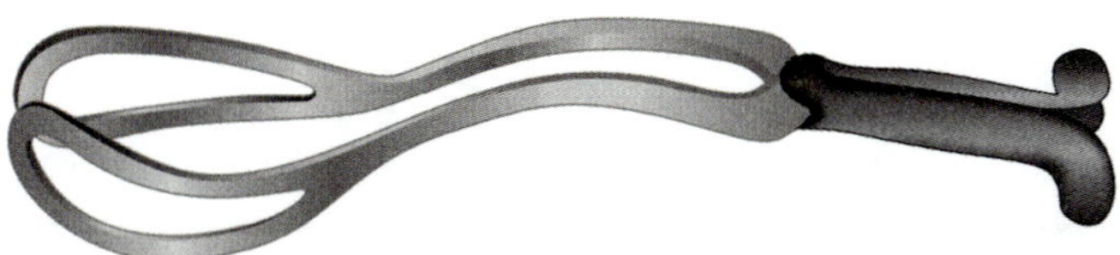

Fig. 21.8: Piper's forceps

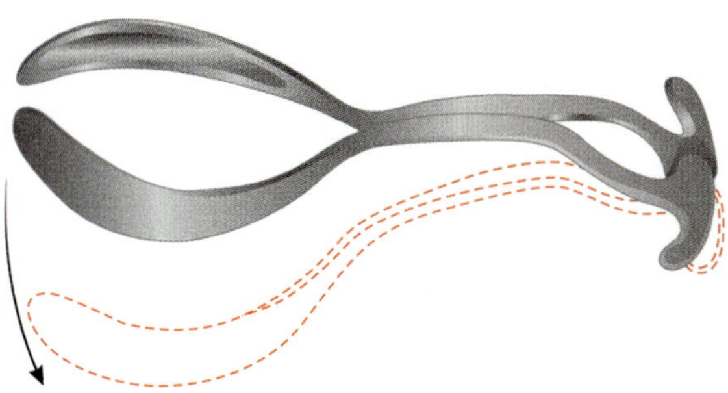

Fig. 21.9: Laufe's forceps

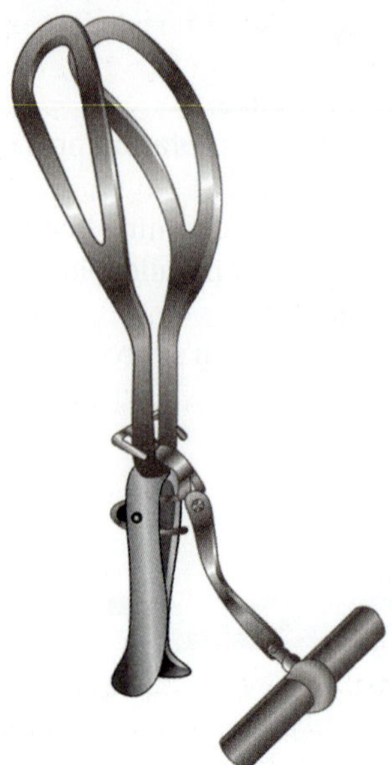

Fig. 21.10: Barnes-Neville forceps

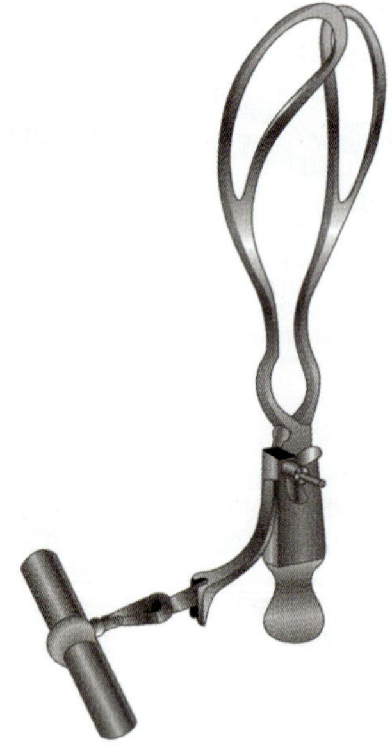

Fig. 21.11: Haig-Ferguson's forceps

Functions of Forceps

- **Traction:** This is the most important function. Pull required in a primigravida is 18 kg and in a multipara it is 13 kg.

- **Compression effect:** This is minimal when properly applied and should not be more than necessary to grasp the head. However, it has some pressure effect on the well-ossified base of the skull.
- **Rotation of head:** This occurs with the use of Keilland's forceps and also in low forceps cephalic application with the occiput in the 2 or 10 'o' clock position.
- **Protective cage:** When applied on a premature baby it protects from the pressure of the birth canal. When applied on the aftercoming head it lessens the sudden decompression effect.
- **As a vectis:** By applying one blade to deliver the head in cesarean section.

Types of Application of Forceps Blades

- Cephalic application
- Pelvic application
  - Cephalic application
    - Blades are applied along the sides of the head, grasping the biparietal diameter in between the widest part of the blades.
    - The long axis of the blades correspond to the occipitomental plane.
    - The ends of the blades lying over the posterior cheeks.
    - The blades should lie symmetrically on both sides of the head.
    - The sagittal suture of the fetal head will be in the middle, and the blades will be equidistant from the sagittal and occipital sutures.
    - At no time should any part of the forceps cover any midline structure.
    - The forceps should lock easily without any force and stand parallel to the plane of the floor.
    - The appropriateness of application should be confirmed before applying traction.
    - The correct cephalic application is with the head in the occiput-anterior (OA) position (Fig. 21.12).
  - Pelvic application.
- The most crucial point of forceps delivery is precise knowledge of the presentation position of the fetus.
- The term pelvic application is used when the left blade is applied on the left side of the pelvis and the right blade is applied on the right side of the pelvis, regardless of the fetal position.
- A pelvic application may be appropriate in some instances, as in a direct occiput posterior presentation.
- Pelvic application is never to be used as a substitute for exact knowledge of the fetal position.
- Inappropriate pelvic application may cause significant harm.
- Serious compression effect on the cranium can occur, so it should be avoided.

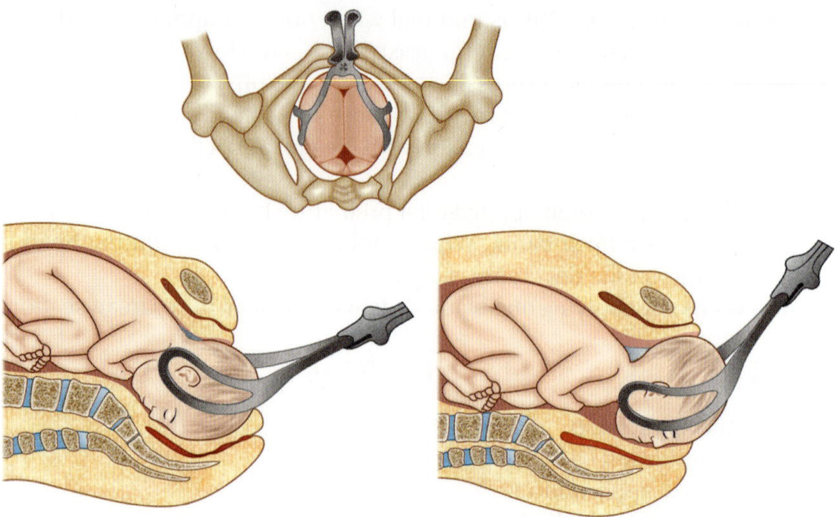

Fig. 21.12: Cephalic and pelvic applications of forceps

When the head is sufficiently rotated, pelvic and cephalic applications naturally coincide and so pelvic application is only justified in low forceps operations.

Traction with Forceps

- During a forceps delivery, traction is applied during contractions.
- The instrument may be used to maintain the station of the fetal head between contractions.
- In an emergency, applying continuous traction may be necessary until the fetal head delivers.
- After confirming proper forceps application, traction starts parallel to the plane of horizon and is then elevated to an almost vertical position as the fetal head extends.
- The amount of traction should be the least necessary to accomplish safe fetal head descent.
- The angle of traction is as important as the force applied in effecting delivery.
- Knowing when to stop and abandon the procedure is a matter of experience.
- Assuming that everything has been done according to proper protocols and no progress is observable in 3 traction attempts, operative vaginal delivery should be discontinued and preparation for abdominal delivery should start as soon as possible (Fig. 21.13).

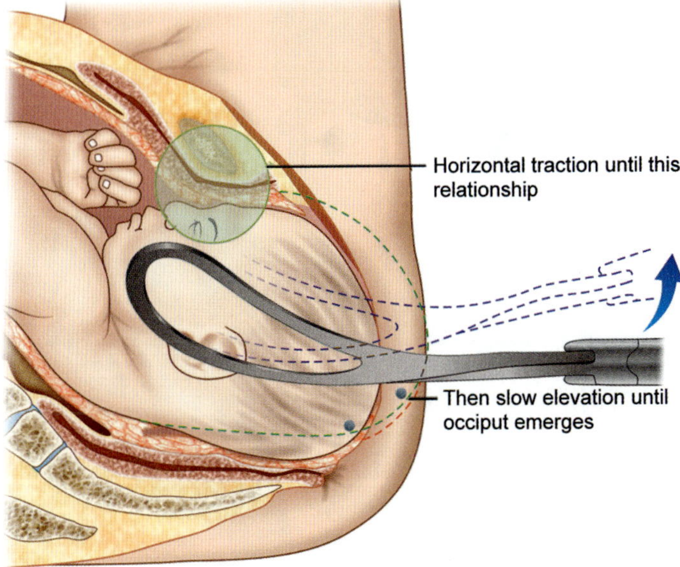

Fig. 21.13: Direction of traction applied during forceps delivery

"ABCDEFGHIJ" Mnemonic for Forceps

A - Address the patient
Ask for help
Anesthesia adequate
B - Bladder empty
C - Cervix fully dilated
D - Determine position
E - Equipment ready
F - Forceps applied
G - Gentle traction
H - Handle elevated to follow the J-shaped pelvic curve
I - Evaluate for Incision for episiotomy when the perineum distends
J - Remove forceps when Jaw is reachable.

Technique of Outlet Forceps

1. Identification of blades and their application:
   - The instrument should be placed in front of the pelvis with the tip pointing upwards and pelvic curve forwards.
   - First the left blade should be applied guided by the right hand (Fig. 21.14).
   - Then the right blade with the left hand (Fig. 21.15).
2. Locking of blades (Fig. 21.16):
   - The blades should articulate with ease indicating correct application.

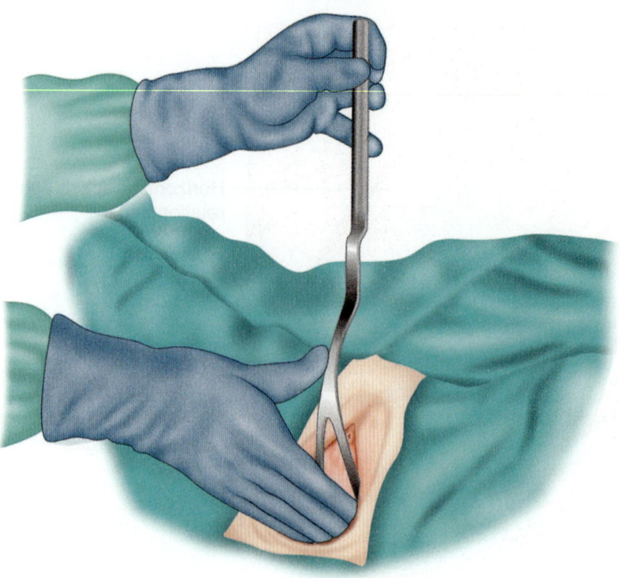

Fig. 21.14: Application of left blade

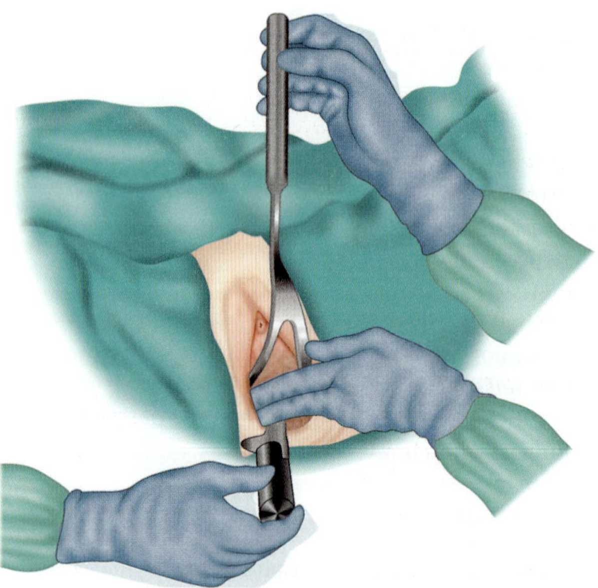

Fig. 21.15: Application of right blade

3. Clinical checks for correct forceps application:
   - Saggital suture lies in the midline of the shanks.
   - The operator is unable to place more than a fingertip between the fenestration of the blade and the fetal head on either side.

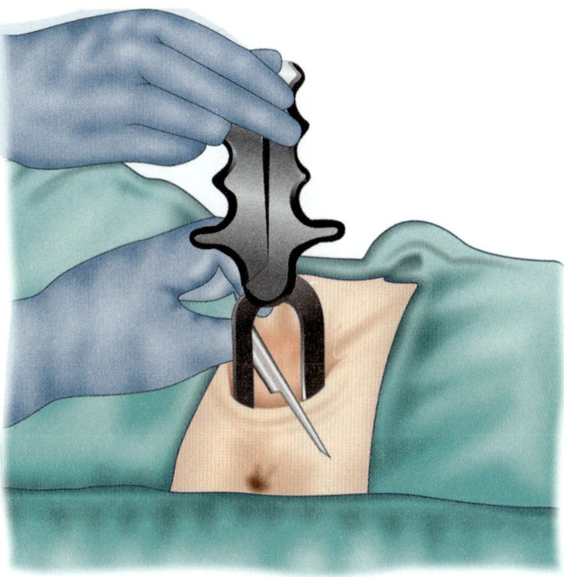

Fig. 21.16: Locking of blades

   - Posterior fontanel is not more than one finger breadth above the plane of the shanks of the forceps.
4. Traction (Figs 21.17 and 21.18):
   - Steady and intermittent traction to be applied during contraction, first downwards (horizontal), backwards, forwards and lastly upwards.
   - In outlet forceps—Only two fingers are to be introduced. Traction is applied straight horizontal, upward and then forwards.
5. Removal of blades—Right blade should be removed first (Fig. 21.19).
6. In occipitoposterior position:
   - Blades are to be applied as usual but they should be equidistant from sinciput and occiput
   - Traction—Horizontal till the root of the nose is under the pubic symphysis, then upward till the occiput emerges over the perineum and finally downwards.
   - This is the easiest and often the best method of delivering an infant with the head in the direct OP position.
   - If the head is low in the pelvis it is likely to be deliverable with very little traction and the fetus is spared the risks of manipulation.
   - A large episiotomy is necessary.

Trial of Forceps

- Knowing that a certain degree of disproportion at mid pelvis may make the procedure incompatible, low/mid forceps delivery is attempted, abandoning it at the earliest in favor of cesarean section.
- So, it should be done only in the OT, keeping everything ready for CS.

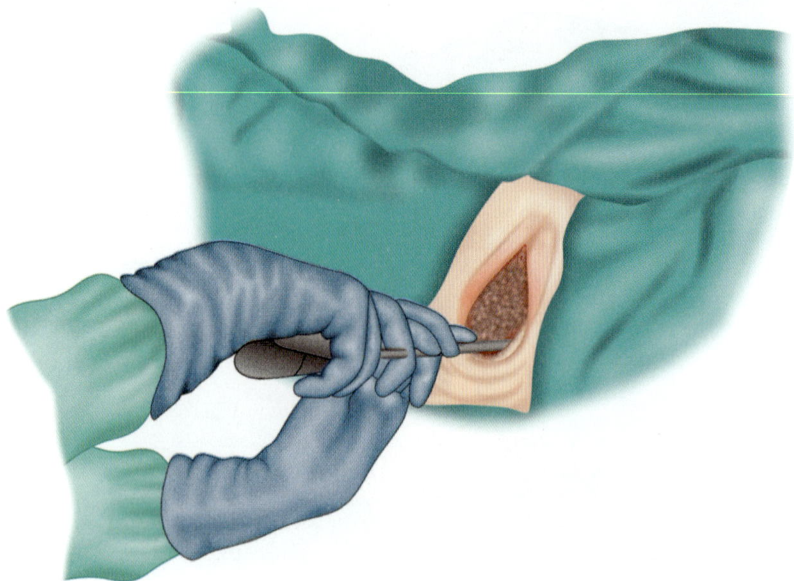

Fig. 21.17: Use of downward traction

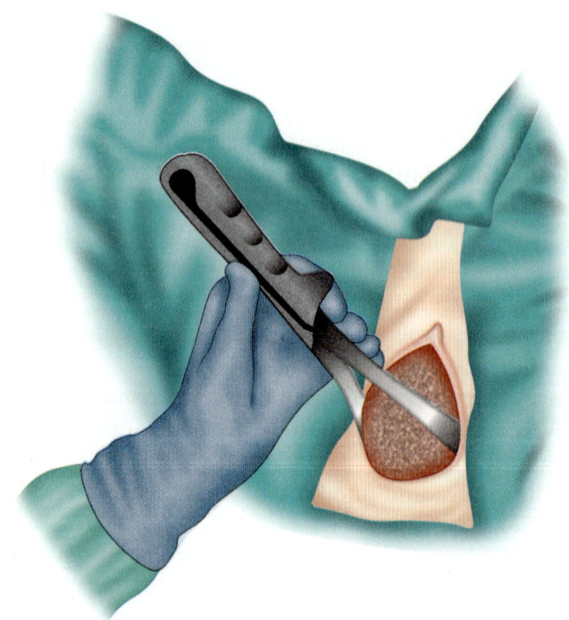

Fig. 21.18: Use of upward traction

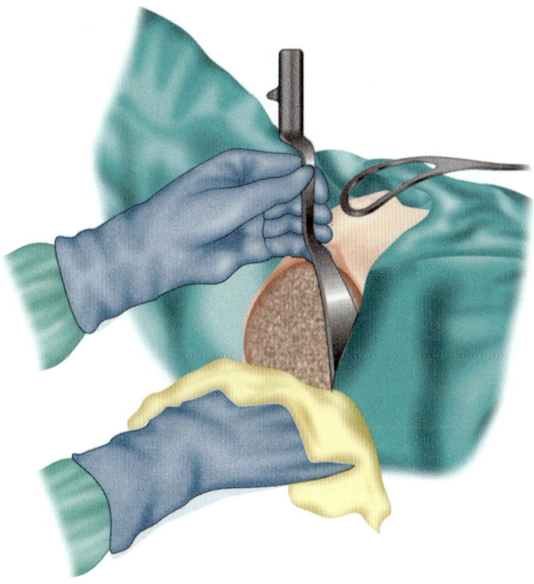

Fig. 21.19: Removal of blades and delivery of the head

Failed Forceps

- When an unsuccessful attempt is made with the forceps resulting in fetal or/and maternal injury.
- Mostly it is due to lack of obstetric skill and poor clinical judgment.
- Factors responsible are:
  - Disproportion,
  - Incomplete cervical dilatation
  - Malposition of fetal head.

Outcome and Prognosis

- The ultimate outcome of forceps deliveries depends on numerous factors.
- Among the most important of these remain the skill and judgment of the operator.
- The operator must be supported by a skilled team, including anesthesia and nursing staff.
- The presence of a person skilled in newborn resuscitation is also mandatory for operative vaginal deliveries.

Complications

Complications of forceps delivery are mostly due to faulty technique rather than the instrument.

- Maternal complications
  - Injury

    - Extension of the episiotomy involving anus and rectum or vaginal vault.
    - Vaginal lacerations and cervical tear if cervix was not fully dilated.
  - Postpartum hemorrhage
    - Due to trauma, atonic uterus or anesthesia.
  - Shock
    - Due to blood loss, dehydration or prolonged labor.
  - Sepsis
    - Due to improper asepsis or devitalization of local tissues.
- Anesthetic hazards.
- Delayed or long-term sequelae
  - Chronic low backache
  - Genital prolapse
  - Stress incontinence.
  - Anal sphincteric dysfunction
- Fetal complications/Dangers
  - Asphyxia.
  - Trauma.
    - Intracranial hemorrhage.
    - Cephalic hematoma.
    - Facial/Brachial palsy.
    - Injury to the soft tissues of face and forehead.
  - Skull fracture.
  - Remote-cerebral palsy.
  - Fetal death-around 2%.

VACUUM/VENTOUSE

Originally, vacuum devices had a rigid metal cup devised by Malstromme (Fig. 21.20) with a separate suction catheter attached laterally and connected to a foot-operated pedal.

Modern day vacuum cups can be soft or rigid and can be different shapes and sizes. Examples of different types of cups include soft or rigid anterior cups and rigid posterior cups (Table 21.6). Posterior cups (Kiwi omnicup (Figs 21.21A to C), Mityvac M-cup, and Bird or O'Neil cups) have been designed for occipito-posterior and asynclitic deliveries.

The flatter cup allows for better placement at the flexing position on the fetal head, which is usually much further back in the sacral hollow during occipitoposterior presentation.

Newer devices allow for an assistant to hand-pump suction using a separate device or for the user to hand-pump suction with a single hand-held device. These hand-held devices are ideally intended for single use and are disposable.

A Cochrane review of nine trials comparing soft and rigid cups showed that soft cups were significantly more likely to fail to achieve vaginal delivery

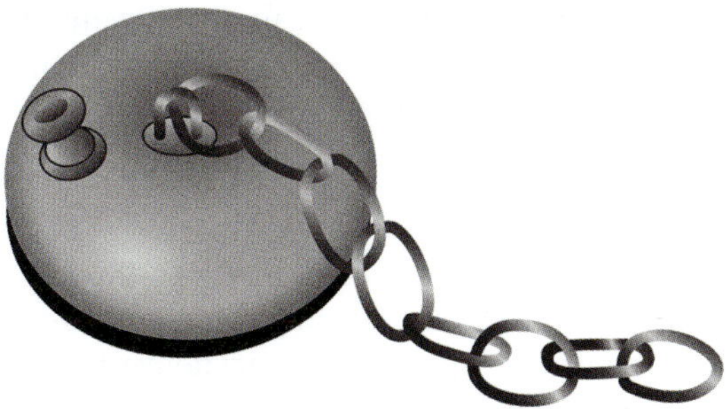

Fig. 21.20: Rigid metal Malstromme cup

TABLE 21.6: Types of vacuum devices
• Rigid/metal
– Malstromme
– Bird
– Modifications
• Silastic
– Kobayashi
• Plastic
– Bell
– Mushroom
– Soft

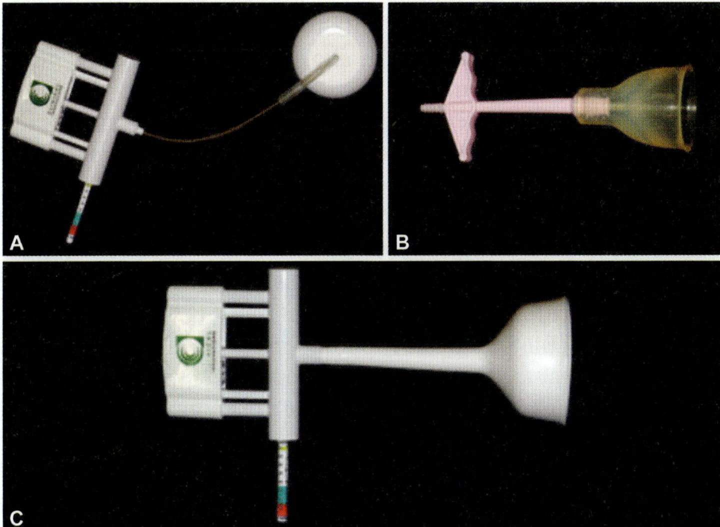

Figs 21.21A to C: Examples of newer vacuum devices; the cups can vary in shape and size. (A) The Kiwi Omnicup is a rigid plastic cup that is disc-shaped and modeled after the original Bird posterior cup; it is suited for occipitoposterior deliveries. Newer devices allow (B) for an assistant to hand-pump suction using a separate device or (C) for the user to hand- pump suction with a single handheld device

(or = 1.65; 95% CI, 1.19 to 2.29). Failure rates were 10% with rigid cups and 22% with soft cups. Soft cups were associated with less scalp injury (or = 0.45; 95% CI, 0.15 to 0.60). There were no significant differences in maternal injury.[17]

Using the "ABCDEFGHIJ" Mnemonic for Vacuum

The mnemonic "ABCDEFGHIJ" is used to describe the steps performed in vacuum extraction.[18] Practicing the techniques on mannequins can provide an introduction to the skills of operative vaginal delivery.

Address the patient and discuss the risks and benefits of operative vaginal delivery.

- ***A***ssistants should be on hand for delivery and for neonatal resuscitation, and should be made aware of the use of instruments.
- ***A***nalgesics should be administered, if needed. Regional or pudendal anesthesia is recommended for forceps delivery; however, vacuum delivery without regional or pudendal anesthesia is not uncommon.
- ***B***ladder should be emptied to avoid risk of injury.
- ***C***ervix should be completely dilated.
- ***D***etermine the position of the fetal head.
- ***E***quipment should be checked to ensure the vacuum and adequate suction.
- ***F***lexion point: With the suction off, the center of the cup should be applied 3 cm anterior to the posterior fontanel, centering the sagittal suture under the vacuum (Figs 21.22A and B). The edge of the cup will be over the posterior fontanel (most cups have a diameter of 5–7 cm). This point, located in the midline along the sagittal suture, approximately 3 cm in front of the posterior fontanel and approximately 6 cm from the anterior fontanel, is called the ***F***lexion point. The flexion point is an important point in maximizing traction and minimizing detachment of the cup. Checking for placement of the cup by using the anterior fontanel as the landmark may be easier because the cup will obscure the posterior fontanel. No maternal tissue, including the vagina, should be under the cup. The risk of subgaleal hemorrhage increases if the cup edge is placed on the sagittal suture. Improper application appears to be common with attempted vacuum-assisted delivery and is thought to be a primary factor in unsuccessful attempts.
- ***G***entle traction: The physician should increase the vacuum suction with the manometer at the recommended range and apply ***G***entle traction at right angles to the plane of the cup during the contraction (Fig. 21.22C).
- ***H***alt: Use of vacuum should be ***H***alted when there are three disengagements of the vacuum (or "pop-offs"), more than 20 minutes have elapsed, or three consecutive pulls result in no progress or delivery. Cephalohematoma rates, as well as brachial plexus injuries, increase with longer application times.
- ***I***ncision for episiotomy: Although it is in the original mnemonic, performing an ***I***ncision for episiotomy increases the risk of perineal trauma

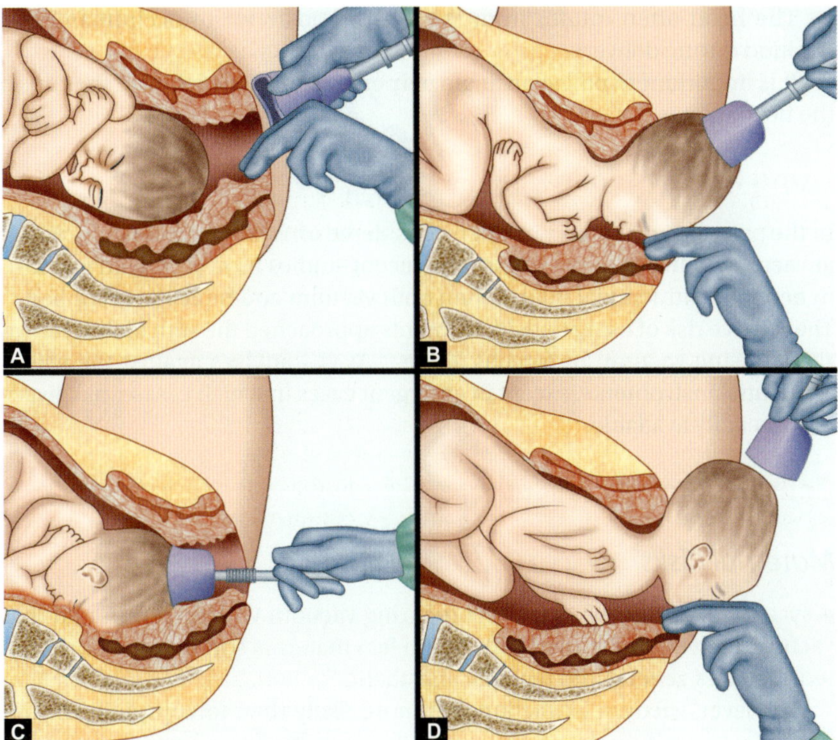

Figs 21.22A to D: Using the vacuum device for delivery.After determining position of the head, (A) insert the cup into the vaginal vault, ensuring that no maternal tissues are trapped by the cup. (B) Apply the cup to the flexion point 3 cm in front of the posterior fontanel, centering the sagittal suture. (C) Pull during a contraction with a steady motion, keeping the device at right angles to the plane of the cup. In occipitoposterior deliveries, maintain the right angle if the fetal head rotates. (D) Remove the cup when the fetal jaw is reachable.

and, therefore, is no longer recommended. Compared with nulliparous women who have spontaneous vaginal delivery without episiotomy, the odds of having a severe (third- or fourth-degree) perineal laceration are increased in women who have vacuum delivery without episiotomy (or = 3.1; 95% CI, 1.9 to 4.3). The odds of a severe perineal laceration are even higher in women who have vacuum delivery with episiotomy (or = 13.7; 95% CI, 10.1 to 17.3).[19] Similar results were noted in multiparous women.

- ***J***aw-the vacuum can be removed when the fetal ***J***aw is reachable (Fig. 21.22D).

Fetal Position and Vacuum-assisted Vaginal Delivery

Vacuum devices can be used when the fetal head is in the occipitoposterior position. However, in one study, the rates of anal sphincter lacerations with the use of forceps and vacuum for occipitoposterior deliveries were greater compared with occipitoanterior deliveries.[20]

The head often rotates from the occipitoposterior to occipitoanterior position during delivery.

It is important to pull at an angle perpendicular to the plane of the cup as the head rotates.

Using Forceps Following Failed Vacuum Delivery

In the past, use of forceps was often considered after an unsuccessful attempt at vacuum delivery. However, several recent studies have shown an increase in neonatal intracranial injury when both vacuum and forceps are applied.[21] The relative risk of using both instruments approached the sum of the relative risk of using vacuum or forceps alone.[22] ACOG advises against the use of sequential instruments, except in emergent cases in which cesarean delivery is not readily available.[23]

Complications of Vacuum

Maternal Risks

A systematic review of 10 trials comparing vacuum with forceps found that vacuum deliveries were associated with less maternal soft-tissue trauma and required less general and regional anesthetic.[16]

However, vacuum extraction was more likely than forceps deliveries to fail.[16]

Neonatal Risks

Vacuum delivery increases the rates of neonatal cephalohematoma and retinal hemorrhage compared with forceps delivery.[16] Hemorrhages typically resolve without sequelae within four weeks of birth, but cephalohematoma can lead to hyperbilirubinemia (Figs 21.23A and B).

Operative vaginal delivery is a risk factor for shoulder dystocia, and it appears to be more common with vacuum delivery than with forceps delivery.[24]

Intracranial hemorrhage and subgaleal or subaponeurotic hematomas are rare but serious events reported with the use of vacuum (Table 21.7).

In 1998, the US Food and Drug Administration issued a warning about the potential risk of serious intracranial injury or death with the use of vacuum devices.[25] The report cited a five-fold increase in reports of fetal death and serious injury that could likely be attributed to the increasing use of vacuum rather than an actual change in the risk of complications. Specific recommendations were made for the use of vacuum, including applying steady traction instead of using a rocking motion, as well as notifying participants in the initial neonatal care that a vacuum was used so that appropriate monitoring could occur.[25]

A study reviewing 583,340 live births showed increased rates of cerebral hemorrhage with operative vaginal delivery compared with spontaneous

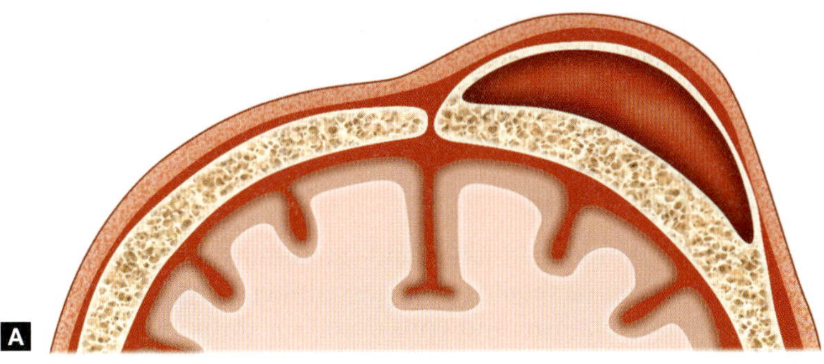

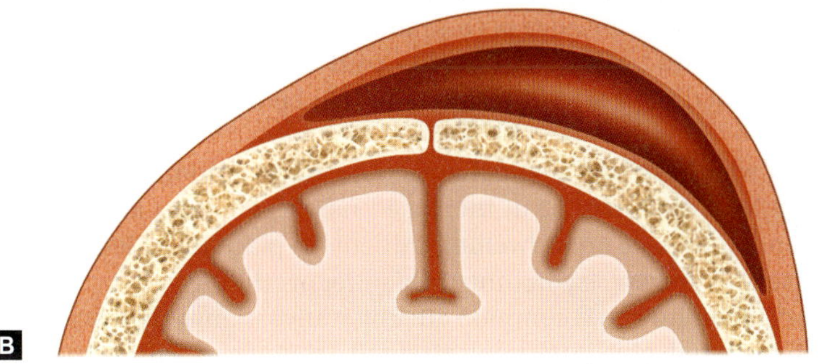

Figs 21.23A and B: Cephalohematoma versus subgaleal hematoma. (A) Cephalohematomas are limited to suture lines. (B) In subgaleal hematomas, the bleeding crosses suture lines, causing diffuse swelling that can indent on palpation

TABLE 7: Signs and symptoms of serious intracranial injury in a neonate
Intracranial hemorrhage
• Bradycardia
• Bulging fontanel
• Convulsions
• Irritability
• Lethargy
• Poor feeding
Subgleal hematoma
• Diffuse head swelling that shifts with repositioning and indents on palpation
• Signs of hypovolemic shock (hypotension, pallor, tachycardia, tachypnea)
• Swelling not limited by suture lines (unlike cephalohematoma)

NOTE: *Signs or symptoms may not appear until several hours after birth.*

vaginal birth, but no statistical difference in the rates of hemorrhage with use of vacuum, forceps, or cesarean delivery; this suggests that abnormal labor may contribute more to intracranial hemorrhage than does method of delivery.

POST-DELIVERY CARE

Mid-cavity delivery, prolonged labor and immobility are risk factors for thromboembolism.Women should be reassessed after delivery for risk factors for venous thromboembolism and considered for thromboprophylaxis if necessary.[26]

Regular paracetamol and diclofenac should be offered after an operative vaginal delivery in the absence of contraindications.

The timing and volume of the first void urine should be monitored and documented. A post-void residual should be measured if retention is suspected.

Women who have had a spinal anesthetic or an epidural that has been topped up for a trial may be at increased risk of retention and should be recommended to have an indwelling catheter in place for at least 12 hours post-delivery to prevent asymptomatic bladder overfilling.

Urinary incontinence is common after operative vaginal delivery. Women should be offered physiotherapy-directed strategies to prevent urinary incontinence.[27]

The woman should be reviewed by the obstetri-cian who conducted the delivery prior to hospital discharge to discuss the indication for operative delivery, management of any complications and the prognosis for future deliveries.

Operative vaginal delivery can be associated with fear of subsequent childbirth and in a severe form may manifest as a post-traumatic stress-type syndrome termed tocophobia.[28] Follow-up of a cohort at 3 years following operative delivery reported that 50% of women did not plan on having a further child and almost half of these women reported fear of childbirth as the main reason for avoiding pregnancy.[29]

Women who have experienced an operative vaginal delivery should be encouraged to aim for spontaneous vaginal delivery in a subsequent pregnancy. The likelihood of achieving a spontaneous vaginal delivery is approximately 80% even for women who have required more complex operative vaginal deliveries in theatre.[29]

Women who sustain a third- or fourth-degree perineal tear should be counseled regarding the risk of recurrence and implications for future childbirth.[30]

TRAINING IN OPERATIVE VAGINAL DELIVERY

The danger of instrumental deliveries depends more on the operator's skills than on the instrument itself.

Training must ensure that obstetricians can identify indications and contraindications, choose the appropriate instrument, use it correctly and know the principles applied to operative vaginal delivery.

The training program must include simultaneous training in both forceps use as well as vacuum extraction. Knowledge of obstetric mechanics should be imparted.

Traditional training may be completed with simulations. This simulation training method also helps to resolve a situation that only extensive experience in a large number of procedures would have helped resolve. This extensive experience is desirable but difficult to attain in real life.

Assessment of training should involve both teachers and trainees.

Sessions to evaluate professional practices should be performed and cover quality criteria associated with operative vaginal deliveries. Such a procedure by involving obstetricians, may improve practices.[31]

FUTURE OF OPERATIVE VAGINAL DELIVERY

Information developed in the 1980s suggests that fetal outcome may be poor after at least some forceps deliveries. Other data suggest that long-term compromise of the maternal rectal sphincter is a common sequel of forceps delivery. In present day, when the ACOG has advocated cesarean delivery on demand for preservation of maternal pelvic musculature, the place of forceps deliveries in obstetrical practices has been questioned. Concerns about the appropriateness of forceps delivery have led to increased concern among practitioners about the medicolegal liability involved in forceps delivery.

Among other effects, this has led to a marked decrease in the training of new physicians to perform these deliveries. Given these trends, forceps deliveries may easily become extinct within the next generation.

Forceps delivery may offer advantages over cesarean section, but only if short-and long-term health benefits can be shown, including the potential for future uncomplicated spontaneous vaginal deliveries.

The challenge for obstetricians is to make sure that options for safe delivery are not limited for women who experience complications in labor. Practice guidelines and protocols may help to ensure safe and consistent obstetric practice.

REFERENCES

1. Bailey PE. The disappearing art of instrumental delivery: time to reverse the trend. Int J Gynaecol Obstet. 2005;91(1):89-96.
2. Royal College of Obstetricians and Gynecologists Clinical Effectiveness Support Unit. National Sentinel Caesarean Section Audit Report. London: RCOG Press; 2001 [*http://www.rcog.org.uk/files/rcog-corp/uploaded-files/nscs_audit.pdf*].
3. Information and Statistics Division, Scottish Health Statistics. Births in Scotland report 2002. Births and babies (Births 1976–2008) [*http://www.isdscotland.org/isd/1612.html; accessed 11 November 2009*].

4. Martin JA, Hamilton BE, Sutton PD, Ventura SJ, Men- acker F, Kirmeyer S. Births: final data for 2004. Natl Vital Stat Rep. 2006;55(1):1-101.
5. PowellJ,GiloN,FooteM,GilK,LavinJP. Vacuum and forceps training in residency: experience and self-reported competency. J Perinatol. 2007;27(6):343-6.
6. US Food and Drug Administration. Food and Drug Administration Public Health Advisory: Need for CAUTION When Using Vacuum Assisted Delivery Devices. 1998 [*http://www.fda.gov/MedicalDevices/Safety/AlertsandNotices/PublicHealthNotifications/UCM062295*]
7. American College of Obstetricians and Gynecologists.ACOG Practice Bulletin No. 17: Operative vaginal delivery. Washington, DC, USA:ACOG; 2000.
8. National Collaborating Centre for Women's and Children's Health. Clinical Guideline No. 55: Intrapartum care: care of healthy women and their babies during childbirth. London: RCOG Press; 2007 [*http://www.gserve.nice.org.uk/nicemedia/ pdf/IntrapartumCareSeptember2007mainguideline.pdf*].
9. British Columbia Reproductive Care Program. Obstetric Guideline 14:Assisted vaginal birth:the use of forceps or vacuum extractor. Vancouver, Canada: BCRCP; 2001 [*http://www.csh.org.tw/Dr.TCJ/Educartion/Guideline/OB%20g uideline/Assist.Delivery%20Guideline.pdf*].
10. Vacca A.The trouble with vacuum extraction. Curr Obstet Gynaecol. 1999;9:41-5.
11. Rosemann GWE.Vacuum extraction of premature infants. S Afr J Obstet Gynaecol. 1969;7:10-2.
12. Royal Australian and New Zealand College of Obstetricians and Gynaecologists. College Statement C-Obs 16: Instrumental vaginal delivery. Melbourne,Australia: RANZCOG; 2009 [*www. ranzcog.edu.au/publications/statements/C-obs16.pdf*].
13. Royal Australian and New Zealand College of Obstetricians and Gynaecologists. College Statement C-Obs 13: Guidelines for use of rotational forceps. Melbourne,Australia: RANZCOG; 2009 [*www.ranzcog.edu.au/publications/statements/C- obs13.pdf*].
14. Cargill YM, MacKinnon CJ, Arsenault MY, Bartellas E, Daniels S, GleasonT, et al.; Clinical Practice Obstetrics Committee. Guidelines for operative vaginal birth. J Obstet Gynaecol Can. 2004;26:747-61.
15. Revah A, Ezra Y, Farine D, Ritchie K. Failed trial of vacuum or forceps - maternal and fetal outcome. Am J Obstet Gynecol. 1997;176:200-4.
16. Johanson RB, Menon V. Vacuum extraction versus forceps for assisted vaginal delivery. Cochrane Database Syst Rev. 1999;(2):CD000224.
17. Johanson R, Menon V. Soft versus rigid vacuum extractor cups for assisted vaginal delivery. Cochrane Database Syst Rev 1999;(4):CD000446.
18. Damos JR, Bassett R. Chapter H: assisted vaginal delivery. In: Advanced Life Support in Obstetrics (ALSO) Provider Syllabus, 4th edn. Leawood, Kan.: American Academy of Family Physicians; 2003:3-8.
19. Kudish B, Blackwell S, McNeeley SG, et al. Opera- tive vaginal delivery and midline episiotomy: a bad combination for the perineum. Am J Obstet Gynecol. 2006;195(3):749-54.
20. Damron DP, Capeless EL. Operative vaginal delivery: a comparison of forceps and vacuum for success rate and risk of rectal sphincter injury. Am J Obstet Gynecol. 2004;191(3):907-10.

21. Towner D, Castro MA, Eby-Wilkens E, Gilbert WM. Effect of mode of delivery in nulliparous women on neonatal intracranial injury. N Engl J Med. 1999;341(23): 1709-14.
22. Gardella C, Taylor M, Benedetti T, Hitti J, Critchlow C. The effect of sequential use of vacuum and forceps for assisted vaginal delivery on neonatal and maternal out- comes. Am J Obstet Gynecol. 2001;185(4):896-902.
23. American College of Obstetricians and Gynecologists. Operative vaginal delivery. Clinical management guidelines for obstetrician-gynecologists. Int J Gynaecol Obstet. 2001;74(1):69-76.
24. Demissie K, Rhoads GG, Smulian JC, et al. Operative vaginal delivery and neonatal and infant adverse out- comes: population based retrospective analysis [published correction appears in BMJ. 2004;329(7465):547]. BMJ. 2004;329(7456):24-29.
25. US Food and Drug Administration, Center for Devices and Radiological Health. FDA public health advisory: need for CAUTION when using vacuum assisted delivery devices. Rockville, Md.: U.S. Food and Drug Administra- tion; 1998. *http://www.fda.gov/cdrh/fetal598.html.* Accessed November 26, 2007.
26. Royal College of Obstetricians and Gynaecologists. Green-top Guideline No. 37: Reducing the risk of thrombosis and embolism during pregnancy and the puerperium. London: RCOG; 2009 [*http://www.rcog.org.uk/files/rcog-corp/GT37ReducingRiskThrombo.pdf*].
27. Zaki MM, Pandit M, Jackson S. National survey for intrapartum and postpartum bladder care: assessing the need for guidelines. BJOG 2004;111:874-6.
28. Murphy DJ, Pope C, Frost J, Liebling RE. Women's views on the impact of operative delivery in the second stage of labour: qualitative interview study. BMJ. 2003;327:1132.
29. Bahl R, Strachan B, Murphy DJ. Outcome of subsequent pregnancy three years after previous operative delivery in the second stage of labour: cohort study. BMJ. 2004;328:311-4.
30. Royal College of Obstetricians and Gynaecologists. Green-top Guideline 29: The management of third- and fourth-degree perineal tears. RCOG: London; 2007 [*http://www.rcog.org.uk/files/rcog-corp/uploaded- files/GT29ManagementThirdFourthDegreeTears2007.pdf*].
31. Vayssière C, Beucher G et al. Instrumental delivery: Clinical practice guidelines from the French College of Gynaecologists and Obstetricians. Eur J Obstet Gynecol Reprod Biol. 2011;159(1):43-8.

22

Obstetric Hysterectomy

Ganpat Sawant, Aaradhana Wagh

INTRODUCTION

In no other gynecological or obstetrical surgery is the surgeon in as much a dilemma as when deciding to resort to an emergency hysterectomy. On one hand it is the last resort to save a mother's life, and on the other hand, the mother's reproductive capability is sacrificed. Many times it is a very difficult decision and requires good clinical judgement.

INCIDENCE

The incidence of obstetric hysterectomy varies from 1 in 350 to 1 in 7000 deliveries and is associated with maternal death rate of 0–30%. Compared to vaginal delivery there is strong association between cesarian section and emergency hysterectomy.

The need for blood transfusion, intensive care and associated risk of trauma to bladder and ureter make this one of the marker for severe maternal morbidity and potential mortality.

INDICATIONS

Emergency obstetric hysterectomy is usually required for complications of delivery associated with hemorrhage.

In most cases it is undertaken when other conservative measures fail.

Main Indications for Obstetric Hysterectomy

- *Abnormal placentation*: The incidence of placenta previa and placenta accreta increases in subsequent pregnancy due to increased rate of cesarean section. In these cases total hysterectomy with placenta *in situ* would be preferred, as removal of placenta causes torrential hemorrhage and shock compromising maternal condition.

- Abruptio placentae causing couvelaire uterus usually responds to oxytocics but on rare occasions hysterectomy may be required in case of uterine atony.
- *Uterine atony*: Occasionally uterus may be refractory to all the available oxytocic agents. Commonly found in patients with prolonged labor, anomaly of uterus, uterine fibroid, etc.
- *Uterine rupture*: Commonly associated with previous uterine scar that is previous cesarean section and in intact uterus reasons being inappropriate use of oxytocic drugs or trauma during manipulation, internal version and instrumental vaginal delivery, etc. Even external trauma such as domestic violence, fall can rarely cause rupture of uterus.
- *Sepsis*: It is an uncommon indication for obstetric hysterectomy, e.g. post partum myometrial abscesses refractory to antibiotics or uterine scar infection in cesarean delivery.
- *Ectopic pregnancy*: Rare varieties of ectopic pregnancy that is cornual and cervical pregnancy may require hysterectomy to control hemorrhage.

SURGICAL CONSIDERATION

- Anatomical and physiological changes in pregnancy create potential difficulties in obstetric hysterectomy as compared to gynecological hysterectomy that is the uterus is largely enlarged and adjacent pelvic tissue is edematous and friable. Even the uterine and collateral vessels are engorged.
- The choice of abdominal incision depends on the circumstances. If the obstetric hysterectomy is being done following a cesarean section then incision is likely to be pfannenstiel incision, but if laparotomy is being performed with anticipation of hysterectomy following vaginal delivery then lower midline incision is preferred for greater pelvic access.
- Choice of total/subtotal hysterectomy depends on the indication of the procedure and the skill of the operating surgeon.
- Subtotal hysterectomy can be performed rapidly with less risk of trauma to ureter and bladder as it is difficult to define the limits of the soft cervix. So, it can be done if trauma and bleeding is confined to upper uterine segment.
- Total hysterectomy has to be performed if cervix and paracolpos is involved and is causing hemorrhage.
- The vascular pedicles are thick and edematous so all the pedicles should be double clamped.

SURGICAL TECHNIQUE

- Uterus is lifted out through the incision and on each side straight clamp is applied at the cornual end of uterus across the adnexal structures that is round ligament, utero ovarian ligament and fallopian tube.

- Anterior leaf of the broad ligament is incised inferomedially. If lower segment cesarean section has been performed this joins the lateral aspect of dissected uterovesical fold of peritoneum.
- The pedicle containing the utero-ovarian ligament and fallopian tube is now secured, clamped and cut to transfix it. Same procedure is repeated on other side.
- This dissection of bladder is limited laterally to avoid the vascular bladder pillars.
- The level of placement of uterine clamps is at junction of cervix with isthmus of uterus and from now onwards all clamps are placed medially to uterine clamp to avoid ureteric damage.
- Large curved clamps placed across the lower uterine segment at the junction of cervix on each side, allows excision of body of uterus.
- If bleeding is due to uterine atony or trauma in upper segment of uterus —hemorrhage should now be controlled and sub-total hysterectomy should suffice.
- If bleeding involves cervix, bladder will have to be further dissected from anterior part of cervix and identification of rim of cervix is done.
- Vaginal cuff can either be closed with continuous locking sutures or interrupted sutures. Perioperative antibiotic prophylaxis should be given.
- During hysterectomy, identification of ureter is essential as it is particularly vulnerable for injury at three sites:
    1. While clamping infundibulopelvic ligament lateral to tube and ovary.
    2. While clamping uterine vessels as ureter is very close as it runs beneath the vessels.
    3. When ureter enters the bladder.

Once the initial postoperative recovery is secured, the whole sequence of events should be reviewed and discussed with her and her relatives and appropriate follow-up should be done.

CONCLUSION

Emergency obstetric hysterectomy is a life saving procedure. The maternal outcome greatly depends on timely decision and good clinical judgement because unnecessary delay can cost life and undue haste can cause morbidity.

Internal Iliac Artery Ligation in Obstetrics

23

Adi E Dastur, Ameya C Purandare

A stitch in time, saves nine

—***an English Proverb***[1]

INTRODUCTION

The major blood supply to the uterus and pelvis comes from the internal iliac artery (also called as hypogastric artery). Bilateral ligation of this artery can effectively control bleeding and thus prevent need for hysterectomy and permanent sterilization. Indeed, it is a life-saving procedure.

SURGICAL ANATOMY

The common iliac artery bifurcates over the sacroiliac joint into external and internal iliac arteries. The internal iliac artery measures 4 cm and enters the pelvis along the medial border of the psoas muscle.

ANATOMIC RELATIONS OF INTERNAL ILIAC ARTERY

- *Anteromedial*: It is covered by peritoneum and on the right side the terminal ileum and cecum may overlie.
- *Anterior*: Ureter crosses over it from lateral to medial side at its origin.
- Posterolateral: External iliac vein and obturator nerve.
- *Posteromedial*: Internal iliac vein.
- *Lateral*: It lies over the psoas muscle.

COLLATERAL CIRCULATION

Internal iliac artery ligation was first performed by Kelly in 1884, who thought that the pelvic blood flow would be completely stopped following bilateral ligation. However, collateral circulation develops in no time and even after simultaneous ligation of both arteries.

Main arterial group having collateral circulation with internal iliac artery are:

- Branches from aorta.
- Braches from external iliac artery.
- Branches from femoral artery.

The anastomoses occur in each hemipelvis both vertically (ipsilaterally) and horizontally (across the midline). After bilateral ligation, the vertical system is most important and there is little transmission across the midline.

The pathways of collateral circulation are the following:

- The uterine artery branching from the hypogastric artery anastomoses with the ovarian artery, branches of aorta.
- The middle hemorrhoidal branch of the hypogastric artery anastomoses with the superior hemorrhoidal artery arising from the inferior mesenteric. The middle hemorrhoidal artery anastomoses with the inferior hemorrhoidal, which is a branch of the internal pudendal artery, which again is a branch of the hypogastric artery.
- The obturator artery, branching from the hypogastric artery, gives off pubic branches, which anastomose with the inferior epigastric artery arising from the external iliac artery.
- The inferior gluteal artery from the hypogastric artery anastomose with the circumflex and perforating branches of the deep femoral artery (this is known as cruciate anastomosis).
- The superior gluteal artery and iliac branch of iliolumbar artery from the hypogastric artery anastomose with deep circumflex iliac (branch of the external iliac artery) and lateral circumflex iliac arteries (branches of femoral artery).
- The iliolumbar arteries from the hypogastric anastomose with the lumbar arteries from the aorta.
- The vesical arteries which supply the bladder are both branches of the hypogastric artery, and they anastomose with the uterine arteries, also from the hypogastric, and under with vaginal arteries.
- Lateral sacral artery branches of hypogastric artery anastomose with middle sacral artery from the aorta.
- Internal pudendal artery, branch of hypogastric, anastomosis with superficial and deep external pudendal artery, branch of femoral artery (this is known as perineal anastomosis).

HEMODYNAMIC CONSEQUENCE OF INTERNAL ILIAC LIGATION

Following ligation of the internal iliac artery, pulsation virtually ceases in arteries distal to ligation. Burchell (1964), Burchell et al. (1966 and 1968) observed the following hemodynamic changes after internal iliac artery ligation (Table. 23.1).

TABLE 23.1 Average percent decrease

Site of ligation	*Pulse pressure*	*Mean pressure*	*Blood flow*
Bilateral	85	24	48
Same side	77	22	49
Opposite side	14	10	–

The changes are thus primarily unilateral, any collateral effect is minimal.

The cardinal hemostatic effect is due to the rapid decrease in pulse pressure. This is due to the small diameter of anastomosis between pairs of arteries involved in collateral circulation. The net effect of ligation is a transformation of effective pelvic arterial circulation into a venous system. However, even though the mean pressure remains greater than the venous pressure, the 'trip hammer' effect of arterial circulation is vertically eliminated.

Thus, it is possible for a stable clot to develop and persist, ensuring effective hemostasis.

INDICATIONS OF INTERNAL ILIAC LIGATION

- *Atonic PPH*: If all the conventional procedures fail, it is performed as an alternative to hysterectomy. One should always remember that the bleeding is coming from multiple open sinuses and it is indeed questionable as to the extent of control of hemorrhage one can achieve following internal iliac and ovarian artery ligation.
- Broad ligament hematoma, following rupture uterus or extension of uterine incision laterally during lower segment cesarean section (LSCS) or cervical tear/colporrhexis, which persistently bleed in spite of attempting hemostatic suturing. Perhaps in these conditions, unilateral ligation may suffice.
- Morbidly adherent placenta, where bleeding continues even after oxytocic use or intrauterine plugging. Internal iliac artery ligation serves as an alternative to hysterectomy.
- Secondary PPH, from the uterine scar where hemostasis cannot be effectively achieved because of friable tissues.

SUCCESS RATE OF INTERNAL ILIAC ARTERY LIGATION

This has been shown in Table 23.2 (Clark et al. 1985).

TECHNIQUE

Site of Ligation

Hemorrhage is usually controlled by ligating the anterior division just distal to its origin and proximal to the point where its first branch arises.

TABLE 23.2: Success rate of internal iliac artery ligation

Indication	*No. of successful*	*No. of unsuccessful*	*Total*
Uterine atony	6	9	15
Lateral extension of a low transverse uterine incision	1	2	3
Placenta accreta	1	0	1
Totals	8	11	19

Approach

In emergency obstetrics, the preferable route is the transabdominal infraumbilical longitudinal. Vertical incision is preferable as it offers a better exposure and is much quicker.

Surgical Steps

- The common iliac artery and its bifurcation into external and internal iliac arteries are palpated and visualized through the peritoneum.
- The peritoneum is opened on the lateral side of the common iliac artery near its bifurcation and extending for 4–6 cm. This incision should be lateral to the ureter. The internal iliac artery is posterior and medial to the external iliac artery.
- Anterior division is clearly identified.
- The areolar tissue joining the posterior wall of the internal iliac artery to the anterior wall of the vein is carefully separated by blunt dissection.
- A Babcock's forceps is used to hold the internal iliac artery and is elevated from the anterior surface of the internal iliac vein.
- A Mixter's forceps is passed below the artery.
- No. 1 Linen (or any non-absorbable suture material) is used for ligation. Double ligation avoids recanalization.
- The artery should not be transected between the ligatures, as there is chance of retraction and subsequent bleeding.
- The peritoneum is closed with interrupted catgut sutures.
- The pulsations of the femoral artery are felt prior to ligation of the internal iliac artery (to make sure that the external iliac is not accidentally ligated) and after ligation. Should the pulsation disappear prior to ligation then one should re-examine the anatomy and confirm the location of the internal iliac artery and then only should one proceed with the ligation.

EFFICACY

Clark and associates (1985) reported on the successful control of bleeding in 8 (42%) of 19 women who underwent hypogastric artery ligation. In a review of hypogastric artery ligation from three series (Table 23.3), Clark (1988) reported that this procedure prevented hysterectomy in about half

TABLE 23.3: Efficacy of internal iliac artery ligation in avoiding hysterectomy for obstetric hemorrhage (Clark, 1988)

Indication	*No. of patients*	*Success*	*Percentage*
Atony	21	8	43
Placenta accerta	7	4	57
Lacerations	8	1	36
Other	4	4	100
Totals	41	18	44

the cases associated with uterine atony and placenta accreta. Interestingly, in the series by Clark and associates, the success of this procedure did not appear to be related directly to conditions for which it was performed. It must be noted, however, that the number in each category is small. Mengert et al. (1969) reported a case of a successful pregnancy following prior bilateral hypogastric, as well as ovarian artery ligation.

COMPLICATIONS

The potential complications of internal iliac artery ligation are following:

- Injury (laceration) of internal iliac and external iliac vein.
- Injury to the ureter.
- Ligation of the external iliac artery.
- Spasm of the external iliac artery can result from placing a ligation on the internal iliac artery close to the bifurcation of the common iliac artery.
- Formation of a clot in the posterior trunk and its subsequent ascent into the external iliac artery, obliterating its lumen creating a vascular crisis.
- Postischemic motor neuron damage.
- Ischemia of the central pelvic area followed by tissue break-down is rare unless lateral circulation is destroyed.

The complications during surgical procedure are important, the rest are transitory and minimal.

RECENT ADVANCES

Chin (1989), described the technique of angiographic embolization for intractable puerperal hematomas (vulvovaginal hematoma) with occlusion of branches of internal iliac artery. Alvarez et al. (1992) have reviewed the indication for embolization and described several cases in which this technique was employed prophylactically in women at high risk of various types of postpartum hemorrhage.

Greenwood et al. (1987), have described the use of gelfoam and other similar substances for successful control of obstetric bleeding. It must be remembered, however, that the techniques are the best performed under elective conditions or at least in hemodynamically stable women.

Hypovolemic, actively bleeding women may not be easily (or safely) transferred or transported to an angiographic facility.

Hence, even though it is a theoretically possible option, its practical utility is limited in a crisis situation.

CONCLUSION

Although this procedure is successful in only about 50% of cases, it is not technically easy to perform and requires special expertise and skill.

BIBLIOGRAPHY

1. Alvarez M, et al. Prophylactic and emergent arterial catheterization for selective embolization in obstetric hemorrhage. Am J Perinatol. 1992;9:441.
2. Burchell RC. Internal iliac artery ligation-hemodynamics. Obstet & Gynaecol. 1964;24:737.
3. Burchell RC, et al. Internal iliac artery ligation-aortograms. Obstet & Gynaecol. 1966;94:117.
4. Burchell RC. Physiology of internal iliac artery ligation. Jr Obstet & Gynaecol Br Commonwealth. 1968;75:642.
5. Chin HG. Angiographic embolizaion of intractable puerperal hematomas. Am Jr Obstet & Gynaecol. 1989;63:365.
6. Clark SL, et al. Uterine and hypogastric artery ligation. In: Phelan JP, Clark SL (Eds). Cesarian delivery. New York, Elsevier; 1988.pp.238.
7. Clark SL, et al. Hypogastric artery ligation for obstetric hemorrhage. Obstet & Gynaecol. 1985;66:353.
8. Greenwood LH, et al. Obstetric and non gynecological bleeding-treatment with angiographic embolization. Radiology. 1987;164:155.
9. Mengert WF, et al. Pregnancy after bilateral ligation of internal iliac and ovarian arteries. Obstet & Gynaecol. 1969;34:664.

24

Laparoscopic Myomectomy

S Krishnakumar, Pratik Tambe

Abstract

Uterine fibroids, the most common neoplasm of reproductive-aged women, can have a significant impact on quality of life, and may affect fertility and pregnancy outcomes. Although it is generally accepted that submucous fibroids are of clinical significance, the effect of intramural and subserous fibroids, and the benefit of surgical removal remains an area of active debate.

We review the current evidence for an association of fibroids and subfertility, and assess the impact of surgical management on fertility outcomes. We also discuss details of operative techniques and their evolution over the past decade. We review the controversy over tissue morcellation and the various options available that promise further refinements to the surgical steps of laparoscopic myomectomy.

INTRODUCTION

We present the recent evidence pertaining to laparoscopic myomectomy, the controversy surrounding power morcellation and focus on the impact on fertility enhancement.

INDICATIONS

Myomectomy is useful for the treatment of symptomatic fibroids and in selected women with infertility. Symptomatic submucous fibroids are classically treated by hysteroscopic resection, using a bipolar resectoscope. Symptomatic intramural and subserous fibroids may be treated by myomectomy, either by laparotomy or laparoscopy depending on their number and size.[1]

Prophylactic myomectomy is not recommended for preventing obstetric complications or the risk of leiomyosarcoma. Although fibroids can have a negative effect on fertility, only the removal of submucous fibroids has been consistently shown to improve spontaneous fertility or outcomes of assisted reproduction technology, while removal of intramural and subserous fibroids for improving fertility still remains controversial.

Uterine fibroids are the most common benign tumor of the female genital tract. They affect a significant proportion of women in the reproductive age group. While some women are asymptomatic, others can suffer from excessive menstrual bleeding and it can adversely affect reproductive outcomes.

Myomectomy is the most suitable surgical option for women who desire preservation of their fertility potential. However, only a selected group of women of childbearing age will benefit from surgery. Furthermore, the consequences of myomectomy on reproductive function have remained controversial.

We review the laparoscopic surgical approach for myomectomy and discuss evidence-based indications for myomectomy in women with fibroids, especially with regards to its impact on reproductive outcomes.

OPERATIVE PROCEDURE

Using a multiport approach, the location, size, shape of the myomas is identified. An elliptical incision is usually preferred, after injection of dilute vasopressin or aqua-dissection using normal saline. The myoma is enucleated from the pseudo-capsule using a combination of blunt and sharp dissection, with traction being applied using a myoma screw. Hemostasis is achieved in the myoma bed using bipolar energy where indicated (Fig. 24.1).

The incision is closed using delayed absorbable No 1 polyglactin 910 sutures in one or two layers as per the depth. Horizontal mattress sutures may be used to achieve better compression of the flaps and obliterate dead space. Simple, continuous or figure-of-8 sutures are preferred for approximating the superficial layers. Barbed or V-lock sutures may afford the advantage of

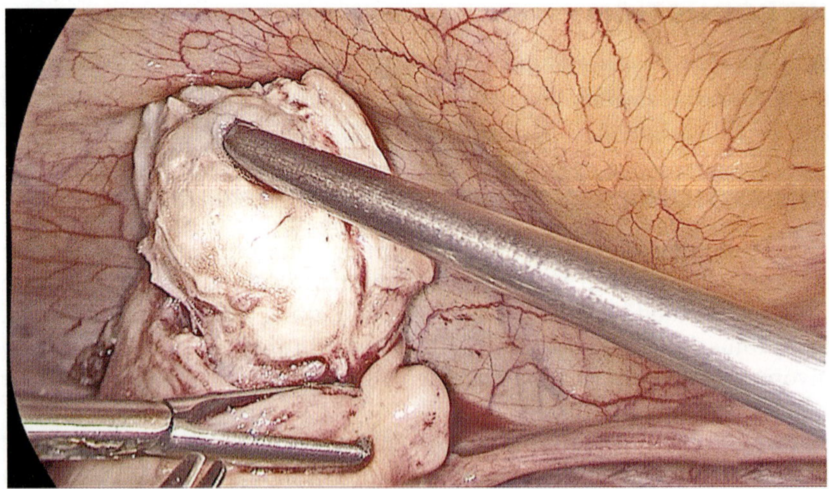

Fig. 24.1: Fibroid enucleation

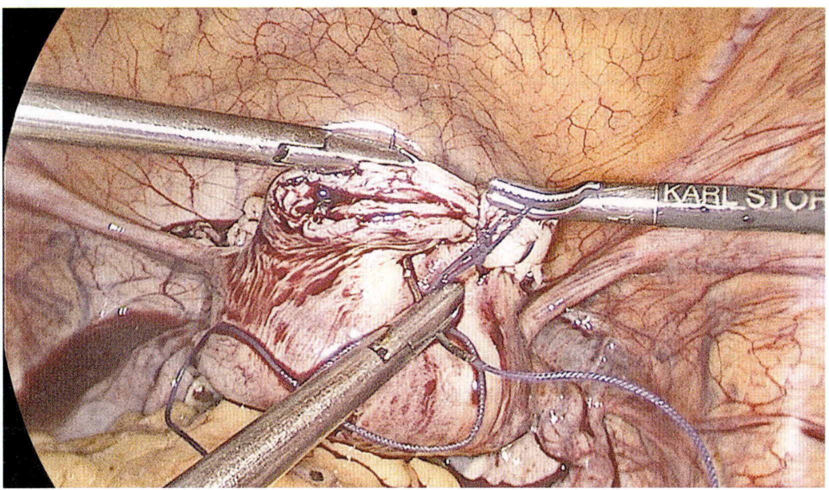

Fig. 24.2: Endosuturing

shorter operating time, though some studies report subsequent omental and bowel adhesions with their usage. A thorough lavage is usually performed using normal saline or Ringer's lactate and a tube drain may be kept in the Pouch of Douglas, brought out via the right lower port (Fig. 24.2).

Retrieval of the myoma specimen has been traditionally performed via a minilaparotomy incision, incision in the POD or via a laparoscopic tissue morcellator. The Karl Storz Rotocut and the Ethicon Gynecare systems are excellent examples of such morcellators. However, there has been some controversy over their use in recent times with fears of dissemination of undiagnosed leiomyosarcoma tissue and secondary peritoneal dispersal of tissue leading in rare cases to peritoneal leiomyomatosis.

Since the US FDA has issued a cautionary notice on use of morcellation, the American Association of Gynecologic Laparoscopists (AAGL) has come out with its own position statement on the same. To circumvent these regulations, specialized tissue retrieval systems in the shape of disposable bags are being introduced to perform in-bag morcellation. These are still in the research stage and promise exciting avenues ahead for refining the operative techniques of laparoscopic myomectomy.

Hemostatic Techniques

In a very recent paper, Hickman LC et al. reported on an evidence based approach for decreasing blood loss during surgery.[2] Myomectomy offers significant quality of life and fertility-sparing benefit for patients affected by uterine leiomyomas but with a risk of substantial intraoperative blood loss. This risk of hemorrhage not only leads to an increased transfusion rate but also to the need for hysterectomy and other potential operative complications. Numerous medical and surgical techniques have been developed to minimize potentially significant blood loss during abdominal, laparoscopic, and robotic-assisted myomectomies. These include injection of vasopressin, peri-cervical tourniquet and uterine artery embolization. Combined with judicious preoperative assessment, these techniques substantially enhance patient safety during myomectomy and outcomes during recovery.

LAPAROSCOPIC VS HYSTEROSCOPIC APPROACH

Wang H et al. 2016 compared the advantages of laparoscopic vs hysteroscopic approach for type II submucous myomas.[3]

A retrospective analysis was performed of those who underwent hysteroscopic or laparoscopic myomectomy from January 2008 to January 2013. The patients were divided into three subgroups according to the myomas diameter (namely, myomas diameter 3-4 cm; 4-5 cm and ≥50 mm). Clinical data such as operation time, amount of bleeding, postoperative hospital stay and complications were collected.

There was no significant difference regarding operation time and amount of bleeding in two groups. They found significant difference in hysteroscopic group (within-subgroup) difference regarding operation time and amount of bleeding, whereas no significant difference in the laparoscopic group and significant differences between-subgroup regarding operating time.

They concluded that both techniques are feasible for type II submucous myomas. Laparoscopic surgery has higher advantages in type II submucous myomas of greater than 4 cm in diameter whereas hysteroscopic approach has greater advantages in type II submucous myomas of less than 4 cm in diameter.

Uterine Fibroids and Subfertility

Brady PC et al. 2013 assessed the role of myomectomy with respect to fertility.[4] Recent analyses of patients with intramural fibroids have reported an increase in pregnancy loss and reduction in pregnancy and livebirth rates. However, when analyzing studies with high quality diagnostic methods for assessing the endometrial cavity, no significant impact on reproductive outcomes was observed, and no benefit of myomectomy was consistently demonstrable.

Myomectomy for submucosal fibroids greater than 2 cm and for intramural fibroids distorting the endometrial contour likely confers improvement of fertility outcome. They concluded that submucous fibroid location and distortion of the endometrial cavity (either submucous or deeply infiltrating intramural fibroids) are most predictive of impaired fertility and probable benefit of surgical removal, and warrant consideration of myomectomy in the subfertile patient.

Cochrane Meta-analysis

Metwally M et al. 2012 performed a systematic review of the surgical treatment of fibroids in subfertility.[5] They specifically sought to address the issue of fertility outcomes following myomectomy. Their findings were as follows:

One study examined the effect of myomectomy on reproductive outcomes and showed no evidence for a significant effect on the clinical pregnancy rate for intramural (OR 1.88, 95% CI 0.57 to 6.14), submucous (OR 2.04, 95% CI 0.62 to 6.66), combined intramural and subserous (OR 2.00, 95% CI 0.40 to 10.09) and combined intramural submucous fibroids (OR 3.24, 95% CI 0.72 to 14.57).

Similarly, there was no evidence for a significant effect of myomectomy for any of the described types of fibroids on the miscarriage rate (intramural fibroids OR 0.89 (95% CI 0.14 to 5.48), submucous fibroids OR 0.63 (95% CI 0.09 to 4.40), combined intramural and subserous fibroids OR 0.25 (95% CI 0.01 to 4.73) and combined intramural submucous fibroids OR 0.50 (95% CI 0.03 to 7.99).

Two studies compared open versus laparoscopic myomectomy and found no evidence for a significant effect on the live birth rate (OR 0.80, 95% CI 0.42 to 1.50), clinical pregnancy rate (OR 0.96, 95% CI 0.52 to 1.78), ongoing pregnancy rate (OR 1.61, 95% CI 0.26 to 10.04), miscarriage rate (OR 1.31, 95% CI 0.40 to 4.27), preterm labor rate (OR 0.68, 95% CI 0.11 to 4.43) and cesarean section rate (OR 0.59, 95% CI 0.13 to 2.72).

They concluded that there is currently insufficient evidence from randomized controlled trials to evaluate the role of myomectomy to improve fertility. Regarding the surgical approach to myomectomy, current evidence from two randomized controlled trials suggests there is no significant difference between the laparoscopic and open approach regarding fertility performance. This evidence needs to be viewed with caution due to the small number of studies. Finally, there is currently no evidence from randomized controlled trials regarding the effect of hysteroscopic myomectomy on fertility outcomes.

Power Morcellation and Occult Malignancy

The American College of Obstetricians and Gynecologists issued a special report on power morcellation and occult malignancy in May 2014.[6]

They suggested that there is a continuing need to develop technology, devices and techniques to improve patient safety in gynecologic surgery. The inability to diagnose leiomyosarcoma preoperatively with certainty illustrates and confirms the need for further research to develop reliable diagnostic tools. It is important to develop more effective and safer methods to reduce the risk of disseminating tissue associated with power morcellation, e.g. use of intraperitoneal bags; appropriate training and credentialing are also important considerations.

The annual incidence of leiomyosarcoma in the US is 0.64 per 100,000 women. 1:350 women undergoing hysterectomy or myomectomy will have an unsuspected sarcoma.

FDA Safety Communication

The USFDA issued an advisory on April 17, 2014 which was updated on November 24, 2014 regarding power morcellation. Their recommendations are as follows:[7]

If laparoscopic power morcellation is performed in women with unsuspected uterine sarcoma, there is a risk that the procedure will spread the cancerous tissue within the abdomen and pelvis, significantly *worsening* the patient's long-term survival. While the specific estimate of this risk may not be known with certainty, the FDA believes that the risk is higher than previously understood.

Laparoscopic power morcellators are contraindicated for removal of uterine tissue containing suspected fibroids in patients who are peri- or postmenopausal, or are candidates for en bloc tissue removal, for example, through the vagina or mini-laparotomy incision.

Laparoscopic power morcellators are contraindicated in gynecologic surgery in which the tissue to be morcellated is known or suspected to contain malignancy.

Be aware of the following new boxed warning recommended by the FDA: The FDA warns that uterine tissue may contain unsuspected cancer. The use of laparoscopic power morcellators during fibroid surgery may spread cancer, and decrease the long-term survival of patients. This information should be shared with patients when considering surgery with the use of these devices.

Carefully consider all the available treatment options for women with uterine fibroids. Thoroughly discuss the benefits and risks of all treatments with patients. Be certain to inform the small group of patients for whom laparoscopic power morcellation may be an acceptable therapeutic option that their fibroid(s) may contain unexpected cancerous tissue and that laparoscopic power morcellation may spread the cancer, significantly worsening their prognosis. This population might include some younger women who want to maintain their fertility or women not yet peri-menopausal who wish to keep their uterus after being informed of the risks.

Insufflated Isolation Bag

Cohen SL et al. in 2014 reported the approach of contained power morcellation within an insufflated isolation bag.[8]

Over the study period of January 2013 to April 2014, 73 patients underwent morcellation of the uterus or myomas within an insufflated isolation bag at the time of minimally invasive hysterectomy or myomectomy. This technique involves placing the specimen into a large plastic bag within the abdomen, exteriorizing the opening of the bag, insufflating the bag within the peritoneal cavity, and then using a power morcellator within the bag to remove the specimen in a contained fashion.

Surgical specimen morcellation within an insufflated isolation bag was successfully used in all cases. The median operative time was 114 minutes (range 32–380 min), median estimated blood loss was 50 mL (range 10–500 mL), and the median specimen weight was 257 g (range 53–1,481 g). There were no complications related to the contained morcellation technique nor was there visual evidence of tissue dissemination outside of the isolation bag.

They concluded that morcellation within an insufflated isolation bag is a feasible technique. Methods for morcellating uterine tissue in a contained manner may provide an option to minimize the risks of open power morcellation while preserving the benefits of minimally invasive surgery.

PRACTICE GUIDELINES

The Society of Obstetrics and Gynecology of Canada (SOGC) published a review on treatment of uterine leiomyomas in 2015.[9] The relevant points are as follows:

Uterine fibroids are common, appearing in 70% of women by age 50; the 20% to 50% that are symptomatic have considerable social and economic impact in Canada. (II-3)

Concern about possible complications related to fibroids in pregnancy is not an indication for myomectomy except in women who have had a previous pregnancy with complications related to these fibroids. (III)

Myomectomy is an option for women who wish to preserve their uterus or enhance fertility, but carries the potential for further intervention. (II-2)

RECOMMENDATIONS

Women with asymptomatic fibroids should be reassured that there is no evidence to substantiate major concern about malignancy and hysterectomy is not indicated. (III-D)

Treatment of women with uterine leiomyomas must be individualized based on symptomatology, size and location of fibroids, age, need and desire of the patient to preserve fertility or the uterus, the availability of therapy, and the experience of the therapist. (III-B)

In women who do not wish to preserve fertility and/or their uterus and who have been counseled regarding the alternatives and risks, hysterectomy by the least invasive approach possible may be offered as the definitive treatment for symptomatic uterine fibroids and is associated with a high level of satisfaction. (II-2A)

Hysteroscopic myomectomy should be considered first-line conservative surgical therapy for the management of symptomatic intracavitary fibroids. (II-3A)

Surgical planning for myomectomy should be based on mapping the location, size, and number of fibroids with the help of appropriate imaging. (III-A)

When morcellation is necessary to remove the specimen, the patient should be informed about possible risks and complications, including the fact that in rare cases fibroid(s) may contain unexpected malignancy and that laparoscopic power morcellation may spread the cancer, potentially worsening their prognosis. (III-B)

Selective progesterone receptor modulators and gonadotropin-releasing hormone analogs are effective at correcting anemia and should be considered preoperatively in anemic patients. (I-A)

Use of vasopressin, bupivacaine and epinephrine, misoprostol, pericervical tourniquet, or gelatin-thrombin matrix reduce blood loss at myomectomy and should be considered. (I-A)

Uterine artery occlusion by embolization or surgical methods may be offered to selected women with symptomatic uterine fibroids who wish to preserve their uterus. Women choosing uterine artery occlusion for the treatment of fibroids should be counselled regarding possible risks, including the likelihood that fecundity and pregnancy may be impacted. (II-3A)

In women who present with acute uterine bleeding associated with uterine fibroids, conservative management with estrogens, selective progesterone receptor modulators, antifibrinolytics, Foley catheter tamponade, and/or operative hysteroscopic intervention may be considered, but hysterectomy *Smart Obstetrics and Gynecology Handbook* may become necessary in some cases. In centers where available, intervention by uterine artery embolization may be considered. (III-B).

CONCLUSION

Uterine fibroids are the most common benign tumor of the female genital tract, affecting a significant proportion of women in the reproductive age group. While some women are asymptomatic, others can suffer abnormal uterine bleeding and can adversely affect reproductive outcomes. The laparoscopic approach to myomectomy offers the benefits of shorter hospital stay and quick recovery with earlier return to work.

Surgical planning for myomectomy should be based on mapping the location, size, and number of fibroids with the help of appropriate imaging. Selective progesterone receptor modulators and gonadotropin-releasing hormone analogs are effective at correcting anemia and should be considered preoperatively in anemic patients. Use of appropriate agents to reduce blood loss during surgery should be considered.

When morcellation is necessary to remove the specimen, the patient should be informed about possible risks and complications, including the fact that in rare cases fibroid(s) may contain unexpected malignancy and that laparoscopic power morcellation may spread the cancer, potentially worsening their prognosis.

A cochrane meta-analysis has concluded that there is currently insufficient evidence from randomized controlled trials to evaluate the role of myomectomy to improve fertility. However, this evidence needs to be viewed with caution due to the small number of studies included.

REFERENCES

1. Wong L, Brun JL. Myomectomy: technique and current indications. Minerva Ginecol. 2014;66(1):35-47.
2. Hickman LC, Kotlyar A, Shue S, Falcone T. Hemostatic techniques for myomectomy: an evidence based approach. J Minim Invasive Gynecol. 2016;8 pii: S1553-4650(16) 00075-3. doi: 10.1016/j. jmig.2016.01.026. [Epub ahead of print]
3. Wang H, Zhao J, Li X, Li P. The indication and curative effect of hysteroscopic and laparoscopic myomectomy for type II submucous myomas. BMC Surg. 2016;16(1):9.
4. Brady PC, Stanic AK, Styer AK. Uterine fibroids and subfertility: an update on the role of myomectomy. Curr Opinion Obstet Gynecol. 2013;25(3):255-9.
5. Metwally M, Cheong YC, Home AW. Surgical treatment of fibroids for subfertility. Cochrane Database Syst Rev. 2012;11:CD003857.
6. American College of Obstetricians and Gynecologists. Power morcellation and occult malignancy in gynecologic surgery: a special report. May 2014. ACOG Press.
7. Updated laparoscopic uterine power morcellation in hysterectomy and myomectomy: FDA Safety Communication. Available online at *http://www. fda. gov/MedicalDevices/Safety/AlertsandNotices/ ucm424443.htm*
8. Cohen SL, Einarsson JI, Wang KC, Brown D, et al. Contained power morcellation within an insufflated isolation bag. Obstet Gynecol. 2014;124:491-7. DOI: 10.1097/ AOG.0000000000000421
9. Vilos GA, Allaire C, Laberge PY, Leyland N. The management of uterine leiomyomas. J Obstet Gynaecol Can. 2015;37(2):157-81.

25

Surgical Management of Endometriosis

Nagendra Sardeshpande

"The world owes its forward progress to men ill at ease"
—***Nathaniel Hawthorne***

INTRODUCTION

Endometriosis is a benign, estrogen dependent gynecological disease affecting 5–10% of women of reproductive age [20–40% of women undergoing assisted reproductive technology (ART)] with symptoms including chronic pain, dysmenorrhea, dyspareunia and infertility.

Endometriomas are endometriotic implants involving to ovary and occur in 17% of subfertile women and in 17–44% of women with endometriosis. Approximately 28% of women with endometriomas have bilateral cysts. Interestingly 1.06% of women with endometriomas have no other clinically detectable endometriotic implants.[1,2]

Endometriosis causes inflammation, dense pelvic adhesions, distorts anatomical relationships between the urogenital structures and bowel and destroys ovarian tissue. Surgery for endometriosis is probably the most challenging surgery in gynecology demanding extensive knowledge of pelvic anatomy and highest level of laparoscopic and microsurgical skills.

INDICATIONS FOR SURGERY

Surgery for endometriosis is indicated in the following situations:

- Primary treatment of a disease diagnosed on radiological evaluation since endometriosis tends to be progressive disease.
- Symptoms related to disease (pain, dyspareunia, infertility).
- Complicated endometriosis (involving bowel, rectum, bladder, ureter, etc.).
- Recurrent symptomatic disease expect possibly in case of recurrent endometriomas in women with infertility.
- Suspected malignant transformation.

WHY SURGERY?

Surgery remains the mainstay of primary treatment of endometriosis. Surgery confirms diagnosis of endometriosis, helps staging, reduces the volume of disease, helps restore reasonably normal pelvic anatomical relationships, reduces or relieves symptoms, improves pregnancy rates (both spontaneous and following ART) and in select cases reduces risk of recurrence.[2]

Medical therapy is useful as for long-term suppression of disease and reduce risk of recurrence and symptoms. In fact, in infertile women, it delays return to fertility. There seems to be no difference in pregnancy rates between expectant management and medical therapy.[2]

WHY ENDOSCOPIC SURGERY?

Laparoscopy remains the gold standard approach for treatment of endometriosis.

The advantages of laparoscopy in endometriosis include:

- Direct access to the posterior and deeper aspects of the pelvis.
- Better planes of dissection due to the pressure of gas (carbon dioxide) as it forces itself between tissues and use of hydrodissection.
- Reduced postoperative adhesion formation.
- Better illumination and magnified view of the pelvis helps detect small lesions.
- Tactile feel (transmitted through instruments) allows palpation of deep infiltrating lesions (advantage over robotic surgery).
- All other advantages of laparoscopy itself (cosmesis, reduced postoperative morbidity, etc.).

PREOPERATIVE EVALUATION

Transvaginal ultrasound can detect endometriomas which appear as cyst with homogeneous internal echoes with thick walls and peripheral blood flows. Ground glass echogenicity of the cyst fluid is the single best variable (sensitivity 73% and specificity 94%). Endometriomas appear as bright lesions on MRI but this expensive investigation offers little benefit. Transvaginal scan (TVS) can also detect pelvic adhesions (reduced mobility between bowel and uterus, probe tenderness and adhesions bands seen during menstruation or midcycle where some fluid is present in the pelvis).[3,4]

A combination of transvaginal and transrectal ultrasound can diagnose rectovaginal adenomyosis with a sensitivity and specificity of 77% and 84% respectively. MRI with echoendoscopy is the most sensitive and specific method of diagnosing bowel and rectovaginal endometriosis.[4]

STEPS OF SURGERY FOR ENDOMETRIOSIS

Adhesiolysis

Endometriosis may present with a few intraperitoneal lesions and ovarian cysts to extensive pelvic disease with total obliteration of the pelvis by dense adhesions.

Since adhesions involve vital structures such as the rectosigmoid and terminal ileum and structures important from view of fertility (Fallopian tube and the ovary), it is of essence to avoid thermal damage to these structures.

Hydrodissection aids surgery. Dilute vasopressin solution (20 units in 100–200 mL of normal saline) can be infiltrated in the adhesions.

The dissection begins at the lateral aspect of the pelvic brim on one side or the other. At the level or slightly above the root of the infundibulopelvic ligaments. Here there are either no or flimsy adhesions. After separating the adhesions, the lateral peritoneum is retracted and the descending colon is retracted medially to create a plane of cleavage. With a combination of blunt and sharp dissection, the lateral aspect of the pelvis can be entered to expose the ovary and Fallopian tube. The ovary and Fallopian tube are tracted away from the ovarian fossa. Sweeping the active blade of the ultrasonic scalpel in the fast mode helps quickly release the adhesions, minimize lateral thermal spread and reduce bleeding. Once the ovary and Fallopian tube is separated from the ovarian fossae on either side, all the uterosacral ligaments can be visualized on either side with a central band of adhesions connecting the rectosigmoid to the uterus, cervix and vagina (Figs 25.1A to C).

Rectal Dissection

Rectal dissection begins by identifying the uterosacral ligaments on either side. At this stage the ovarian fossa may be opened and the ureter identified or isolated.

The plane between the uterosacral ligaments and the rectum is infiltrated with dilute vasopressin solution. The peritoneum between the uterosacral ligaments and the rectum is opened up cranially in the pelvis in a relatively disease-free area on either side. The incision is extended caudally to the junction of the rectum with the cervix. A plane is identified between the uterosacral ligaments laterally and the perirectal pad of fat and a space is created with blunt and sharp dissection. This is extended caudally till on reaches the lateral aspect of the cervix and vagina. This helps the surgeon orient and identify the central plane between the rectum and cervix/vagina. This is the area of the most dense adhesions. Using a sharp scissors and keeping the curve parallel to the anterior surface of the rectum and descending colon, the adhesions are divided sharply till a disease free area in the pouch of Douglas is entered (Figs 25.2A to E).

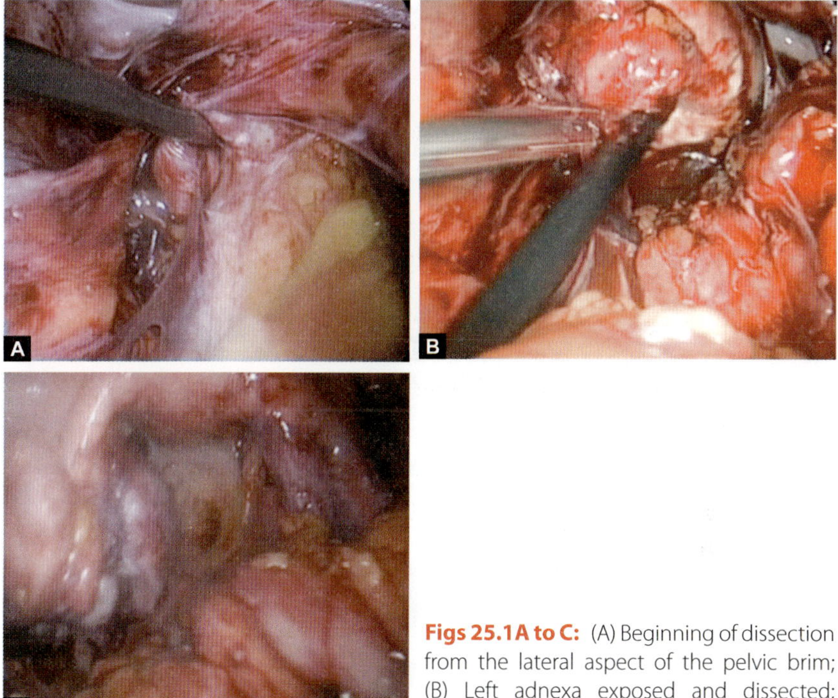

Figs 25.1A to C: (A) Beginning of dissection from the lateral aspect of the pelvic brim; (B) Left adnexa exposed and dissected; (C) Pelvic adhesiolysis completed

Identification and Separation of Ureter

Before excising or ablating implants inside the pelvis, the ureter should be visualized as it enters the pelvis below the infundibulopelvic ligament and passes nearly parallel and close to the uterosacral ligaments. Although the ureters may not be involved in the disease, inflammation, scarring and puckering of the peritoneum will bring the ureter close to the root of the infundibulopelvic ligament and to the ovary (especially important during oophorectomy), tether it to peritoneum (increasing the risk of thermal damage), uterosacrals (endangering it during excision of deep infiltrating disease) and the parametrium and lateral aspect of vagina (potentially increasing risk of delayed injury during hysterectomy). It may be necessary to expose the ureter retroperitoneally and even dissect it off the peritoneum before proceeding with surgery for endometriosis. This can be done by accessing the ureter either through the triangle between the round ligament and infundibulopelvic ligament or by incising the peritoneum at the pelvic brim below the infundibulopelvic ligament and entering the retroperitoneum through the ovarian fossa (Figs 25.3A and B).

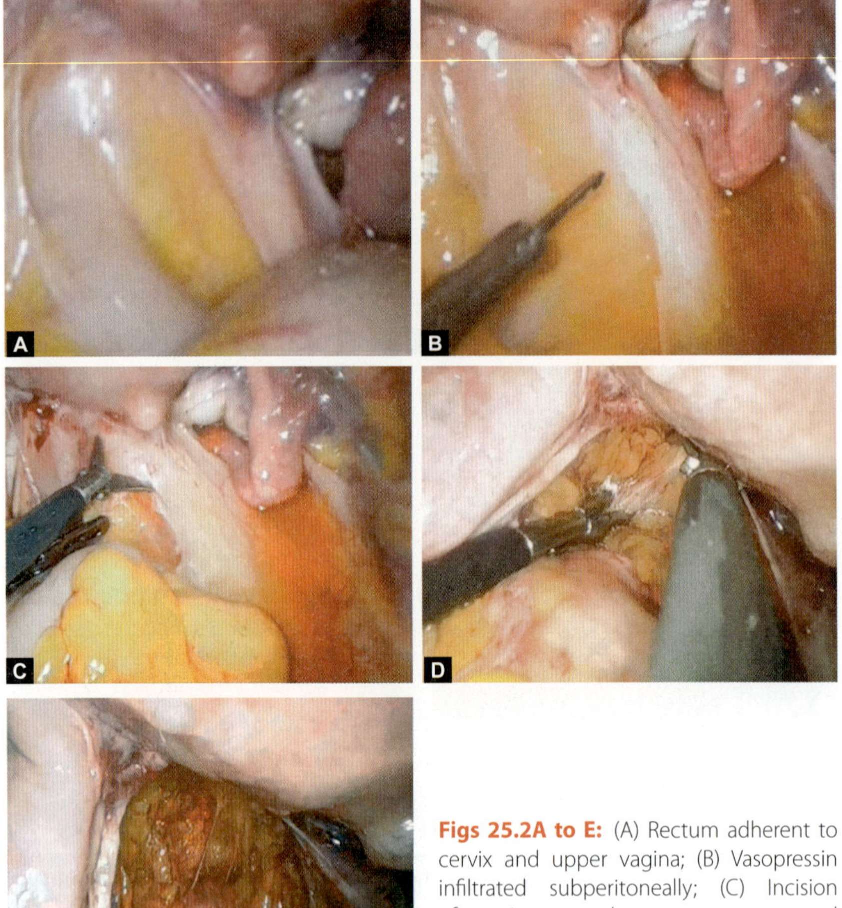

Figs 25.2A to E: (A) Rectum adherent to cervix and upper vagina; (B) Vasopressin infiltrated subperitoneally; (C) Incision of peritoneum between rectum and uterosacral ligaments; (D) Rectum grasped and adhesions cut sharply; (E) Pouch of Douglas freed of adhesions

Excision and Ablation of Endometriotic Implants

Excising endometriotic implants allows removal of deeply infiltrating peritoneal lesions and reduces risk of recurrence. Palpation of lesions, although not foolproof, may help detect subperitoneal lesions and guide dissection. Superficial lesions such as the vesicular and red flame like lesions may be fulgurated. Narrow band imaging technology detects areas of abnormal vascularization in the peritoneum and these can be biopsied to excise and diagnose early endometriosis.[5]

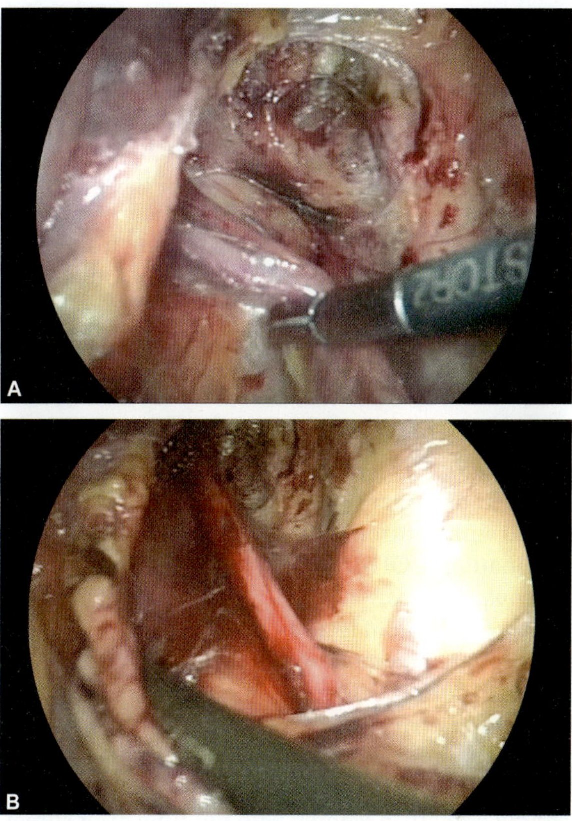

Figs 25.3A and B: (A) Ureter adherent to inflamed and puckered peritoneum; (B) Ureter dissected away from operating field

SURGERY FOR DEEP INFILTRATING ENDOMETRIOSIS

Deep infiltrating endometriosis is defined as peritoneal invasion over 5 mm in depth and occurs in 20% of women with endometriosis. In decreasing order, it affects the uterosacral ligaments, rectosigmoid colon, vagina and urinary tract. It presents with a variety of symptoms including bowel symptoms (hematochezia and tenesmus) and urinary symptoms.[4]

These lesions are usually adenomyotic nodules from stimulation of Müllerian remnants in the retroperitoneum. Hence, surgical excision with a margin of healthy tissue is the best option.

In case of rectovaginal endometriosis, the nodule is first isolated from its vaginal attachment with sharp dissection. Ultrasonic energy reduces blood loss along with use of dilute vasopressin infiltration. The vagina may be entered in the process. This defect can be sutured after excising the nodule. The rectal aspect of the nodule usually infiltrates the superficial serosa or occasionally the superficial muscularis layer. This nodule can be shaved off the rectosigmoid without an enterotomy. The superficial defect in the rectosigmoid can be sutured with interrupted sutures of 2-0 or 3-0 Polyglactin 910 in a single layer.

For lesions involving full thickness of the rectum or sigmoid colon, the circumferential extent of involvement is noted. If the lesion involves less than one half of the circumference, the lesion is completely excise and the enterotomy closed transversely with No. 2-0 0r 3-0 Polyglactin 910 in 2 layers of continuous sutures. For lesions involving more than one half of the bowel circumference or presence of multiple lesions, resection anastomosis is mandatory (Figs 25.4A to D).

Interestingly, improved pregnancy rates varying from 44% to 72% have been noted following surgery for deep infiltrating endometriosis.[6]

DECISION MAKING IN ENDOMETRIOSIS ASSOCIATED WITH INFERTILITY

- **Stage I/II Endometriosis**
  - *Asymptomatic/undiagnosed*
    - No benefit of surgery
    - Proceed with controlled ovarian hyperstimulation—intrauterine insemination (COH-IUI)[2]
  - *Laparoscopic diagnosis*
    - Ablation/excision of lesions
    - Expectant management or IUI for women below 35 years and in vitro fertilization (IVF) for women above 35 years[2]
- **Stage III/IV endometriosis**
  - Conservative surgery improves fertility outcomes
  - Surgery should be followed by IVF
  - IVF without surgery in women with multiple prior surgeries and poor ovarian reserve
  - GnRH analogs 3–6 months prior to IVF[2]

SURGICAL MANAGEMENT OF ENDOMETRIOMAS

Conventional Treatment of Endometriomas

Ovarian cystectomy is the standard treatment for ovarian endometriomas. Endometriomas by themselves are associated with 33–66% reduction in ovarian follicles compared to benign ovarian cysts and a contralateral normal ovary. Ovarian endometriomas are also associated with reduced follicles with stimulation, fewer oocyte retrieved and reduced implantation rates. This is because of associated inflammation and oxidative stress which increases apoptosis in adjacent oocytes.[7,8]

Laparoscopic cystectomy has the benefits of a reduced recurrence (9.6–45%), histopathological sampling and increased spontaneous pregnancy rates (14–54%). Conversely, cystectomy damages ovarian cortex and follicles [reduced anti-Müllerian hormone (AMH)], increases risk of ovarian failure (2.3–3.03%), induces inflammation and scarring, increases risk of periovarian and peritubal adhesions and increases oxidative stress. A waiting period of 6–12 months has also been recommended prior to ART.[9, 10]

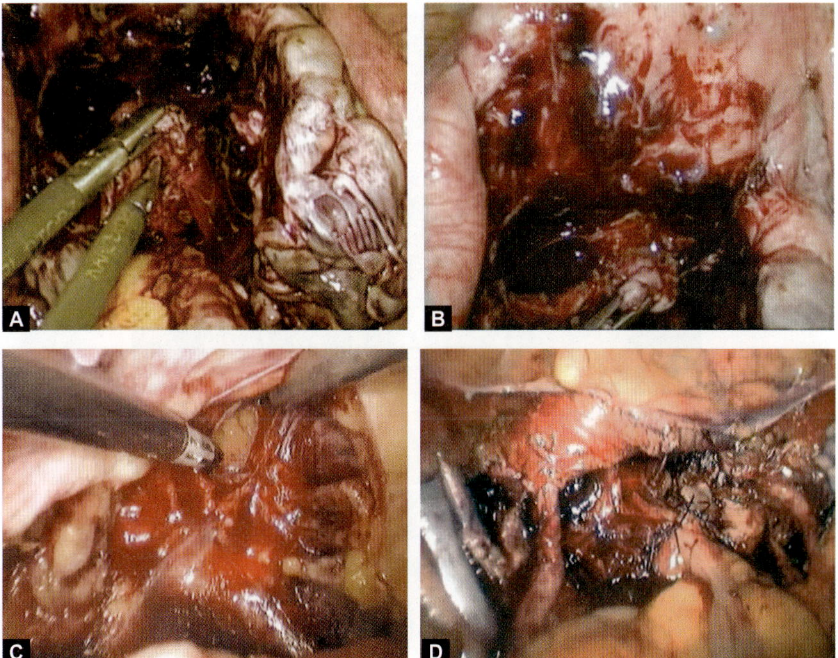

Figs 25.4A to D: (A) Rectovaginal nodule; (B) Nodule shaved off the rectum; (C) Enterotomy during excision of deep infiltrating endometriosis; (D) Rectal suturing completed

Alternatives to Ovarian Cystectomy

- *Nonintervention*: Nonintervention increases risk of spontaneous rupture (Figs 25.5A and B), puncture during oocyte retrieval (2.8%), increase in size during infertility treatment and inability to rule out a malignancy (0.7%).[11]
- *Aspiration*: Repeated aspiration is associated with reduced recurrence (5.4%) compared with single aspiration (91.5%). Cumulative pregnancy rates of 43.4–73.2% with 78% spontaneous conception rates have been noted. However, the risk of pelvic inflammatory disease (PID) following aspiration has to be considered (Figs 25.6A and B).[12]
- *Laparoscopic ablation*: KTP laser ablation of endometriomas has been associated with a 24.4% recurrence, 48.9% spontaneous pregnancy rates and 50% IVF pregnancy rates.[13]
- *Combined ablation and cystectomy*: Donnez proposed removal of 80–90% of cyst wall followed by ablation of the base of the cyst. He noted no difference in volume between the normal and affected ovary, 8.2% recurrence and 41% pregnancy rate. Risk of thermal damage to the normal ovary persists.[14]
- *Three stage procedure*: Donnez also proposed cyst drainage and GnRH analog therapy for 3 months followed by ovarian cystectomy. Treatment is lengthy with risk of thermal damage but there was less reduction in AMH and a higher AFC in the affected ovary.[15]

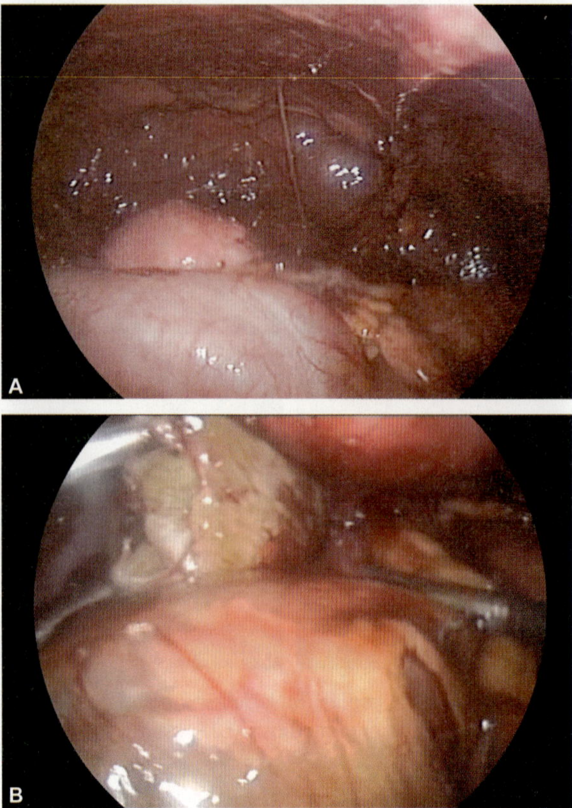

Figs 25.5A and B: (A) Endometriotic fluid in abdomen due to spontaneous leakage of endometrioma; (B) Spontaneous rent in an endometrioma

- *Aspiration with sclerotherapy using 95% ethanol or methotrexate 30 mg/3 mL NS*: This short procedure is associated with lesser recurrence (14%) compared to simple aspiration (45%) and may be associated with moderately increased oocyte count, fertilization/implantation/pregnancy rates.[16]
- *Novel therapies*: Ovarian/oocyte cryopreservation during primary surgery and autotransplantation of cryopreserved or fresh ovarian tissue.[17]

Decision Making during Management of Endometriomas

Decision for ovarian cystectomy especially in women with infertility is made on the following:

- *Laterality*: Surgery for bilateral endometriomas is associated with increased risk of reduced ovarian reserve (10.6% versus 1.2%) and premature ovarian failure (3.03% versus 0%). Hence, surgery is best delayed or avoided.[18]

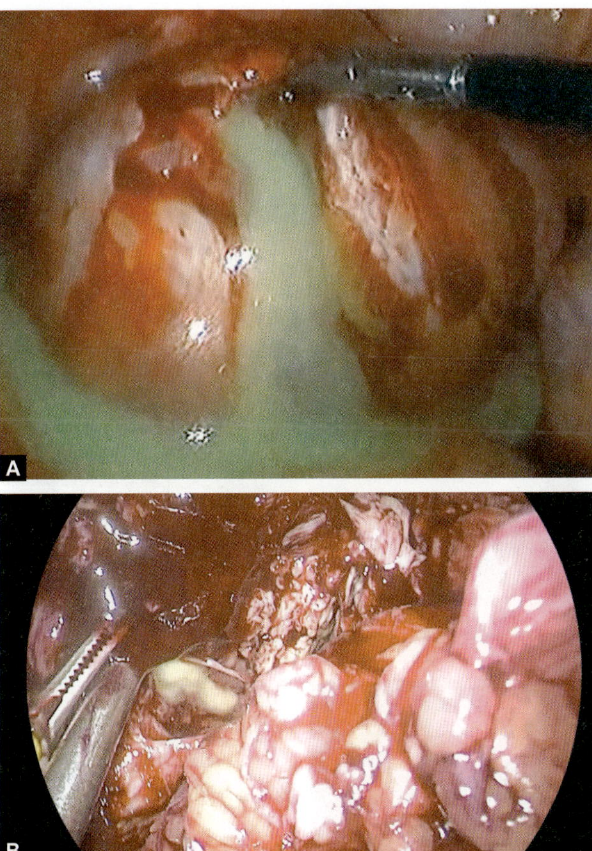

Figs 25.6A and B: (A) Infected endometrioma; (B) Pelvic inflammatory disease (PID) following aspiration of an endometrioma

- *Size, location and hindering effects of the cyst*: Cystectomy is recommended for endometriomas larger than 4 cm and those which may interfere with ovum pickup.[19]
- *Age of woman*: Elderly women have lesser inflammation associated with endometriomas but have already reduced ovarian reserve. Hence, surgery should be considered with caution.[20]
- *Prior surgical treatment*: There is 45.1% recurrence within 20 months of repeat surgery and lower pregnancy rates have been noted at 12 and 24 months after repeat surgery (13 and 22% respectively) compared to primary surgery (25 and 30% respectively).[21]

Ovarian Tissue Conservation during Cystectomy

In view of potential for damage and loss of follicles during ovarian cystectomy leading to a fall in ovarian reserve and also possibility of periovarian adhesion formation, certain precautions should be taken during ovarian cystectomy (Figs 25.7A to F).

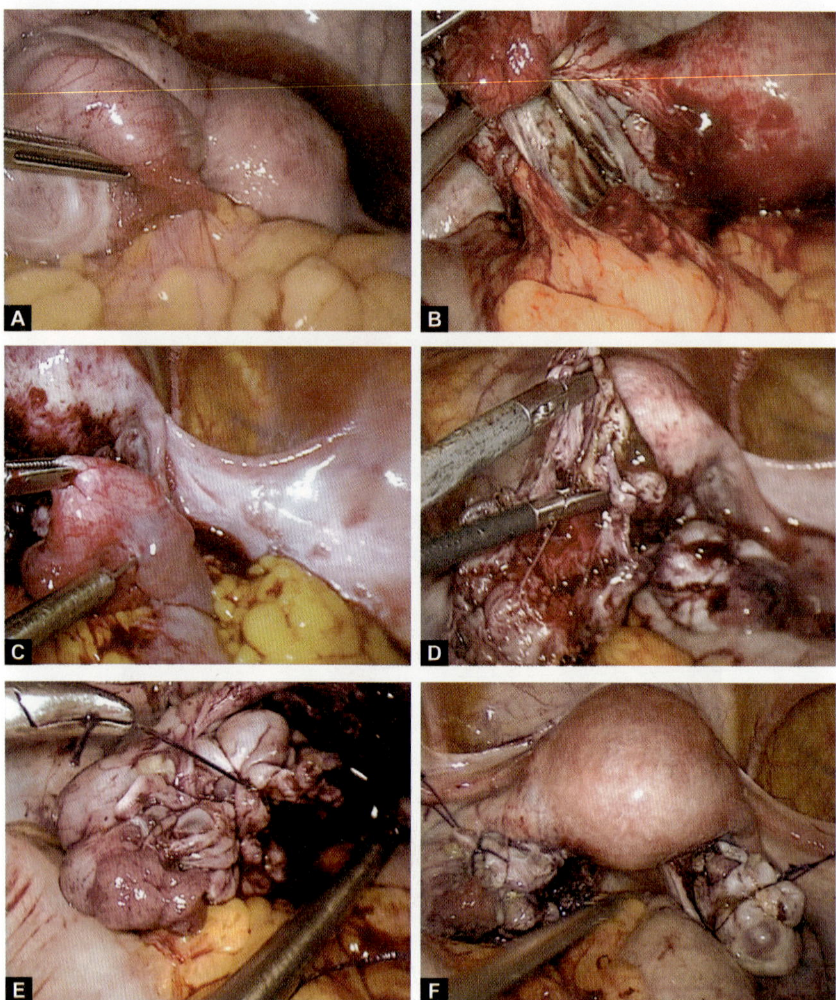

Figs 25.7A to F: (A) Left ovarian endometrioma; (B) Endometrioma drained; (C) Vasopressin infiltration in the ovary; (D) Ovarian cystectomy performed; (E) Ovarian bed approximated with interrupted sutures; (F) Ovarian suspension done

- *Avoid use of energy sources:* Since any energy source has potential for lateral thermal damage to normal functional ovarian tissue, it is wise to avoid use of energy sources during ovarian cystectomy. The endometrioma is drained by making a cut in the most prominent portion and insertion of a suction cannula. This cut can be extended by grasping the two sides with Allis graspers and carefully stretching the tissue. The cyst wall can be enucleated by finding a correct plane between the ovarian tissue and the cyst capsule.
- *Hemostatic agents:* Infiltration of dilute vasopressin (20 units in 100–200 mL of normal saline) or saline adrenaline solution (1:300000 concentration) along with intravenous tranexamic acid (1 g) preoperatively minimizes

bleeding from the ovarian bed. About 10 mL dilute hemostatic solution is infiltrated either prior to cyst drainage or following cyst drainage and before cystectomy. In addition to hemostasis, it facilitates finding a plane of cleavage between the ovarian tissue and the cyst capsule. Since the major blood supply to the ovaries are from the ovarian arteries, compression of the infundibulopelvic ligament for about 5 minutes with a atraumatic graspers allows cessation of oozing from the ovarian bed.[22]

- *Closure of the ovarian bed:* The ovarian bed can be closed with interrupted or internal purse-string sutures of 2-0 or 3-0 polyglactin. This provides hemostasis and internalizes the raw are of the ovarian cortex.
- *Ovarian suspension:* Postoperative adhesions between the ovary and the ovarian fossa results in loss of normal anatomical tubo-ovarian relationship and entraps growing follicles in the adhesions. This prevents ovulation and results in functional entrapped ovarian cysts. A technique proposed is to passed a simple nonabsorbable suture of No.1-0 or 2-0 nylon or prolene through the ovary and bring it out through the abdominal wall. This can be removed after 5–7 days. Alternatively, for women not willing for this procedure, a rapidly absorbable suture such as rapidly absorbable polyglaction 910 can be used to gently suspend the ovary to the ipsilateral round ligament. The intention is to lift the ovary away from the ovarian fossa during the healing phase. Care is taken to bring the ovary close to the fimbrial end, not lift it out of the pelvis (it should always remain below the pelvic brim) and avoid kinking or constriction of the ipsilateral Fallopian tube. Once the suture is autolyzed, the ovary remains or returns to its normal anatomical position in the pelvis.[23]

ROLE OF ADHESION BARRIERS

A number of adhesion barriers have been used to reduce perioperative adhesions. The two commonly used ones are oxidized cellulose and hyaluronic acid membranes or films (Fig. 25.8). Newer ones such as Adept solution or Sprayshield solutions are on the horizon. While adhesion barriers do reduce the intensity and number of adhesions, it is not yet certain if use of these barriers translate into improved pregnancy rates. Hence, adhesions barriers are an adjunct but not an alternative to use of microsurgical principles (gentle tissue handling, minimize use of energy sources, repeated irrigation of tissue with lactated Ringer solution and use of fine least reactive sutures) during surgery for endometriosis.[24]

SURGICAL MANAGEMENT OF OTHER COMMON FORMS OF ENDOMETRIOSIS

Bowel Endometriosis

Bowel endometriosis is the most frequent site of extragenital endometriosis (5.4–12%). Bowel endometriosis occurs due to peritoneal dissemination of endometrial tissue. This commonly involves the appendix and terminal ileum (Figs 25.9A and B).

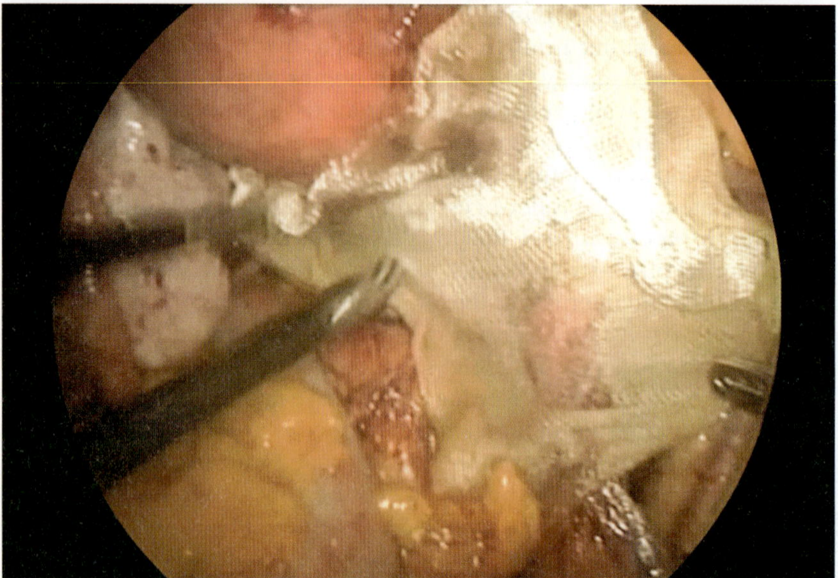

Fig. 25.8: Oxidized cellulose adhesion barrier

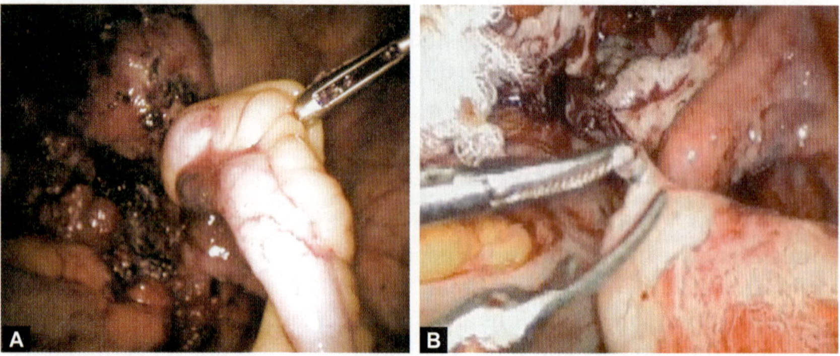

Figs 25.9A and B: (A) Endometriotic nodule on the appendix; (B) Bowel endometriosis

The principles of surgical treatment is the same that of rectosigmoid disease. Radical excision improves symptoms in 91–100% of women and pregnancy rates of 43–45% have been noted following surgery.[25]

Urinary Tract Endometriosis

Urinary tract endometriosis is a variation of retroperitoneal deeply infiltrating endometriosis. It involves adenomyotic nodules infiltrating the bladder and pelvic (especially terminal portion) part of ureter. Bladder endometriosis commonly usually infiltrates the muscularis dome and trigonal aspect of the bladder usually not invading the mucosa although the nodule with push and protrude into the cavity of the urinary bladder. It causes ulceration of the bladder mucosa leading to cyclical hematuria and dysuria although it a large number of women it tends to be asymptomatic. The nodule usually is an extension of endometriosis along the lateral parametrium hence is usually asymmetrically placed on the bladder. The lesion should be biopsied to differentiate it from bladder malignancy. Ureteric endometriosis occurs because of proximity of the terminal ureters to the uterosacral ligaments. The adenomyotic tissue infiltrates the parametrium and completely or partially encircles the ureters constricting them. These lesions are usually unilateral. The endometriosis usually does not infiltrate the seromuscular layer of the ureters.

Excision of bladder endometriosis usually requires stenting of the one or both ureters depending on the size and location of the lesion. The bladder is cut vertically to expose the cavitary aspect of the lesion and also visualize the ureteric orifices. The nodule is excised with approximately 1cm of healthy tissue to reduce recurrence. The defect in the bladder wall is closed with 2 layers of continuous sutures of 2-0 or 3-0 Polyglactin 910 (Figs 25.10A to C).

Treatment of ureteric endometriosis involves release of ureteric tissue from the fibrous tissue encircling it after stenting the dissection starts at the pelvic brim where the dilated proximal portion of the ureter guides dissection. Care should be taken to proceed parallel to the ureter to reduce thermal damage and avoid transection of the afflicted portion of the ureter. Since the disease often involves the terminal portion of the ureter, the dissection has to extend up to the insertion of the ureter into the bladder. The round ligament may be cut and the uterine artery clipped and cut to access the distal portion of the ureter. The ureter has to be completely freed from all aspects to release it from the endometriotic tissue and the diseased parametrial tissue completely excised to reduce recurrence. Excision of ureter with end to end anastomosis or re-implantation is rarely needed. This is considered with extensive involvement of the ureter with endometriosis in terms of length or infiltration of the seromuscular layer causing irremediable constriction for the lumen.

Following surgery, the ureteric catheter is removed after 6–8 weeks and ureteric wall integrity confirmed by fluoroscopy.

Vaginal Endometriosis

Vaginal nodules may be found in women with rectovaginal adenomyosis. These are usually found in the posterior fornix and rarely lower down in the cul de sac. Occasionally large nodules may infiltrate the vaginal wall and extend laterally into the paravaginal, pararectal and periurethral region. These require a combined vaginal and laparoscopic approach. Laparoscopically, the disease is shaved off the adjacent structures including bladder and rectum. The through a vaginal incision the entire nodule is excised. Sometimes the vaginal defect is so large as to exclude repair with sutures. The defect is packed to achieve hemostasis. The vagina almost always heals spontaneously by epithelialization over the defect.

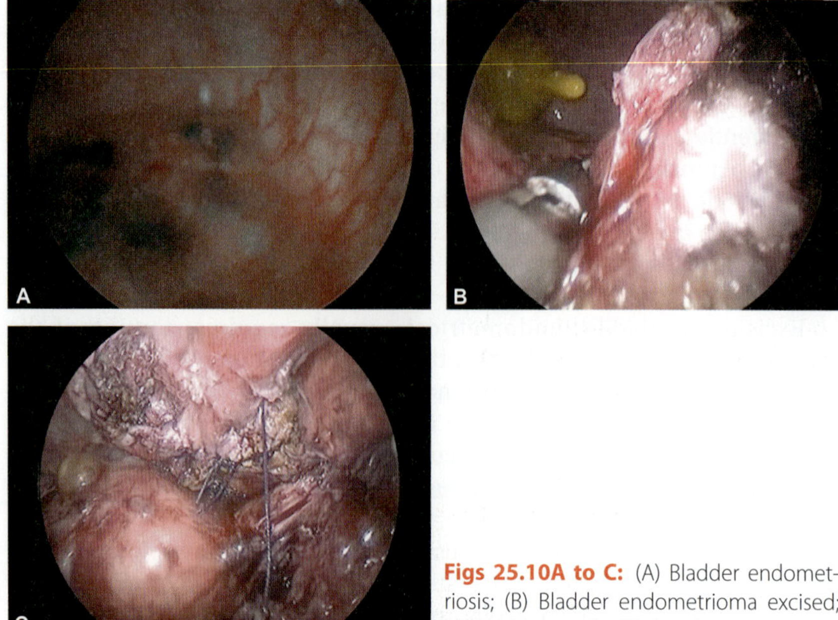

Figs 25.10A to C: (A) Bladder endometriosis; (B) Bladder endometrioma excised; (C) Bladder repaired in two layers

Cutaneous or Scar Endometriosis

The incidence of cutaneous or scar endometriosis is increasing. This is associated most commonly with cesarean delivery and occasionally with surgery for pelvic endometriosis. The endometriotic (or adenomyotic) tissue extends the full thickness of the abdominal wall including subcutaneous tissue, rectus sheath, muscle and peritoneum) and is associated with cyclical swelling and pain in the scar.

Cutaneous endometriosis can also occur in the umbilicus and over the mons pubis (probably tracking down the round ligament).

Treatment involves wide excision fo the mass including 1–2 cm margin of healthy tissue. The excision has to extend right up to the peritoneum. Laparoscopic evaluation at the time of surgery allows visualization of any intraperitoneal extension and associated pelvic and abdominal endometriosis. A small abdominal wall defect can be closed with conventional layered suturing. However, larger defects may require tension sutures and even application of a mesh to close the defect in the rectus sheath.

OTHER SITES OF ENDOMETRIOSIS

Endometriosis can be occasionally be found at other sites abdominally (spleen, kidney, etc.) and extra-abdominally (thorax, pericardium, nose, brain, etc.). These are rare lesions and require multispecialty management. They may be quiescent and asymptomatic and are incidentally diagnosed during surgery for other pathology or may have symptoms suggestive of endometriosis (catamenial nose bleeds) or mimic symptoms of other disease (pleural effusion or chest pain or unexplained space occupying cerebral lesion or intracranial bleed).

PAIN RELIEF FOR SYMPTOMATIC ENDOMETRIOSIS

Women with endometriosis often present with chronic pelvic pain or severe dysmenorrhea. The cause of pain is multidimensional and includes inflammation, fibrosis, and infiltration of the pelvic nerves with endometriosis.

Whereas laparoscopic uterine nerve ablation does not seem to often significant relief (except in adenomyosis), presacral neurectomy offers significant relief from pelvic pain.

The surgery involves exposure and isolation of the superior hypogastric plexus over the sacral promontory. A 3 cm segment of the nerves is cauterized and excised.

The procedure may be associated with bladder and bowel dysfunction (symptoms of retention). The long-term benefit of the procedure is not known.[26]

PERIOPERATIVE MANAGEMENT

Preoperative treatment with suppressive therapy [Dienogest or gonadotropin-releasing hormone (GnRH) analog] does not seem to benefit surgery. There may be some reduction in vascularity but smaller lesion may be masked and, hence, missed during surgery. Fibrosis following suppressive therapy may hamper dissection during surgery.

GnRH analog therapy following surgery has no benefit with regards to fertility. However, 3–6 months of GnRH analog therapy may improve pregnancy rates in ART for grade III and IV endometriosis.

Long-term suppressive treatment with GnRH analogs (with add back therapy), dienogest and the LNG-IUD reduces incidence of recurrence of endometriosis.[2]

HYSTERECTOMY FOR ENDOMETRIOSIS

Hysterectomy is considered for women who have completed childbearing, have severe symptoms of endometriosis (pain and dysmenorrhea), complicated endometriosis (urinary tract, rectovaginal or bowel endometriosis), recurrent disease, malignant transformation (usually well differentiated endometrioid adenocarcinomas or clear cell carcinomas) or associated pathology (adenomyosis, uterine fibroids, ovarian cysts, etc.).

The decisive treatment for symptomatic endometriosis is hysterectomy with bilateral salpingo-oophorectomy and excision of endometriotic implants. Any compromise in terms of incomplete excision of endometriosis or ovarian conservation increases risk of recurrence (62% with 6 fold risk of recurrent pain and 8 fold risk of reoperation with ovarian conservation).[27]

Approximately 18% of hysterectomies are done for endometriosis.[28] *Hysterectomy in the setting of endometriosis is fraught with danger because of the following reasons:*

- Deeper level of dissection to remove the cervix.
- Previous surgeries with recurrent or progressive disease.
- Proximity of ureter to the ovaries, infundibulopelvic ligament and vagina and fixation of ureters to the peritoneum.
- Fixation of rectum, descending colon and, at times, the terminal ileum, appendix and cecum to the uterus and adnexae with loss of fascial planes.
- Bladder may be adherent to the uterus and cervix because of endometriosis or previous cesarean delivery.

A few principles may be followed to reduce risk of injury the bowel, bladder or ureter during surgery:

- The importance of exposing and isolating the ureters prior to dissection can not be over emphasized.
- The uterine arteries can be clipped, ligated or cauterized at their origin from the internal iliac arteries prior to dissection. This is done by opening the peritoneum between the infundibulopelvic ligaments and round ligament (lateral approach) or by opening the anterior leaf of the broad ligament and tracing the uterine artery retrograde to its origin (retrograde approach).
- Follow principles of adhesiolysis and rectal dissection.
- Bladder dissection is commenced from the lateral aspect anterior to the uterine vessels and lifting the bladder off the the cervix and vagina from the lateral aspect where the adhesions are the least before cutting the central pillar of adhesions between the bladder and the cervix (lateral window technique).
- In case of extensive pelvic dissection, a drain may be placed in the pelvis. Alternatively, the vagina may be closed with interrupted or figure of 8 sutures. The vagina, thus, acts, as a drain and prevents collection of inflammatory or hemorrhagic fluid in the peritoneal cavity.

CONCLUSION

The treatment of endometriosis, whether medical or surgical, invites debate. Inspite of improved understanding of the disease and advances in medical therapy, surgery remains the primary line of management. With modifications in surgical technique and more precise energy sources, this complex surgery has become far safer than ever before. Thus, in the modern era of gynecological surgery, we can offer a range of individualized treatment options to offer relief to women suffering from endometriosis.

"Any path which narrows future possibilities may become a trap. Humans are not threading their way through a maze; they scan a vast horizon filled with unique opportunities"

—Kevin Anderson

REFERENCES

1. Guidice LC, Kao LC. Endometriosis. Lancet. 2004;364(9447):1789-99.
2. Practice Committee of the American Society for Reproductive Medicine. Endometriosis and Infertility: a committee opinion. 2012;98(3):591-8.
3. Holland TK. Ultrasound mapping of pelvic endometriosis: does the location and number of lesions affect the diagnostic accuracy? A multicentre diagnostic accuracy study. BMC Women's Health. 2013;13:43.
4. Bazot M, Lafont C, et al. Diagnostic accuracy of physicals examination, transvaginal sonography, rectal endoscopic sonography and magnetic resonance imaging to diagnose deep infiltrating endometriosis. Fertility Sterility. 2009;92(6):1825-33.
5. Jacobson TZ, et al. Cochrane Database Systematic Review. 2007;4:CD001398.
6. Fuchs F, Raynal P, et al. Reproductive outcome after laparoscopic treatment of endometriosis in an infertile population. J Gynecol Obstet Biol Reprod. 2007;36(4):354-9.
7. Kuroda M, Kuroda K, et al. Histological assessment of impact of ovarian endometrioma and laparoscopic cystectomy on ovarian reserve. J Obstet Gynecol Res. 2012;38(9):1187-93.
8. Matsuzaki S, Schubert B. Oxidative stress status in normal ovarian cortex surrounding ovarian endometriosis. Fertil Steril. 2010;93(7):2431-2.
9. Carmona F, et al. Ovarian cystectomy versus laser vaporization in the treatment of ovarian endometriomas: a randomized clinical trial with a five year follow up. Fertil Steril. 2011;96(1):251-4.
10. Hayasaka S, et al. Risk factors for recurrence and re-recurrence of ovarian endometriomas after laparoscopic excision. J Obstet Gynecol Res. 2011;37(6):581-5.
11. Kennedy S, et al. ESHRE Special Interest group for Endometriosis and Endometrium Guideline Development. ESHRE guideline for the diagnosis and treatment of endometriosis. Hum Reprod. 2005;20 (10):2698-704.
12. Zhu W, et al. Repeat transvaginal ultrasound-guided aspiration of ovarian endometrioma in infertile women with endometriosis. Am J Obstet Gynecol. 2011;204(1):61e1-61e6.
13. Roman H, et al. Ovarian endometrioma ablation using plasma energy versus cystectomy: a step towards better preservation of the ovarian parenchyma in women wishing to conceive. Fertil Steril. 2011;96:1397-400.
14. Donnez J, et al. Laparoscopic management of endometriomas using a combined technique of excisional (cystectomy) and ablative surgery. Fertil Steril. 2010;94(1):28-32.
15. Tsolakidis D, et al. The impact on ovarian reserve after laparoscopic ovarian cystectomy versus three-stage management in patients with endometriomas: a prospective randomized study. Fertil Steril. 2010;94(1):71-7.
16. Shawki HE. The impact of in situ methotrexate after transvaginal ultrasound-guided aspiration of ovarian endometriomas on ovarian response and reproductive outcomes during IVF cycles. Middle East Fertil Soc. 2012;17:82-8.
17. Matthews Ml, et al. Cancer, fertility preservation and future pregnancy: a comprehensive review. Obstet Gynecol Int. 2012.pp.937-53.

18. Hirokawa W, et al. The post-operative decline in serum anti-Mullerian hormone correlates with the bilaterality and severity of endometriosis. Hum Reprod. 2011;26(4):904-10.
19. Tulandi T, Marzai A. Redefining reproductive surgery. JMIG. 2012;19(3):296-306.
20. Romualdi D, et al. Follicular loss in endoscopic surgery for ovarian endometriosis: quantitative and qualitative observation. Fertil Steril. 2011.pp.374-8.
21. Vercilleni .pp., et al. The second time around: reproductive performance after repetitive versus primary surgery for endometriosis. Fertil Steril. 2009;92(4):1253-5.
22. Carnahan M, et al. Ovarian endometrioma: Guidelines for selection of cases for surgical treatment or expectant management. Expert Rev Obstet Gynecol. 2013;8(1):29-55.
23. Serrachioli R, et al. The role of ovarian suspension in endometriosis surgery: a randomized controlled trial. JMIG. 2014;21(6):1029-35.
24. Ahmed G, O'Flynn H, et al. Barrier agents for adhesion prevention after gynaecological surgery (review). Cochrane Database Sys Review (Wiley Online library). 2015;CD000475.
25. Bediawy MA, Barker NM. Evidence based surgical management of endometriosis. Middle East Fertil Soc J. 2012;17:57-60.
26. Triolo O, Lagana AS, Sturlese E. Chronic pelvic pain in endometriosis: an overview. J Clin Med Res. 2013;5(3):153-63.
27. Rizk B, et al. Recurrence of endometriosis after hysterectomy. Facts Views Vis ObGyn. 2014;6(4):219-27.
28. Malinowski A, Makowska J, Antosiak B. Total laparoscopic hysterectomy-indications and complications in 158 patients. Ginekologia Polska. 2013;84(4):252-7.

Index

Page numbers followed by *f* refer to figure and *t* refer to table.